Natural Toxins

Animal, plant, and microbial

Natural Toxins

Animal, plant, and microbial

EDITED BY

JOHN B. HARRIS

Professor of Experimental Neurology,
University of Newcastle upon Tyne, and Director,
Muscular Dystrophy Group Research
Laboratories, Newcastle General Hospital

Assisted by
D. A. Chapman, R. Pain, A. Panchen,
and M. Sussman

CLARENDON PRESS · OXFORD
1986

Oxford University Press, Walton Street, Oxford OX2 6DP

Oxford New York Toronto
Delhi Bombay Calcutta Madras Karachi
Petaling Jaya Singapore Hong Kong Tokyo
Nairobi Dar es Salaam Cape Town
Melbourne Auckland

and associated companies in
Beirut Berlin Ibadan Nicosia

Oxford is a trade mark of Oxford University Press

Published in the United States
by Oxford University Press, New York

British Library Cataloguing in Publication Data
Harris, John B.
Natural toxins: animal, plant, and microbial.
1. Toxins
I. Title
615.9'5   QP631
ISBN 0-19-854173-2

Library of Congress Cataloging in Publication Data
Natural toxins.
"This volume is the formal record of the plenary
lectures delivered during the Eighth World Congress on
Animal, Plant, and Microbial Toxins, held during
August 1985 in the University of Newcastle upon Tyne,
UK" — Pref.
Includes bibliographies and index.
1. Toxins — Physiological effect — Congresses.
2. Antitoxins — Congresses. I. Harris, John B. (John
Buchanan), 1940–   . II. World Congress on Animal,
Plant, and Microbial Toxins (8th : 1985 : University of
Newcastle upon Tyne)
QP631.N38 1986 615.9'5 86-18228
ISBN 0-19-854173-2

Set by Computerised Typesetting Services Ltd, London
Printed in Great Britain by Butler & Tanner Ltd,
Frome, Somerset

Preface

Poisonous animals and plants have been known to mankind for centuries. Their poisons have been used to add power to our weapons, to help immobilize prey and to drug and torture our enemies. In many societies, the use of such poisons resulted in the emergence of a special class of druggist, skilled both in the preparation of poisons and in the concoction of remedies to protect against poisoning.

The serious scientific study of animal, plant, and microbial poisons probably began with the works of Redi and Fontana published during the latter half of the seventeenth and the early eighteenth centuries. This was a period when cures for poisoning by animals and plants were being sought, and when viper fat, cautery, olive oil, eaù de Luce, and ammonia were all being strongly recommended. The prevalence of such nonsense, still appearing in the midst of serious scientific work in the latter half of the twentieth century, led to the formation of the International Society on Toxinology in the early 1960s. This Society has stimulated a large increase in the amount of research being undertaken on natural poisons by producing a journal specifically designed for the publication of such work — *Toxicon* — and by sponsoring regular international meetings of toxinologists. This volume is the formal record of the plenary lectures delivered during the Eighth World Congress on Animal, Plant, and Microbial Toxins held during August 1985 in the University of Newcastle upon Tyne, UK.

Although this publication presents new and original findings in many topical fields of toxinology, it is intended to provide the reader with a sound review of the field and should provide an authoritative statement for several years. It is also my hope that the publication will convey some of the excitement generated by the gathering of such an eclectic group of international experts.

I am indebted to all those who helped in the organization of the Congress, and in particular I should thank Professors Pain and Sussman and Drs Panchen and Chapman, who gave editorial assistance during the preparation of this book. I would also like to thank the Oxford University Press for their helpfulness and patience.

Newcastle upon Tyne   J. B. H.
1986

Contents

Part III Biochemical studies on the metabolism of natural toxins

18 The use of monoclonal antibodies to elucidate the antigenic structure and the mechanisms of neutralization of snake toxins　　332

André Ménez, Jean-Claude Boulain, Jean-Marc Grognet, Eric Gatineau, Jacques Couderc, Alan Harvey, and Pierre Fromageot

Plates 2.1–2.4 fall between pages 32 and 33, and Plates 4.1–4.2 between pages 64 and 65.

Contributors

Black, A. R.
Department of Biochemistry, Imperial College, London SW7 2AZ, UK.

Black, J. D.
Department of Biochemistry, Imperial College, London SW7 2AZ, UK.

Boulain, Jean-Claude
Service de Biochimie du Département de Biologie, CEN Saclay, 91191 Gif-sur-Yvette, France.

Busam, L.
Department of Chemistry, Hannover School of Veterinary Medicine, D-3000 Hannover, Federal Republic of Germany.

Couderc, Jacques
Université INSERM 20, Hôpital Broussais, 75014 Paris, France.

Dolly, J. O.
Department of Biochemistry, Imperial College, London SW7 2AZ, UK.

Dougan, Gordon
Bacterial Genetics Group, Molecular Biology, Wellcome Research Laboratories, Beckenham, Kent BR3 3BS, UK.

Evans, Nigel
Consultant Paediatrician, Royal Alexandra Hospital for Sick Children, Brighton, UK. Visiting Research Fellow, University of Sussex, Brighton, UK.

Freer, J. H.
Department of Microbiology, University of Glasgow, Glasgow G11 6NU, UK.

Fromageot, Pierre
Service de Biochimie du Département de Biologie, CEN Saclay, 91191 Gif-sur-Yvette, France.

Gatineau, Eric
Service de Biochimie du Département de Biologie, CEN Saclay, 91191 Gif-sur-Yvette, France.

Grognet, Jean-Marc
SPI de Biochimie du Département de Biologie, CEN Saclay, 91191 Gif-sur-Yvette, France.

Habermehl, G. G.
Department of Chemistry, Hannover School of Veterinary Medicine,
    D-3000 Hannover, Federal Republic of Germany.

Halliwell, J. V.
MRC Neuropharmacology Research Group, School of Pharmacy, London
    WC1 1AL, UK.

Harvey, Alan
University of Strathclyde, Glasgow G1 1XW, UK.

Liener, Irvin I.
Department of Biochemistry, University of Minnesota, St Paul, Minnesota
    55108, USA.

Lüthy, J.
Institute of Toxicology, Swiss Federal Institute of Technology and the
    University of Zurich, CH-8603 Schwerzenbach, Switzerland.

Ménez, André
Service de Biochimie du Département de Biologie, CEN Saclay, 91191 Gif-
    sur-Yvette, France.

Minton, Sherman, A.
Department of Microbiology and Immunology, Indiana University School
    of Medicine, Indianapolis, Indiana 46223, USA.

Nukina, M.
Department of Chemistry, University of Hawaii at Manoa, Honolulu 96822,
    USA.

Olsnes, Sjur
Norsk Hydro's Institute for Cancer Research, Montebello, 0310 Oslo 3,
    Norway.

Pelchen-Matthews, A.
Department of Biochemistry, Imperial College, London SW7 2AZ, UK.

Rosenberg, Philip
Section of Pharmacology and Toxicology, University of Connecticut,
    School of Pharmacy, Storrs, Connecticut 06268, USA.

Sandvig, Kirsten
Norsk Hydro's Institute for Cancer Research, Montebello, 0310 Oslo 3,
    Norway.

Sanyal, Suhas C.
Department of Microbiology, Institute of Medical Sciences, Bararas Hindu
    University, Varanasi 221005, India.

Scheuer, P. J.
Department of Chemistry, University of Hawaii at Manoa, Honolulu 96822, USA.

Shirmizu, Y.
Department of Pharmacognosy and Environmental Health Sciences, College of Pharmacology, University of Rhode Island, Kingston, Rhode Island 02881, USA.

Stone, Bernard F.
CSIRO, Division of Tropical Animal Science, Long Pocket Laboratories, PMB3, Indooroopilly, Queensland 4068, Australia.

Strichartz, G. R.
Anaesthesia Research Laboratories, Brigham and Women's Hospital, and Department of Pharmacology, Harvard Medical School, Boston, Massachussets 02115, USA.

Tachibana, K.
Department of Chemistry, University of Hawaii at Manoa, Honolulu 96822, USA.

Theakston, R. D. G.
WHO Collaborative Centre for Control of Antivenoms, Liverpool School of Tropical Medicine, Pembroke Place, Liverpool L3 5QA, UK

Warrell, David A.
Nuffield Department of Clinical Medicine, John Radcliffe Hospital, Headington, Oxford OX3 9DU, UK.

Part I

The Redi lecture

1

Origins of poisonous snakes: evidence from plasma and venom proteins

Sherman A. Minton

Introduction

Snakes are reptiles whose basic feeding strategy involves subjugation of relatively large prey that is swallowed without dismemberment or mastication. While mechanical methods such as constriction can overcome prey, oral and other digestive secretions are essential for swallowing and digestion. Moreover, the latter process is facilitated if the digestive secretion can be introduced into prey before death and distributed by the prey animal's circulation. Grooved or hollow teeth associated with oral glands producing digestive enzymes and cofactors are a way to accomplish this. If one postulates toxicity for some of the enzymes and cofactors (Ivanov and Ivanov 1979), the snake gains an alternative and versatile method for prey subjugation; it becomes venomous. Savitsky (1980) considers this a key adaptation determining the success of modern snakes, for it allowed snakes to evolve a variety of body forms and locomotor mechanisms while retaining their ability to prey on comparatively large animals. This may have been associated with the spread of more open habitats in the Miocene Period, which seems to have been an exceptionally active era in snake evolution.

Most contemporary snakes probably are venomous in the sense that they have toxic oral secretions and some dental modification for their injection. The oldest fossil snake teeth and teeth of the most primitive living snakes are ungrooved and more or less equal in size (Fig. 1.1). Enlargement of anterior maxillary teeth is common among boas and pythons, and in more advanced snakes. Kardong (1980, 1982) points out that the anterior teeth of snakes function primarily in prey capture and thus are often long and recurved. Elongate posterior teeth, seen in many snakes, are more likely to be heavy and blade-like. Their function is one of holding prey and manipulating it into position for swallowing. Some snakes such as *Dinodon* of eastern Asia and *Trimorphodon* of Middle America display both types. Grooves on anterior or lateral surfaces of maxillary teeth appear in numerous lineages of advanced snakes, in some cases involving only the posterior teeth and in

3

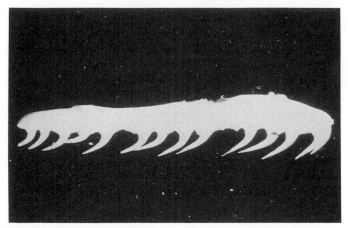

Fig. 1.1 Maxilla of typical colubrid snake (*Elaphe obsoleta*), showing numerous, more or less equal, solid teeth.

other cases virtually all the teeth. Grooved posterior teeth are usually enlarged. Species with grooved and ungrooved teeth may be very closely related by most other criteria. Closure of the anterior face of the groove to form a hollow fang has occurred in several snake lineages. Development of this type fang is nearly always associated with loss of maxillary teeth and shortening of the maxilla. This permits development of larger and more mobile fangs.

Snakes have numerous types of oral glands (Taub 1966; Kochva 1978, Bdolah 1979). The effectiveness of their secretion in lubrication is evident to anyone who has watched a snake feed. Secretions have also been reported to have antibacterial activity (Jansen 1983) and a cleansing action (Gans 1978). A digestive function for pit viper venom has been demonstrated experimentally by Thomas and Pough (1979), but is speculative for oral secretions of other groups. Strydom (1979) proposed a phylogeny of snake venom toxins based on amino-acid sequences in which the ancestral proteins are digestive phospholipases and ribonucleases. Pathways of molecular evolution are better indicated for the proteroglyphs than for the viperids. Kochva (1978) recognized four principal types of venom-producing glands: the venom glands of the elapids or proteroglyphs, the viperids, and the atractaspidids, and Duvernoy's gland of the colubrid snakes. The former three types show greater similarity one with another than with Duvernoy's gland.

Production and injection of venom are obviously the *sine qua non* of a poisonous snake, but Underwood (1979) states:

Poisonous snakes have bedevilled the classification of higher snakes in general. Because people sometimes die when bitten by snakes, the venom apparatus and in particular the dentition have attracted much interest. The classification and evolution of . . . snakes came to be seen in terms of a progression from harmless forms with simple teeth and no venom glands through various intermediate stages to the vipers with their elaborate venom injection apparatus. Much snake taxonomy to this day rests upon dentition and external features to the neglect of other aspects.

This chapter will attempt to analyse the origins and relationships of the major groups of snakes that are known to be venomous. If there is evidence from immunological or biochemical studies of plasma proteins or venom it will be used; however, these data are not inherently more reliable than data from morphology or zoogeography. Snake plasma proteins are probably less subject to selection pressures and to evolutionary parallelism and convergence than are dentition, scale arrangements, and colour pattern, but they are relatively fragile materials, and techniques for their identification and measurement are relatively difficult and not well standardized. Venoms are better known biochemically than are plasma proteins and often are more readily available; however, they may show considerable variation ontogenically and geographically. In a study of venoms of the genus *Vipera*, Saint Girons and Detrait (1978) concluded that differences in venom proteins can evolve more rapidly than morphological features in small isolated populations. This was not the case in large panmictic populations.

Despite Underwood's strictures, dentition does provide a convenient and more or less natural way to divide the venomous snakes into three large groups. One has grooved or hollow fangs at the anterior end of a maxilla that may be reduced but still retains its horizontal orientation with respect to the palatine and pterygoid bones, has limited capacity for rotation, and may bear additional posterior teeth (Fig. 1.2). In a second group, grooved fangs are at the posterior end of a maxilla that usually is long and bears numerous teeth anterior to the fang (Fig. 1.3) but in extreme cases may be much

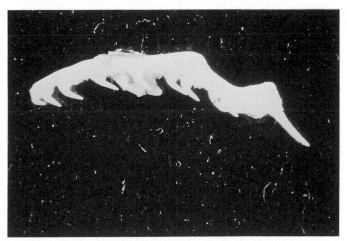

Fig. 1.2 Maxilla of opisthoglyph colubrid (*Malpolon*), showing enlarged posterior tooth which is grooved on its anterior surface.

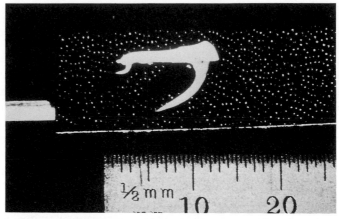

Fig. 1.3 Maxilla of the large proteroglyph *Oxyuranus scutellatus*, showing large anterior hollow fang. The proteroglyph maxilla is elongate and often bears teeth posterior to the fangs.

reduced and otherwise toothless. In the third group, a hollow fang is the only tooth on the maxilla which is greatly reduced and can be rotated until it is at least perpendicular to the palatine and pterygoid bones (Fig. 1.4).

One automatically looks to the lizards for clues to the origins of venomous snakes, but the evidence is very scant and equivocal. Only one lizard family, the Helodermatidae, is venomous, and it appears in no way ancestral to snakes. Its known fossil history extends no further in time than that of many

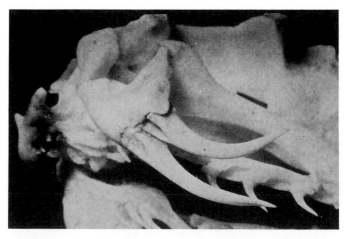

Fig. 1.4 Greatly reduced maxilla of a viperid (*Crotalus*), here shown with two functional fangs. However the lateral fang will be replaced by the medial. (Provided by John Tashjian.)

snake families. The two living species, *Heloderma suspectum* and *H. hor-ridum*, occur in North America. The venom apparatus consists of grooved teeth and venom glands, but these are located in the lower rather than the upper jaw. Like snake venoms, *Heloderma* venoms are mixtures of enzymes and toxic polypeptides. Mebs (1970) and Minton (1974) reported *H. suspectum* venom non-reactive in immuno-electrophoresis and immunodiffusion against snake antivenoms; however, more recently I have observed what appear to be immunoprecipitin lines between freshly-collected *H. horridum* venom and five commercial snake antivenoms.

There is no evidence that the oral secretions of primitive snakes of the families Anomalopidae, Typhlopidae, Leptotyphlopidae, Loxocemidae, Xenopeltidae, Aniliidae, Uropeltidae, Boidae, Acrochordidae, Trop-idophiidae, and Bolyeriidae are toxic, but there have been few investiga-tions of this topic. I found an oral secretion collected from the boa, *Epicrates striatus*, definitely reactive in Ouchterlony immunodiffusion preparations against three commercial snake antivenoms, and questionably reactive against three more. At least two antigens were involved (Table 1.1)

The proteroglyphs

Probably the most primitive venomous snakes occurring today are a group that includes *Toxicocalamus* of New Guinea, *Ogmodon* of Fiji, and possibly some species in Australia and the Solomon Islands. In these species, the short anterior grooved fangs are followed, usually without a gap, by four to seven teeth of gradually decreasing size. McDowell (1969) believes this type dentition is a derived rather than a primitive state, but I see these snakes as relics of what may have been a circumtropical group descended from unknown ancestors. They seem to have participated in the Australian radiation of proteroglyph snakes and given rise to the sea kraits (*Laticauda*). Their contribution to proteroglyph radiations in Africa, Asia, and America is unknown. There have been no studies of their plasma proteins or venoms.

Here I avoid the use of the family name Elapidae, for the content of the family is defined quite differently by Dowling (1975), Smith, Smith, and Sawin (1977), and Cogger, Cameron, and Cogger (1983). My own opinion is that the terrestrial elapids represent at least three groups of family rank. A curious little controversy recently centred around the name Elapidae itself. The small African snakes of the genus *Elaps* gave the name to the family and have long been recognized as proteroglyphs; however, McDowell (1968) reclassified them in the colubrid subfamily Aparallactinae, chiefly on the basis of cranial morphology. Kochva and Wollberg (1970) proposed their return to the Elapidae as a result of their study of the venom glands and associated structures. Because of the widespread use of 'elapid' and related words in medical, biochemical, and toxicological literature, Smith and

Table 1.1 Reactions of 11 colubrid and 1 boid oral secretions with 14 commercial snake antivenoms using Ouchterlony immunodiffusion.

Antivenom and source	Snake Species											
	Dispholidus typus	*Boiga cyanea*	*Trimorphodon biscutatus*	*Rhabdophis tigrinus*	*Rhabdophis subminiatus*	*Thamnophis elegans vagrans*	*Thamnophis s. sirtalis*	*Nerodia erythrogaster*	*Nerodia taxispilota*	*Heterodon platyrhinos*	*Elaphe schrencki*	*Epicrates striatus*
Boomslang (*Dispholidus*) South African Inst. Med. Res.	3+	1	0	0	?	0	0	0	0	1	1	0
Tiger Snake (*Notechis scutatus*) Commonwealth Serum Australia	?	2	1+	?	?	0	?	1	0	1	1	?
Cobra, monovalent Razi Inst., Teheran, Iran	1	1	2	0	2	?	1	1	0	0	0	?
Cobra, polyvalent Behringwerke, Germany	3	2+	2	2	1	2	2	2+	0	1	1	1
Mamba, monovalent Institut Pasteur, Paris	1	1+	1+	2	2	1	2	1	1+	1	2	1
Mamba, polyvalent South African Inst. Med. Res.	2+	2+	3+	2	2+	1	2	1	1+	1	2	1
Coral snake Instituto C. Picado, Costa Rica	0	0	0	—	—	—	0	—	—	0	—	—
Bitis, polyvalent Institut Pasteur, Paris	0	0	2	0	—	—	—	?	—	—	—	0
Vipera lebetina Razi Inst., Teheran, Iran	—	0	—	0	—	—	0	0	—	—	—	0
Echis (Saw-scaled viper) South African Inst. Med. Res.	1	2+	2+	1+	2+	?	2	1	?	1+	0	0

Table 1.1 (*continued*)

Antivenom and source	Snake Species											
	Dispholidus typus	*Boiga cyanea*	*Trimorphodon biscutatus*	*Rhabdophis tigrinus*	*Rhabdophis subminiatus*	*Thamnophis elegans vagrans*	*Thamnophis s. sirtalis*	*Nerodia erythrogaster*	*Nerodia taxispilota*	*Heterodon platyrhinos*	*Elaphe schrencki*	*Epicrates striatus*
Echis (Saw-scaled viper) Razi Inst., Teheran, Iran	—	0	1	1	1	0	0	0	—	0	0	—
Habu (*Trimeresurus flavoviridis*) Inst. Infect. Diseases, Tokyo	1	—	—	0	—	—	?	—	—	—	—	0
Thai pit viper Queen Saovabha Inst., Bangkok	—	0	—	0	—	0	—	0	—	0	—	0
Polyvalent crotalid Wyeth Inc., USA	1	0	1	0	0	?	1	1	1	0	0	?

Numerals indicate the number of precipitin lines. The + symbol indicates unusually strong lines; the ? symbol indicates weak lines seen only after staining with amidoschwarz.

Smith (1976) appealed for security for the family name Elapidae, linking it specifically to the American coral snakes. They recommended use of the generic name *Homoroselaps* for the African snakes formerly known as *Elaps* and tentatively assigned them to the Colubridae. Of more fundamental zoological importance is that *Homoroselaps* is a genus showing a mixture of colubrid and proteroglyph traits. Its relationship to the primitive proteroglyphs of New Guinea and *Elapsoidea* of Africa is worthy of further investigation, particularly by immunological studies of the blood and venom proteins.

The numerous and diverse terrestrial proteroglyph snakes of Australia may represent no more than two original stocks as based on serological data reported by Mao, Chen, Yin and Guo (1983) and on work being continued in our laboratory. Of 13 species whose plasma has been available to us for study by immunoelectrophoresis and radial immunodiffusion, 12 are similar enough to belong to a single stock, while one, *Demansia psammophis*, is distinctly different. Coulter, Harris, and Sutherland (1981) report the toxin notexin as being present in the venoms of four species of Australian proteroglyphs and lacking or present only in trace amounts in three others.

Smith *et al.* (1977) recognized seven tribes of Australian terrestrial proteroglyphs. Mengden (1983) has reviewed the taxonomy of this group.
There is good evidence, both from antigens of plasma and venom, that a
lineage of Australian proteroglyphs containing the genera *Notechis, Hemi-
aspis,* and *Austrelaps* gave rise to all of the sea snakes except *Laticauda.*
Laticauda seems to have branched off quite early from primitive proteroglyph stock, probably in the New Guinea region. Immunological cross-
reactivity of transferrin and albumin indicate that its closest relatives are
Australian terrestrial proteroglyphs and other sea snakes, but it shares more
antigenic determinants with more remotely related proteroglyph groups
such as kraits, coral snakes, and some African genera (Mao, Chen, and
Chang 1977; Mao *et al* 1983; Minton, unpublished). Amino-acid sequences
of toxins indicate that *Laticauda* may be more closely related to the Australian terrestrial snakes than to the other sea snakes (Strydom 1973).
Burger and Natsuno (1974) divided the remaining marine proteroglyphs
into three groups. One contains the genera *Hydrelaps, Ephalophis,* and
Parahydrophis, which are small snakes of estuarine habitat. *Aipysurus* and
Emydocephalus, which are larger and characteristic of coral reefs, make up
a second group. The third group consists of 10 genera and at least 35 species
that are variable in morphology and habitat. Serological studies by Minton
and da Costa (1975), Mao *et al.* (1977), and Cadle and Gorman (1981) show
a close relationship among the species of the third group. *Aipysurus* and
Emydocephalus are also closely related to this group according to Mao and
co-workers, but quite distinct according to Cadle and Gorman (1981).

Africa has been the other main centre of proteroglyph evolution, with the
cobras (*Naja* spp.) and mambas (*Dendroaspis* spp.) as the most spectacular
genera. Romer (1956) considered the maxilla of the mambas sufficiently
different to set them apart from other proteroglyphs, and Saint Girons and
Detrait (1980) found mamba venoms markedly different antigenically from
those of other snakes. On the other hand, workers such as Underwood
(1979) tend to group mambas with *Naja* and other cobra-like genera, with
Pseudohaje as a possible connecting genus. Strydom (1979) found some
Dendroaspis toxins distinctive in their amino-acid sequence, while others
were similar to cobra and sea snake toxins. The cobras and cobra-like
African snakes (*Naja, Boulengerina, Hemachatus, Walterinnesia*) are usually treated as a closely related group; however, there are considerable
differences in the toxicity and antigenic make-up of their venoms
(Mohamed, Khalil, and Baset 1977). Strydom (1979) has analyzed the
relationships between the cytotoxins and neurotoxins as based on the study
of amino-acid sequences. The toxins fall into five groups that are not well
correlated with taxonomic categories. There has been no sero-taxonomic
work done on this group.

I consider the Asian *Naja* as relatively recently derived from two African stocks, one with the fangs modified for 'spitting', and one without this modification. With respect to serum albumin and other plasma proteins, Asian *Naja* are very different from *Bungarus*, and from all Australian and marine proteroglyphs as well as *Elapsoidea* of Africa (Mao *et al.* 1983; Minton, unpublished). The king cobra (*Ophiophagus*) is something of an enigma. I prefer to think of it as an autochthonous Asian species. Its serologic relationship to the sea snakes appears remote (Cadle and Gorman 1981).

Three genera, *Calliophis*, *Maticora*, and *Bungarus*, are restricted to Asia. Very little is known of venoms of the first two genera, which appear to be related to each other and perhaps to *Parapistocalamus* of the Solomons (Mengden 1983). *Bungarus* has been comparatively well studied with respect to both serum and venom, and appears to be quite distinct from all other proteroglyphs. Its affinities are somewhat closer to the Australian than to the African radiation.

In America the proteroglyphs are represented by the coral snakes *Micrurus*, with 43 species, and *Micruroides* with one. They appear to represent a single lineage, although inter-species differences in serum albumins (Cadle and Sarich 1981) and venom antigens indicate a fairly long evolutionary history. The most generally accepted hypothesis for their origin is one of migration of a *Calliophis*-like ancestor from Asia in the early or middle Miocene Period; however, the work with serum albumin using complement fixation shows them about equally distant from *Laticauda* and *Pseudonaja* and more remote from *Bungarus* and *Naja* (Mao *et al.* 1983). Our work with radial immunodiffusion and rocket immunoelectrophoresis tends to confirm this. Accordingly, if the coral snakes had an Asian ancestor, it was probably not *Bungarus*, and it leaves open the possibility that they arose from a line of primitive austral proteroglyphs. Their origin from South American xenodontine colubrids appears unlikely (Cadle and Sarich 1981).

The colubrids and atractaspidids

The second major subdivision of venomous snakes probably evolved from snakes with enlarged posterior maxillary teeth that may or may not have been grooved. Snakes with this type dentition make up a substantial segment of the large family Colubridae. There is little agreement among herpetologists as to relationships within the family or between colubrids and snakes of other families. Smith *et al.* (1977) recognized 28 subfamilies of colubrids; however, definition and content of many are uncertain. Using immunological data from comparison of serum albumins, Dowling, Highton, Maha, and Maxon (1983) recognized seven subfamilies in a study involving 30 representative genera and 56 species. McKinstry (1983) listed 93 genera with enlarged, grooved posterior maxillary teeth (opisthoglyphs),

41 genera with enlarged, ungrooved posterior maxillary teeth (aglyphs), and 43 genera with unmodified teeth but a serous or muco-serous Duvernoy's gland. All these snakes are potentially venomous. Human envenomations have been associated with 34 genera, of which 23 are opisthoglyphous and 11 aglyphous or with unmodified teeth (Minton 1979 and unpublished). All McKinstry's groups are polyphyletic. Bailey (1966) commented on opisthoglyphy as a biological phenomenon. Snakes with this dentition are characteristic of South American and South African fauna, are likely to be nocturnal, and, at the species level, are specialized in food choice.

In our laboratory, we have collected Duvernoy's secretion (venom) from 11 colubrid species belonging to eight genera, three of which are opisthoglyphous and five aglyphous or with unmodified teeth. Ouchterlony reactions between these secretions and commercial snake antivenoms show that all are reactive, and more strongly with mamba and cobra antivenoms (Table 1.1). Further immunological studies show these secretions to be antigenically heterogenous. Some have antigens apparently identical with snake serum proteins; others have not. Their antigens are not related to major cobra and mamba toxins. Polyacrylamide gel electrophoresis shows that the venoms of *Dispholidus typus*, *Boiga cyanea*, *Trimorphodon biscutatus*, and *Thamnophis elegans* are quite different, and that they differ from the venoms of *Crotalus atrox*, *Dendroaspis polylepis*, and *Atractaspis bibroni*, which belong to other families. Our results were similar to those obtained by Young and Miller (1974) using cellulose acetate electrophoresis.

Immunological study of plasma proteins has contributed considerably towards an understanding of the relationships within the Colubridae, but less towards relationships with other families. There is evidence from the immunoelectrophoresis of whole plasma that the colubrid *Heterodon* shares more antigens with the viperids *Agkistrodon*, *Crotalus*, and *Vipera* than other colubrids whose plasmas have been tested (Minton and Salanitro 1972; Minton 1978 and unpublished). Earlier data suggesting a relationship between natricine colubrids and sea snakes (Minton and da Costa 1975) has not been confirmed by recent studies using albumin rather than whole plasma. Plasmas of the Asian colubrids *Dinodon rufizonatum* and *Elaphe carinata* react more strongly with antiserum against albumin of the Australian proteroglyph *Pseudonaja textilis* than do other colubrid plasmas. Those of *Heterodon* and several natricine genera are virtually non-reactive. If a generalization can be made from the serologic evidence, it is that proteroglyphs and viperids arose from quite different colubrid stocks.

The Atractaspididae (burrowing asps, mole vipers, side-biting snakes), consisting of about 15 species mostly confined to Africa, are an interesting group of snakes. Uniformly dark in colour with small heads and cylindrical bodies terminating in a short tail, they resemble diverse burrowing snakes the world over. The long hollow fangs on a greatly reduced maxilla are capable of little forward movement but can be moved backwards as the lower jaw is shifted to the side opposite the fang. One fang is used at a time, and the snakes bite with the mouth virtually closed. The venom glands are unique in structure and histochemical reactions (Kochva, Shayer-Wollberg, and Sobol 1967). In some species they extend well back into the body, a situation seen in the oriental proteroglyph genus *Maticora* and in some species of the primitive African viperid genus *Causus*. Atractaspidids share some venom antigens with proteroglyphs and viperids (Minton 1968a); however, they have an apparently unique cardiotoxin as well as other low molecular weight compounds (Kochva, Viljoen, and Botes 1982; Weiser, Wollberg, Kochva, and Lee 1984).

In our laboratory, plasma of *Atractaspis bibroni* shows more arcs with antisera produced against plasmas of *Vipera palaestinae*, *Agkistrodon piscivorus*, and *Pseudechis porphyriticus* than that against plasmas of the colubrids *Boiga dendrophila*, *Elaphe obsoleta*, *Coluber constrictor*, and *Nerodia sipedon*. This does not imply a specially close relationship between atractaspidids and viperids or Australian proteroglyphs, but does seem to exclude atractaspidids from some of the major colubrid groups. Dowling, Highton, Maha, and Maxon (1983) placed them in the colubrid subfamily Lycodontinae, although molecular data did not support this. The restriction of atractaspidids to Africa and small areas of the Middle East and the apparent absence of close relatives in other parts of the world seem to indicate they are a small but possibly ancient offshoot of some African colubrid stock. However, they have accumulated sufficient morphological and physiological differences to justify their recognition as a family.

The viperids

The viperids represent a reasonably well defined group characterized by hollow fangs on a greatly reduced maxilla that is capable of considerable rotation. They apparently evolved from colubrids with enlarged, grooved posterior teeth (Fig 1.5) by suppression of the anterior maxillary teeth, shortening of the bone, and closure of the groove (Edmund 1969). This condition can be seen today in the South American colubrid *Tomodon dorsatus*, which has almost attained viperid dentition, although the fangs remain posterior in position and apparently do not have the range of movement of viperid fangs. Nothing is known of its venom; however, immunological characterization of its serum albumin puts it within the xenodontine group of South American colubrids (Cadle 1984), some of which are distinctly venomous. Other colubrids that approach this condition include *Xenodon* and *Waglerophis* of tropical America, *Heterodon* of North

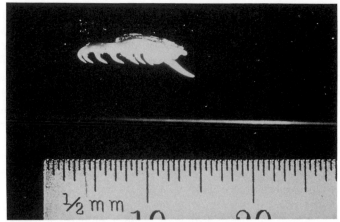

Fig. 1.5 Maxilla of a colubrid with an enlarged rear fang and some shortening of the bone. Further shortening with loss of anterior teeth would produce the viperid maxilla similar to that shown in Fig. 1.4.

America, *Crotaphopeltis* and *Pythonodipsas* of southern Africa, and *Psammodynastes* of south-east Asia. Most of these snakes are viper mimics; some may be viper ancestors. Immunological evidence has been previously mentioned with respect to significant reactivity between *Heterodon* plasma and antisera against viperid plasmas.

Two viperid genera are distinctly colubrid-like in appearance and presumably are primitive. *Causus*, with six species, occurs throughout sub-Saharan Africa, and *Azemiops*, with a single species, inhabits mountainous areas along the China–Burma border. Fangs of *Causus* are short (2.1 mm in a 39 cm specimen) and the venom channel is a groove for about 80 per cent of its length. Except for marked elongation in some species, venom glands are like those of more advanced vipers (Shayer-Wollberg and Kochva 1967). Venoms of *Causus* have received little study. *C. rhombeatus* venom studied in our laboratory showed reactivity in immunodiffusion tests with a wide variety of proteroglyph and viperid commercial antivenoms. Detrait and Saint Girons (1979) also found this venom widely reactive in immuno-electrophoresis against viperid antivenoms. Strongest reactions were with *Bitis arietans* and *Cerastes cerastes*, but these only indicated about 20 per cent common antigens. *Azemiops* has longer and more completely cannulated fangs; however, in cranial morphology and general external characteristics it appears to be more primitive than *Causus* (Liem, Marx, and Rabb 1971). Preliminary studies (Vest and Kardong, unpublished) indicate that the venom of *Azemiops* is not markedly different in antigenic make-up and toxicity from that of other viperids. The serologic affinities of *Causus* and *Azemiops* to other vipers and viper-like colubrids have not been investigated.

The advanced vipers are easily divided into two groups, the crotaline snakes, with heat-sensing loreal pits, and the viperine snakes, without such pits. No morphological intermediates exist, but plasma immuno-electrophoresis indicates that the crotaline *Calloselasma rhodostoma* is as closely related to the viperine *Vipera palaestinae* as to *Agkistrodon piscivorus*, which was formerly considered congeneric with it. The same technique indicates that differences between *V. palaestinae* of Asia and *A. piscivorus* of North America are no greater than those between *V. palaestinae* and *Bitis arietans* of Africa.

Venoms of crotaline and viperine viperids appear to have a fairly large suite of common antigens, although species with pharmacologically aberrant venoms (*Trimeresurus wagleri*, *Crotalus tigris*, *Pseudocerastes fieldi*, *Bitis atropos*) occur in both subfamilies. Evidence seems to favour a dual origin for the viperine snakes with an African lineage arising from a *Causus*-like snake and giving rise to *Bitis*, *Atheris*, *Echis*, *Cerastes*, *Pseudocerastes*, and *Eristicophis*, while *Vipera* appears to be of Asian origin but probably not directly descended from *Azemiops*.

Zoogeographic evidence strongly indicates an Asian origin for the crotaline snakes, although the oldest fossil is from the Miocene Period of Texas (Holman, 1966). The ancestry of the pit vipers is almost wholly unknown other than for an indication that serologically, *Vipera* appears closer to them than do the African genera. Two aberrant and presumably primitive pit vipers are *Calloselasma rhodostoma* and *Trimeresurus wagleri*, both native to south-east Asia. *Calloselasma* is quite different in plasma protein antigens from other pit vipers including *Agkistrodon*, the genus in which it was long included. Its venom antigens are also sufficiently different that there is no cross-neutralization of its venom by other pit viper antivenoms (Kawamura 1974). It has smooth scales, thus differing from all other viperids except *Azemiops* and *Causus*. *T. wagleri* shows a mixture of primitive osteological characters with some specializations, such as keeled gular scales. Brattstrom (1964) considered it the most primitive living pit viper. Its venom contains an apparently unique, low molecular weight, thermostable toxin (Minton 1968b). There is no information on the serum proteins.

Pit vipers apparently moved from Asia to America via a land bridge in the late Oligocene or early Miocene Period, the migration involving stocks related to both *Agkistrodon* and *Trimeresurus*. *Agkistrodon*, because of more limited ecological tolerance or more limited inherent capacity for variation, has remained largely in North America. The three American species are closely related to each other, and, on the basis of serological data, are also close to the Asian *blomhoffi*, *caliginosus*, and *intermedius*. One school of thought derives the rattlesnakes from *Agkistrodon*-like ancestors, principally because of the presence of large head shields in *Agkistrodon* and the more primitive rattlesnakes. This hypothesis is not strongly supported by my work with plasma immunoelectrophoresis, which shows little difference between plasmas of advanced rattlesnakes (*Crotalus atrox*, *C. horridus*, *C. viridis*) and those of primitive rattlesnakes (*Sistrurus catenatus*, *S. ravus*) when reacted with antiserum to plasma of *Agkistrodon piscivorus*.

The palaeotropical *Trimeresurus* and neotropical *Bothrops* show striking superficial similarities and have at times been considered congeneric. Most recent workers have recognized their distinctness, but only a few, such as Brattstrom (1964) and Hoge and Romano-Hoge (1981), have made critical comparisons of considerable numbers of species. Their studies indicate the presence of subgroups in both genera, e.g. the stocky terrestrial *Trimeresurus* typified by *monticola* and *okinavensis* comprise one group, and several arboreal Central American *Bothrops* including *schlegeli*, *nigroviridis*, and *lateralis* comprise another. The large South American *Bothrops*, such as *jararaca*, *atrox*, and *alternatus*, and *B. asper* of Central America, make up a third group of closely related species. The bushmaster, *Lachesis muta*, is a unique pit viper that has been suggested as an ancestor of the rattlesnakes; however, its large size, tuberculate scales, and unusual arrangement of subcaudals mark it as a specialized species, possibly close to the *Trimeresurus*-like pit vipers that migrated from Asia to America in the Miocene Period. As with a large number of *Trimeresurus* species it is oviparous, being unique among American pit vipers in this respect.

My limited work with plasma immunoelectrophoresis indicates that *Trimeresurus mucrosquamatus* and *Bothrops neuwiedi* react to approximately the same degree with *Agkistrodon piscivorus* and *Vipera palaestinae* antisera, but *T. albolabris* is somewhat more reactive with *Vipera*. Reactions between *Agkistrodon* and *Crotalus* are stronger than those between *Agkistrodon* and either *Trimeresurus* or *Bothrops*, while those between *Vipera* and *Crotalus* are weaker than those between *Vipera* and *Trimeresurus* or *Bothrops*.

Detrait and Saint Girons (1979), using immunoelectrophoresis, found 50 per cent of *Trimeresurus flavoviridis* venom antigens developed by *Bothrops lanceolatus* antiserum, which was slightly higher than the percentage of *B. jararaca* and *B. atrox* antigens developed and much higher than those of *Agkistrodon piscivorus*. Using isotachophoresis, Tu, Stermitz, Ishizaki, and Saneo (1980) showed marked differences between *Trimeresurus* and *Bothrops* venoms, although these were not evident with immunodiffusion. Reactions were weak between *T. flavoviridis* antiserum and *Agkistrodon contortrix* venom.

The rattlesnakes (*Sistrurus* and *Crotalus*) appear to represent a group of closely related species. Plasmas of 13 species were all quite similar in their immunoelectrophoresis patterns with *Agkistrodon piscivorus* antiserum; the reaction of *C. durissus* was least distinct. Patterns with *Vipera* antiserum were weak.

Rattlesnake venoms show much variation at the species and population level. For example, venom of *Crotalus tigris* has an antigenic relationship of only about 20 per cent with *C. atrox*. Differences do not reflect phylogeny. *C. atrox* venom has an antigenic relationship of 52 per cent with *Sistrurus miliarius*, a primitive species not closely related to *atrox*, but only 35 per cent with *C. scutulatus*, a closely related species that may occasionally hybridize with *atrox*. With respect to other pit viper genera, both Detrait and Saint Girons (1979) and Tu *et al.* (1980) found venoms of *Bothrops* and *Trimeresurus* closer to *Crotalus* than those of New World *Agkistrodon*. In our laboratory, using immunoelectrophoresis and ELISA, we found the intergeneric relationships of *C. atrox* to be closest with New World *Agkistrodon*, next closest with Central American *Bothrops* (*schlegeli* and *godmani*) and Japanese *Agkistrodon blomhoffi*, third with *Bothrops asper* and *Lachesis*, and least with *Trimeresurus* (*albolabris, flavoviridis*, and *wagleri*) and *Calloselasma* (Minton, Weinstein, and Wilde 1984). In a comprehensive survey of 90 snake venoms for the toxin known as Mojave toxin or K' toxin, Weinstein, Minton, and Wilde (1985) detected it in venoms of 6 of 16 species of *Crotalus* and in *Trimeresurus flavoviridis*. North American rattlesnake populations having the toxin form a geographical mosaic; its presence in South American populations is more general.

Conclusions

The scanty fossil record of snakes indicates an origin in the Lower Cretaceous Period about 130 million years ago. For almost 100 million years they were apparently a group comparatively few in numbers and limited in diversity. The first appearance of venomous species in the fossil record 15 to 20 million years ago indicates that both proteroglyph and viperid lineages were well established at the time. The origins of these groups are highly speculative but probably can be dated near the end of the Oligocene Period, about 30 million years ago. Kardong (1982) proposes the development of both lineages from a presumably opisthoglyph colubrid ancestor. I favour the development of venomous snakes from two stocks, with the proteroglyphs appearing first from ancestors that may have been primitive colubrids or boa-like snakes, and the atractaspidids and viperids appearing later from opisthoglyph colubrids. Evidence from plasma proteins seems to favour this latter hypothesis, while evidence from toxins and other venom components is more in keeping with a monophyletic origin. Students of snake phylogeny have always been more or less in the position of the blind Hindus examining the elephant — each strokes and palpates his own beast and draws his conclusions accordingly. The worker who is at home with amino-acid sequences of toxins may feel uneasy in the world of the palaeontologist and osteologist. Someone who can correlate changes in the serum albumin with the geographical timetable may be uncertain as to the significance of a capitate hemipenis with a deeply forked sulcus spermaticus. Interpreting cranial myology and retinal cell pattern may be easier for some than interpreting data from ecology or zoogeography.

Future work on evolution of snakes and their venoms will probably follow the two approaches that have dominated biology in recent decades, the organismic and the molecular. Methods for identifying antigens have come a long way from the ring precipitin test I learned as a medical student, to ELISA and radioimmunoassay. Techniques for determining amino-acid sequences of toxins, and computer programs for integrating data make possible the construction of elegant phylogenetic trees, incidently without the need for actually looking at a snake. Deciphering the genetic code that governs toxin production has begun. At the level of the organism, new X-ray and cinematographic techniques indicate better how snakes use their peculiar tooth and jaw morphologies. Radiotelemetry gives a much better idea of how poisonous snakes hunt for prey and how often their paths intersect those of people.

Acknowledgements— In the preparation of this chapter I have profited from discussion with many friends and colleagues, but owe special thanks to Kenneth V. Kardong, Scott A. Weinstein, and Madge R. Minton. Some of the ideas expressed were formulated as the result of a visit to Australia funded in part by National Science Foundation Grant INT 79–20007. Research on pit vipers and their venoms was funded in part by a grant from Wyeth Laboratories Inc. Figure 4 was contributed by John Tashjian. For clerical assistance, I wish to thank Karen Coffman.

References

Bailey, J. R. (1966). Modes of evolution in New World opisthoglyph snakes. *Mem. Inst. Butantan Simp. int.* **33**, 67–72.

Bdolah, A. (1979). The venom glands of snakes and venom secretion. In *Snake venoms* (ed. C. Y. Lee), pp. 41–57. Springer, Berlin.

Brattstrom, B. H. (1964). Evolution of the pit vipers. *Trans. San Diego Soc. nat. Hist.* **13** (11), 185–268.

Burger, W. L. and Natsuno, T. (1974). A new genus for the Arafura smooth sea snake and redefinitions of other sea snake genera. *Snake* **6**, 61–75.

Cadle, J. E. (1984). Molecular systematics of neotropical xenodontine snakes: I South American xenodontines. *Herpetologica* **40**, 8–20.

—— and Gorman, G. C. (1981). Albumin immunological evidence and the relationships of sea snakes. *J. Herpetol.* **15**, 329–34.

—— and Sarich, V. M. (1981). An immunological assessment of the phylogenetic position of New World coral snakes. *J. Zool.* **195**, 157–67.

Cogger, H. G., Cameron, E. E., and Cogger, H. M. (1983). *Zoological catalogue of Australia.* Vol. 1, *Amphibia and reptilia.* Australian Government Publishing Service, Canberra.

Coulter, A. R., Harris, R. D., and Sutherland, S. K. (1981). Enzyme immunoassay and radioimmunoassay: their use in the study of Australian and exotic snake venoms. *Proceedings of the Melbourne Herpetology Symposium,* pp. 39–43. Zoological Board of Victoria, Melbourne.

Detrait, J. and Saint Girons, H. (1979). Communautes antigeniques des venins et systematique des viperidae. *Bijdr. Dierk.* **49**, 71–80.

Dowling, H. G. (1975). A provisional classification of snakes. In *Yearbook of herpetology* pp. 167–70. HISS Publications, American Museum of Natural History, New York.

——, Highton, R., Maha, G. C., and Maxon, L. R. (1983). Biochemical evaluation of colubrid snake phylogeny. *J. Zool.* **201**, 309–329.

Edmund, A. G. (1969). Dentition. In *Biology of the reptilia,* (ed. C. Gans, A. Bellairs and T. S. Parsons), Vol. 1, Morphology A, pp. 173–84. Academic Press, London.

Gans, C. (1978). Reptilian venoms: some evolutionary considerations. In *Biology of the reptilia* (ed. C. Gans and K. A. Gans), Vol. 8, Physiology B, pp. 1–42. Academic Press, London.

Hoge, A. and Romano-Hoge, S. A. R. W. L. (1981). Poisonous snakes of the world Part I. Checklist of the pit vipers Viperoidea, Viperidae, Crotalinae. *Mem. Inst. Butantan* **42/43**, 179–310.

Holman, J. A. (1966). A small Miocene herpetofauna from Texas. *Q. J. Fla Acad. Sci.* **21**, 267–75.

Ivanov, C. P. and Ivanov, O. C. (1979). The evolution and ancestors of toxic proteins. *Toxicon* **17**, 205–20.

Jansen, D. W. (1983). A possible function of the secretion of Duvernoy's gland. *Copeia* **1983** (1), 262–4.

Kardong, K. V. (1980). Evolutionary patterns in advanced snakes. *Am. Zool.* **20**, 269–82.

—— (1982). The evolution of the venom apparatus in snakes from colubrids to viperids and elapids. *Mem. Inst. Butantan* **46**, 106–118.

Kawamura, Y. (1974). Study of the immunological relationships between venom of six Asiatic *Agkistrodons. Snake* **6**, 19–26.

Kochva, E. (1978). Oral glands of the Reptilia. In *Biology of the reptilia* (ed. C. Gans and K. A. Gans), Vol. 8, Physiology B, pp. 43–161. Academic Press, London.

—— and Wollberg, M. (1970). The salivary glands of Aparallactinae (Colubridae) and the venom glands of *Elaps* (Elapidae) in relation to the taxonomic status of this genus. *Zool. J. Linn. Soc.* **49**, 217–24.

——, Shayer-Wollberg, M., and Sobol, R. (1967). The special pattern of the venom gland in *Atractaspis* and its bearing on the taxonomic status of the genus. *Copeia,* **1967** (4), 763–772.

——, Viljoen, C. C., and Botes, D. P. (1982). A new type toxin in the venom of snakes of the genus *Atractaspis. Toxicon* **20**, 581–92.

Liem, K. F., Marx, H., and Rabb, G. B. (1971). The viperid snake *Azemiops:* its comparative cephalic anatomy and phylogenetic position in relation to Viperinae and Crotalinae. *Fieldiana Zool.* **59**, 65–126.

McDowell, S. B. (1968). Affinities of the snakes usually called *Elaps lacteus* and *E. dorsalis*. *J. Linn. Soc. Zool.* **47**, 561–78.

—— (1969). *Toxicocalamus*: a New Guinea genus of snakes of the family Elapidae. *J. Zool.* **159**, 443–511.

McKinstry, D. M. (1983). Morphologic evidence of toxic saliva in colubrid snakes: a checklist of world genera. *Herpetol. Rev.* **14**, 12–15.

Mao. S., Chen, B., and Chang, H. (1977). The evolutionary relationships of sea snakes suggested by immunological cross-reactivity of transferrins. *Comp. Biochem. Physiol.* **57**, 403–6.

——, ——, Yin, F. and Guo, Y. (1983). Immunotaxonomic relationships of sea snakes to terrestrial elapids. *Comp. Biochem. Physiol.* **74A**, 869–72.

Mebs, D. (1970). Untersuchungen uber die Wirksamkeit einiger Schlangengift-seren gegenuber *Heloderma*-gift. *Salamandra* **6**, 135–6.

Mengden, G. A. (1983). The taxonomy of Australian snakes: a review. *Rec. Austr. Mus.* **35**, 195–222.

Minton, S. A. (1968a). Antigenic relationships of the venom of *Atractaspis microlepidota* to that of other snakes. *Toxicon* **6**, 59–65.

—— (1968b). Preliminary observations on the venom of Wagler's pit viper (*Trimeresurus wagleri*). *Toxicon* **6**, 93–7.

—— (1974). *Venom diseases*. Charles C. Thomas, Springfield, Illinois.

—— (1978). Serological relationships among some midwestern snakes. *Proc. Indiana Acad. Sci.* **87**, 438–45.

—— (1979). Beware: nonpoisonous snakes. *Clin. Tox* **15**, 259–65.

—— and da Costa, M. (1975). Serological relationships of sea snakes and their evolutionary implications. In *The biology of sea snakes* (ed. W. A. Dunson), pp. 33–55. University Park Press, Baltimore.

—— and Salanitro, S. K. (1972). Serological relationships among some colubrid snakes. *Copeia* **1972**, 246–52.

——, Weinstein, S. A. and Wilde, C. E. (1984). An enzyme-linked immunoassay for detection of North American pit viper venoms. *J. Tox. clin. Tox.* **22**, 303–16.

Mohamed, A. H., Khalil, F. K., and Baset, A. A. (1977). Immunological studies on polyvalent and monovalent snake antivenins. *Toxicon* **15**, 271–75.

Romer, A. S. (1956). *Osteology of the reptiles*. University of Chicago Press, Chicago.

Saint Girons, H. and Detrait, J. (1978). Communautes antigeniques des venins et systematique des viperes Europeénes. Etude immuno-electrophoretique. *Bull. Soc. zool. France* **103**, 155–66.

—— and —— (1980). Communautes antigeniques des venins et systématique des elapinae. *Bijdr. Dierk.* **50**, 96–104.

Savitzky, A. H. (1980). The role of venom delivery strategies in snake evolution. *Evolution* **34**, 1194–204.

Shayer-Wollberg, M. and Kochva, E. (1967). Embryonic development of the venom apparatus in *Causus rhombeatus* (Viperidae, Ophidia) *Herpetologica* **23**, 249–59.

Smith, H. M. and Smith, R. B. (1976). Request for suppression and validation of names related to the Elapidae (Reptilia: Serpentes). *Bull. Zool. Nomencl.* **33**, 73–84.

——, ——, and Sawin, H. L. (1977). A summary of snake classification (Reptilia: Serpentes). *J. Herpetol.* **11**, 115–21.

Strydom, D. J. (1973). Snake venom toxins. Structure–function relationships and phylogenetics. *Comp. Biochem. Physiol.* **44B**, 269–74.

—— (1979). The evolution of toxins found in snake venoms. In (ed. C. Y. Lee) *Snake venoms*, pp. 258–75. Springer, Berlin.

Taub, A. (1966). Ophidian cephalic glands. *J. Morphol.* **118**, 529–42.

Thomas R. G. and Pough, F. H. (1979). The effect of rattlesnake venom on digestion of prey. *Toxicon* **17**, 221–28.

Tu, A. T., Stermitz, J., Ishizaki, H., and Saneo, N. (1980). Comparative study of pit viper venoms of genera *Trimeresurus* from Asia and *Bothrops* from America: an immunological and isotachophoretic study. *Comp. Biochem. Physiol.* **66B**, 249–54.

Underwood, G. (1979). Classification and distribution of venomous snakes in the world. In Snake venoms (ed. C. Y. Lee), pp. 15–40. Springer, Berlin.

Weinstein, S. A., Minton, S. A., and Wilde, C. E. (1985). The distribution among ophidian venoms of a toxin isolated from the venom of the Mojave rattlesnake (*Crotalus s. scutalatus*). *Toxicon* **23**, 825–44.

Weiser, E., Wollberg, Z., Kochva, E., and Lee, S. Y. (1984). Cardiotoxic effects of the venom of the burrowing asp, *Atractaspis engaddensis*. *Toxicon* **22**, 767–74.

Young, R. A. and Miller, D. M. (1974). Comparative study of the venoms of Crotalidae, Elapidae, Viperidae, and Boiginae. *Trans. Ill. State Acad. Sci.* **67**, 444–50.

Part II

Clinical effects of natural poisons
on humans and domestic livestock

2

Tropical snake bite: clinical studies in south-east Asia

David A. Warrell

Introduction: the global importance of snake bite and other types of direct envenoming

As viewed from most Western countries, the clinical problem of direct envenoming may seem too rare or even esoteric to deserve much attention. This may explain the relative neglect of clinical aspects of envenoming as a subject for research compared to the basic biochemical, immunological, and pharmacological properties of animal venoms. However, in an increasing number of tropical countries, venomous bites and stings are becoming recognized as major causes of morbidity and mortality, affecting particularly the rural populations as an occupational risk of farmers and plantation workers. Both under-reporting (Reid and Lim 1957; Warrell and Arnett 1976; Pugh, Theakston, Reid, and Bhar 1980) and errors in epidemiological methods (Pugh and Theakston 1980) have obscured the true incidence of bites and stings and their effects. The following examples can do no more than point to the potential size of the problem. If hypersensitivity to venoms (e.g. of Hymenoptera) is excluded and only direct effects of venoms injected by bites or stings are considered, only snake bites and scorpion stings are sufficiently common and severe to constitute a major medical problem.

Fatal scorpion stings are common in Mexico, Brazil, Trinidad, and parts of north Africa, the Middle East, and India. In Mexico there were thought to be 300 000 cases of scorpion stings each year, with between one and two thousand deaths attributable to *Centruroides* species (World Health Organization 1981). The incidence of fatalities is highest in Colima State (84 deaths per 100 000 population per year) compared to a mere 3 per 100 000 caused by *C. suffusus* in the infamous Durango State (Mazzotti and Bravo-Becherelle 1963). Hospital data from Brazil (Bücherl, 1978) indicate a high incidence of scorpion stings caused mainly by *Tityus* species with case fatalities ranging from 1 per cent in adults to 20 per cent in young children. In Trinidad there were an average of 175 stings by *Tityus trinitatis* and 8 deaths

25

each year (Waterman 1950). In Algeria, there were an average of 1260 stings and 24 deaths per year attributable to *Androctonus australis* (Balozet 1964). In southern Libya, there were 900 stings with 7 deaths per 100 000 population in 1979 (World Health Organization 1981). Reports from India suggest a high mortality, even in adults, following stings by *Buthotus tamulus* (formerly *Buthus tamulus*) (Bawaskar 1982).

Fatal snake bite is even more common, and more widespread than scorpion sting. The estimated annual mortality in Brazil decreased from 4800 in 1929 to about 2000 in 1949 and is now thought to be much lower (Swaroop and Grab 1954). In Venezuela there are an average of 973 bites and 103 deaths per year: *Bothrops atrox* is responsible for 38 per cent and *Crotalus durissus terrificus* for 24 per cent (Dao, 1971). In the savanna region of West Africa, there is a high incidence of bites by *Echis carinatus*. In the Benue Valley of Nigeria, there is an incidence of 497 bites per 100 000 population per year, with a 12.2 per cent case mortality (Warrell and Arnet 1976; Pugh and Theakston 1980). Snake bite is a major cause of death among some hunter–gatherer tribes, such as the Yanomamo of Amazonian Venezuela (2 per cent of all adult deaths) (Chagnon 1968), the Waorani of eastern Ecuador (5 per cent of all deaths) (Theakston, Reid, Larrick, Koplan, and Yost 1981b), the Hadza of Tanzania (Woodburn 1978, personal communication) and the highlanders of Papua New Guinea (Gajdusek 1977). In the 1880s Sir Joseph Fayrer (1882) wrote: '. . . not less than 20 000 persons are destroyed annually by snakes (in British India)'. The recent mortality of snake bite in the whole of India is unknown, but in Maharashtra State alone, there are more than 1000 deaths a year (World Health Organization 1981). In Thailand, more than 10 000 bites are reported each year, but this is undoubtedly an underestimate. It is unlikely, however, that there are now more than about 100 deaths per year. In Burma, the reported annual snake bite mortality exceeded 2000 (15.4 per 100 000 population) in the 1930s and was as high as 36.8 per cent 100 000 population in Sagaing District (Swaroop and Grab 1954). It is still thought to exceed 1000 per year (3.3 per 100 000 population; Aung-Khin 1980) but is probably much higher. It has been the country's fifth most important cause of death. In Sri Lanka, the incidence of snake bite seems to be increasing and currently exceeds 60 000 per year, with more than 900 deaths (de Silva, unpublished).

Clinical research on snake bite in Thailand, Burma, and Sri Lanka

The classical studies of the late Dr H. Alistair Reid were a great stimulus to the systematic clinical investigation of snake-bitten patients in south-east Asia. His work in north west Malaya provided a corpus of reliable clinical observations on the effects of bites by cobras (*Naja kaouthia*), Malayan pit vipers (*Calloselasma rhodostoma*) and sea snakes, on which to base further studies of envenoming by these and related species.

Taxonomy and zoology

The principal species of medical importance are: in Thailand, *Calloselasma rhodostoma*, *Naja kaouthia*, *Vipera russelli*, *Trimeresurus albolabris* and *Bungarus candidus*; in Burma, *V. russelli*, *N. kaouthia*, and *T. erythrurus;* and in Sri Lanka, *V. russelli*, *N. naja*, *B. caeruleus*, and *H. hypnale*. Despite the notable contributions by F. Wall (1921), M. A. Smith (1943) and E. H. Taylor (1965), there remain some taxonomic problems with the venomous terrestrial snakes of this region, which could have important clinical implications. The cobras of south-east Asia have been regarded as subspecies or varieties of a single species *Naja naja* (Linnaeus) (Smith 1943). Deraniyagala (1960–61) and Soderberg (1973) have suggested specific status for the monocellate cobra (*Naja kaouthia*, Lesson in Ferussac 1831) (Fig 2.1). In Thailand and Malaya, cobras capable of 'spitting' their venom are morphologically distinct, lacking the monocellate nuchal marking. These spitting cobras either have no marking at all on the hood (Fig 2.2) or only a vague suggestion of the 'spectacle' of the *forma typica* of *N. naja* in India. Thai spitting varieties, which occur in distinctive black and white and brown phases, should probably be referred to as *N.n. sputatrix* (Boie 1827) as in Malaya (Tweedie, 1983). The clinical importance of distinguishing between *N.n sputatrix* and *N. kaouthia* was indicated by analysis of a new monospecific antivenom raised against Malayan *N.n. sputatrix* venom. Using a standard mouse assay technique (Theakston and Reid 1983), Dr R. D. G. Theakston found that the antivenom was effective against

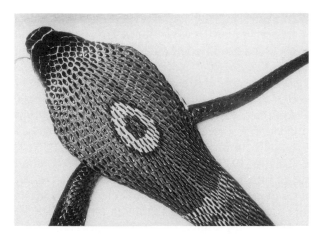

Fig. 2.1 Monocellate cobra (*Naja kaouthia*): specimen from Trang, Thailand. (Copyright © D. A. Warrell.)

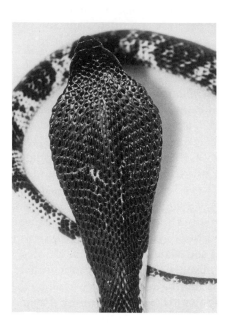

Fig. 2.2 Spitting cobra (*Naja naja sputatrix*), black and white variety: specimen from
Suphanburi, Thailand. (Copyright © D. A. Warrell.)

N.n. sputatrix venom from Malaysia (mean ED_{50} 47 μg per mouse), but was
ineffective against *N. kaouthia* venom from Thailand, and *N. naja* venoms
from India and Sri Lanka (Theakston, R. D. G., unpublished). The second
important area of confusion in Thai herpetology is the identification of the
various species of arboreal green pit viper, genus *Trimeresurus* (Plates 2.1–
2.4). Failure to observe the condition of the nasal and first supralabial scale
has led to the misidentification of *T. macrops* (Kramer 1977; Regenass and
Kramer 1981) as *T. popeorum* by Klemmer (1963), Nootpand (1971), and
Kundert (1974) and of *T. popeorum* as *T.erythrurus* (which does not occur
in Thailand) by Nootpand (1971) and Freiberg and Walls (1984). This
confusion in identification has rendered all the work on *Trimeresurus* venoms in Thailand virtually uninterpretable (Mitrakul 1973, 1979; Mitrakul
and Impun 1973; Talalak 1977). A national survey of venomous snakes
responsible for snake bites, still in progress, has shown that *T. albolabris*
causes far more cases of snake bite than any other member of the genus, and
also produces more severe envenoming, although fatalities are extremely
rare (Looareesuwan *et al.*, unpublished). The only antivenom available for
treatment of Thai green pit viper bites is manufactured by the Queen
Saovabha Memorial Institute (Thai Red Cross Society), Bangkok, which

takes no account of the various species of green *Trimeresurus*. Admixture of venom from *T. macrops*, which is abundant in the Bangkok area, may partially explain the disappointing potency of this antivenom in the treatment of systemic envenoming by *T. albolabris* (Looareesuwan *et al.*, unpublished; Visudhiphan, Dumavibhat, and Trishnananda 1981; Trishnananda, unpublished).

The habits, diurnal and seasonal changes in behaviour, and ecology of the venomous snakes of south-east Asia are virtually unknown. The population density of clinically important venomous species is one of the determinants of snake bite incidence, yet this has never been estimated for any species. The only hint of the size of the snake population is provided by the numbers of snakes brought in response to offers of rewards. For example, 115 921 *Echis carinatus* were killed in 8 days in Ratnagiri, India (Vidal 1890) and 81 251 *Vipera russelli* were killed in one year in Tharrawaddy, Burma (Burma Gazetteer 1959).

Confirmatory immunodiagnosis of the biting species
In most parts of the world, only a minority of snake bite victims bring the dead snake for identification. In the remainder, the diagnosis is conjectural. This is one of the major defects of the snake bite literature. Over the last 30 years, a variety of immunological and other methods have been used to identify the biting species by detecting specific venom or venom components in the serum and other body fluids of the patient (Theakston 1983; Ho, Warrell, Warrell, Bidwell, and Voller 1986). Enzyme-linked immunosorbent assay (ELISA) (Theakston, Lloyd-Jones, and Reid 1977) has been the most widely used. Under some circumstances, this test could produce a result in 30 min or less, which might be useful in directing the management of an acutely envenomed patient. This would be particularly valuable in areas where the venoms of a number of different species produce the same clinical syndrome, but where monospecific antivenoms are used for treatment. The ELISA technique is undoubtedly sensitive, but problems have been encountered when it has been used for the detection of venom antigen and particularly venom antibody in rural communities in the tropics. Thus 36 out of 100 healthy controls with no history of snake bite had sera which were positive for *C. rhodostoma* antigen, and 22 out of 35 similar controls from Lower Burma had sera positive for *Vipera russelli* antigen. These results were shown to be the result of non-specific binding and the problem was partly controlled by addition of 1 per cent normal rabbit serum to the diluent of serum and conjugate (Ho *et al.* 1986). Non-specific reactions are even more of a problem in the detection of venom antibody. Seventy-five per cent of a group of 102 non-bitten healthy controls had sera which showed absorbence values above the negative cut-off point chosen by previous epidemiological surveys using ELISA in Nigeria (Theakston, Pugh, and

Reid 1981a) and Ecuador (Theakston *et al*. 1981b). It is clear from the work of Dr May Ho that the positive:negative threshold for ELISA assays must be based on the mean absorbence value of a large group of non-bitten controls from the same community and socio-economic background as the patient population. In Thailand there is no cross-reactivity between the venoms of the four most important venomous species: *Naja kaouthia*, *Calloselasma rhodostoma*, *Vipera russelli* and *Trimeresurus albolabris*. Between the venoms of *T*. *albolabris* and *T*. *macrops*, the two species of *Trimerusurus* found in the Bangkok area, there is some cross-reactivity, but at levels many-fold lower than the reaction with homologous antibody (Ho *et al*. 1986). However, in Australia, cross-reactions have created problems with the use of the Commonwealth Serum Laboratories' ELISA diagnostic kit (Marshall and Herrmann 1984; McCarthy 1984; Fulde and Smith 1984).

Immunodiagnosis has proved useful in Thailand for revealing unexpected causes of severe or fatal envenoming. Thus the Malayan krait (*Bungarus candidus*) was found to be responsible for a number of cases of fatal or severe neurotoxic envenoming in eastern Thailand (Warrell, Looareesuwan, White, Theakston, Warrell, Kosakarn, and Reid 1983). These results have been confirmed by a survey in north-eastern Thailand (Looareesuwan *et al*., unpublished). A study in Bang Phli, 30 km south-east of the centre of Bangkok, found that the serum of one of four fatal cases of neurotoxic envenoming attributed to *N*. *kaouthia* contained a high concentration of banded krait (*Bungarus fasciatus*) venom (Viravan, Veeravat, Warrell, Theakston, and Warrell 1986). In two surveys of snake bite mortality in Anuradhapura district of Sri Lanka, the common krait (*B*. *caeruleus*) was implicated in 22 and 40 per cent of fatal cases (de Silva 1981; Sawai, Toriba, Itokawa, de Silva, Perera, and Kottegoda 1984). However, the identification was not confirmed in the majority of cases and all the bites occurred at night. In this case, as with the night-biting *B*. *candidus* of south-east Asia and spitting cobra (*Naja nigricollis*) of West Africa, immunodiagnosis is the only way of establishing the true cause of envenoming (Warrell, Greenwood, Davidson, Ormerod, and Prentice 1976; Warrell *et al*. 1983).

Clinical manifestations of envenoming by Russell's viper

Neurotoxic envenoming in Sri Lanka   Russell's viper (*V*. *russelli*) occurs in nine Asian countries: Pakistan, India, Sri Lanka, Burma, Thailand, Kampuchea, southern mainland China, Taiwan, and in several islands of Indonesia. Publications from India, and clinical experience in Thailand, Burma, and Sri Lanka, have revealed a fascinating geographical variation in the clinical effects of the venom of of this snake, which is regarded as a single species throughout its range. These differences, some of them unconfirmed,

Table 2.1 Geographical variation in the clinical manifestations of Russell's viper bite.

	Sri Lanka	India	Burma	Thailand
Renal failure	++	+	++	+
Pituitary haemorrhage	−	+	++	−
Inravascular haemolysis	++	+	−	−
Neuro-mytoxicity	++	+	−	−
Generalized capillary permeability	−	−	+	−
Hypotension	−	+	++	−

are summarized in the Table 2.1. Most striking is the development of neurotoxicity after bites by *V. r. pulchella* (Gray) in Sri Lanka and Southern India. This was first noted by Spaar (1910), who looked after a fatal case in Trincomalee: 'The elevators of the lids exhibited paretic symptoms.' Neurological manifestations and generalized myalgia developed in more than 70 per cent of hospital cases (Jeyarajah 1984). There is ptosis, ophthalmoplegia, inability to open the mouth and protrude the tongue (Fig. 2.3), and paralysis of the muscles of deglutition and respiration, even leading to respiratory distress (Munasinghe and Kulasinghe 1965; Peiris, Wimalaratne, and Nimalasuriya 1969; Visuvaratnam, Vinayagamoorthy and Balakrishnan 1970; Nimalasuriya 1971). These effects seem to be reversible by Haffkine polyspecific antivenom (raised against Indian *V. r. russelli* venom), exchange blood transfusion (Peiris *et al.* 1969), and anticholinesterase (Nimalasuriya 1971). In Sri Lankan victims of *V. r. pulchella*, dark urine has been attributed to haemoglobinuria resulting from massive intravascular haemolysis (Peiris *et al.* 1969). However, in the absence of definite haemoglobinaemia and significant haematuria, the passage of dark red urine suggests myoglobinuria (Jeyarajah 1984). The combination of neurotoxicity, generalized myalgia, and myoglobinuria would imply the presence in *V. r. pulchella* venom of a presynaptic neurotoxin with phospholipase A_2 activity similar to that of some hydrophiid venoms.

Pituitary haemorrhage, 'Sheehan's syndrome', in Burma and India Pituitary dysfunction following snake bite was first described by Wolff (1958) in a man bitten 7 years previously by *Bothrops jararacussu* in Brazil. Panhypopituitarism in three patients suspected of having been bitten by Russell's vipers in southern India was reported by Eapen, Chandy, Kochuvartey, Zacharia, Thomas, and Ipe (1976), who have subsequently observed diabetes insipidus as a late complication of snake bite (Eapen,

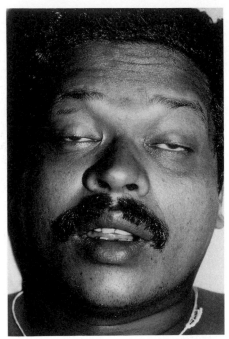

Fig. 2.3 Sri Lankan patient with neurotoxic envenoming caused by *Vipera russelli pulchella*. He is attempting to look up and to the right, to open his mouth and protrude his tongue. (Copyright © D. A. Warrell.)

Chandy, and Joseph 1984). In Burma, pituitary haemorrhage with or without adrenal haemorrhage is a common finding in fatal cases of Russell's viper (*V. r. siamensis*) bite (Maung-Maung-Aye 1976; Hla-Myint, Hla-Mon, Maung-Maung-Khin, and Thet-Win 1982). Haemorrhages are mainly confined to the anterior lobe, pituitary stalk, optic chiasma and the base of the brain (Fig. 2.4). It is interesting that patients with these post-mortem appearances have usually survived the acute coagulopathy: blood coagulability has been restored following treatment with specific antivenom and blood transfusion, but thrombocytopenia and increased fibrinolytic activity may persist. Acute pituitary–adrenal insufficiency has been blamed for the profound and sometimes refractory hypotension that develops soon after severe envenoming (Maung-Maung-Aye 1976; Hla-Myint *et al.* 1982). This condition resembles the acute necrosis of the anterior pituitary associated with post-partum hypotension and haemorrhage (Sheehan 1939). Survivors of *V. r. siamensis* bite in Burma may present in coma during the year after the bite with features of Addisonian crisis, or years later with chronic panhypopituitarism (Hla-Mon, unpublished; Maung-Maung-Aye 1984). These fascinating phenomena are being investigated by the staffs of the

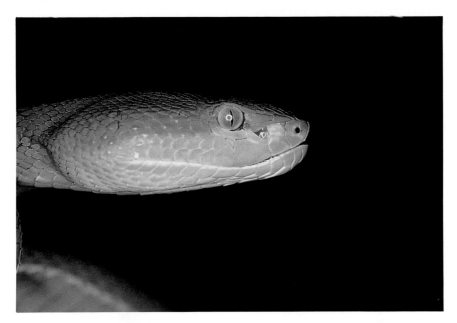

Plate 2.1 *T. albolabris* — a common cause of snake bite throughout Thailand. Note fused nasal and first supralabial scales. (Copyright © D. A. Warrell.)

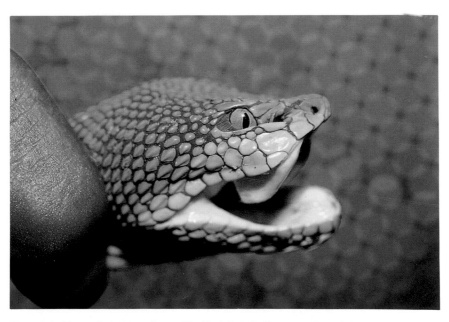

Plate 2.2 *T. erythrurus* replaces *T. albolabris* in Burma where it is responsible for occasional bites. Note keeled temporal scales and fused nasal and first supralabial scales. (Copyright © D. A. Warrell.)

Plates 2.1–2.4 Green pit vipers (genus *Trimeresurus*), showing condition of nasal and first supralabial scales, an important guide to their identification. (Copyright © D. A. Warrell.)

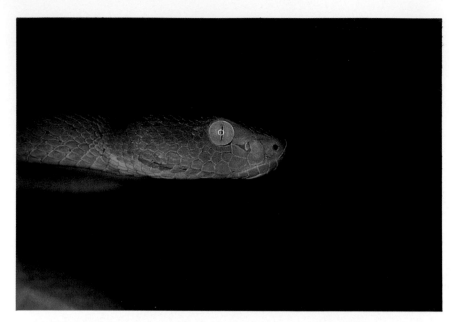

Plate 2.3 *T. macrops* — a common cause of snake bite in Bangkok area. Note fused nasal and first supralabial scales. (Copyright © D. A. Warrell.)

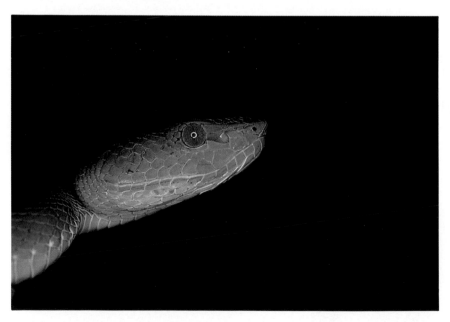

Plate 2.4 *T. popeorum* — an uncommon snake in Thailand, not yet implicated as a cause of snake bite. Note divided nasal and first supralabial scales. (Copyright © D. A. Warrell.)

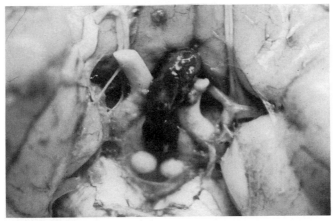

Fig. 2.4 Pituitary haemorrhage in a Burmese patient who died one week after being envenomed by *Vipera russelli siamensis*. (By courtesy of Dr U Hla Mon, Rangoon.)

Department of Medical Research and the Renal Unit, Rangoon General Hospital, Rangoon, Burma.

Generalized increase in capillary permeability in Burma Conjunctival oedema (chemosis) occurs in patients severely envenomed by *V. r. siamensis* in Burma (Maung-Maung Aye 1972) (Fig. 2.5). This sign has not been described from the other countries inhabited by Russell's viper. In Burma, local swelling at the site of the bite is usually quite limited, but there is initial haemoconcentration and a fall in serum albumin during the first few days (Myint-Lwin, Warrell, Phillips, Tin-Nu-Swe, Tun-Pe, and Maung-Maung-

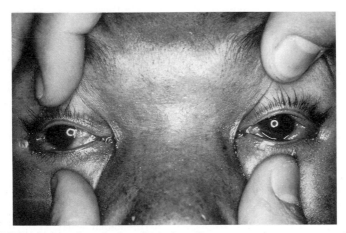

Fig. 2.5 Bilateral conjunctival oedema in a Burmese patient envenomed by *V. r. siamensis*. (Copyright © D. A. Warrell.)

Lay 1985). Taken together with clinical observations of hypovolaemia, serous effusions, pulmonary oedema, and conjuctival oedema, these findings suggest a generalized increase in capillary permeability with leakage of fluid and protein into the tissues. This could be a direct effect of the venom or the result of autopharmacological release of endogenous mediators such as histamine, 5-hydroxytryptamine, kinins, and prostaglandins.

Important clinical manifestations caused by venoms of other south-east Asian species

Malayan pit viper (Calloselasma rhodostoma) (formerly Ancistrodon or Agkistrodon rhodostoma)   The detailed clinical observations reported by the late Dr H. Alistair Reid (Reid, Thean, Chan, and Baharom 1963a; Reid, Chan and Thean 1963b) in Malaya, leave little scope for further work. However, studies of *C. rhodostoma* bite in eastern and southern Thailand (Warrell, unpublished) have revealed some differences from the clinical pattern in Malaya. This species appears to be the commonest cause of snake bite morbidity (but *not* mortality) in Thailand, Laos, Kampuchea, Vietnam, and Java as well as in the northern part of peninsular Malaysia. In Thailand it has been collected in almost every province (Looareesuwan *et al.*, unpublished), but is most uncommon in the areas of highest rainfall in the eastern and southern parts of the country. In Thailand, the gingival sulci and not the lungs are the commonest site of spontaneous systemic haemorrhage. Hypotension ('shock') is very uncommon, and electrocardiographic abnormalities have not been found. Neutrophil leucocytosis and thrombocytopenia are the rule in patients with systemic envenoming. A few deaths do occur from intracranial haemorrhage or massive gastrointestinal haemorrhage during the acute phase of envenoming. However, the clinical picture in Thailand is dominated by local effects of the venom. Massive local swelling, bruising, blistering (Fig 2.6) and extensive necrosis of skin and muscle are not uncommon. Occasionally, the pressure in the anterior tibial compartment is greatly increased and this may contribute to muscle necrosis. Herbal remedies, administered by traditional healers ('moor glang barn') or monks are still popular in most rural areas of Thailand. Patients often present late to hospital with gangrenous limbs after wasting days or weeks undergoing this useless treatment. Secondary infections, including tetanus, are responsible for some deaths.

Cobra bites (Naja kaouthia)   Neurotoxic envenoming seems to be relatively more common in Thailand than in Malaya. Fifty-two per cent of the patients at Bang Phli who had evidence of envenoming showed ptosis or other neurotoxic signs (Viravan *et al.* 1986) compared with 24 per cent of Reid's patients (Reid 1964). In both countries, local necrosis is an important

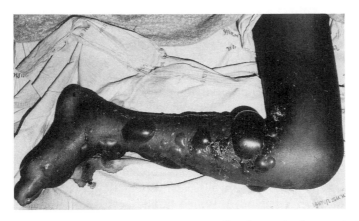

Fig. 2.6 Severe local effects of envenoming by *Calloselasma rhodostoma* in Eastern Thailand. (Copyright © D. A. Warrell.)

consequence of cobra bite. Reid's patients were bitten by cobras with monocellate nuchal markings (*N. kaouthia*) like the ones in Thailand (Fig. 2.1).

Pathophysiological studies

Mechanism of haemostatic disturbances following bites by C. rhodostoma, V. r. siamensis, and T. albolabris The coagulant of *C. rhodostoma* venom, Arvin/Ancrod, has a direct action on fibrinogen which differs from that of physiological thrombin in that only fibrinopeptide A and not fibrinopeptide B is cleaved off and Factor XIII is not activated (Regoeczi, Gergely, and McFarlane 1966). Studies in Trang, southern Thailand (Hutton *et al.*, unpublished) confirmed that the plasma of patients with incoagulable blood contained little or no fibrinogen, while the levels of serum fibrin/fibrinogen degradation products (FDPs) were very high. The small amount of detectable fibrin was mainly not cross-linked.

The fibrin that was cross-linked may have arisen non-specifically or as a result of a weak activator of Factor XIII in the venom itself. The commonly-observed slight fall in Factor XIII, especially in the A subunit (XIII:A) in the absence of any good evidence of thrombin generation also suggests a venom activator. The increasing proportion of cross-linked FDPs (D-dimer) later in the clinical course may be attributable to the greater resistance to fibrinolytic attack of these FDPs, which are therefore degraded after uncrosslinked FDPs have been cleared.

Two mechanisms are responsible for defibrination in victims of *C. rhodostoma*: cleavage of fibrinogen by Arvin, and activation of fibrinolysis causing fibrinogenolysis. It is not clear whether fibrinolysis is activated by a direct action of the venom on plasminogen or whether tissue plasminogen activator is involved. The dramatic effect of monospecific antivenom in reversing the coagulopathy suggests that a direct action of the venom is the principal cause of defibrination. Recent studies of patients bitten by eastern and western diamond-backed rattlesnakes (*Crotalus adamanteus* and *C. atrox*) implicated primarily venom-induced fibrinogenolysis with secondary activation of plasminogen as the cause of defibrination, rather than consumption coagulopathy (Kitchens and Van Mierop 1983; Budzynski, Pandya, Rubin, Brizuela, Soszka, and Stewart 1984). In patients bitten by *C. rhodostoma*, clotting factors, other than fibrinogen, and to a mild extent Factor XIII, are not depleted, and so defibrination is not the result of disseminated intravascular coagulation. Studies carried out in Trang, southern Thailand, revealed thrombocytopenia and inhibition of platelet aggregation. Plasma concentrations of platelet-derived products such as β-thromboglobulin and platelet Factor 4 were not elevated, suggesting that thrombocytopenia had not resulted from platelet activation. Failure of platelet aggregation was attributable to hypofibrinogenaemia and high concentrations of FDPs (Hutton *et al.*, unpublished). Essentially similar results were obtained in patients envenomed by *T. albolabris*.

In patients envenomed by *V. r. siamensis* the pattern of coagulopathy is completely different (Hutton *et al.*, unpublished). Here, there is evidence of disseminated intravascular coagulation (DIC), but Factor V is depleted far more than Factor VIII and Factor X more than Factor IX, reflecting the activity of Factor V and X procoagulants in the venom. If the coagulation system were generally activated, as in 'classical' DIC, these pairs of factors would be expected to be equally depleted. In most patients the other coagulation factors were normal or only slightly reduced. The mean levels of Factors V, X, and XIII:A were significantly lower than Factors VIII and XIII: S (Hutton *et al.*, unpublished). Levels of antithrombin III (AT III) and C_1 esterase inhibitor were occasionally reduced. These did not correlate with the degree of coagulation factor depletion. The C_1 esterase results are not compatible with kallikrein or complement activation. The relatively normal level of AT III is intriguing and has possible therapeutic implications. AT III, a serine protease inhibitor, would be expected to inhibit Factor Xa and be consumed in the process. However, in Russell's Viper envenoming, production of phospholipid from thrombin-activated platelets and Factor Va could protect Factor Xa from inhibition by AT III (Marciniak 1973; Miletich, Jackson, and Marjerus 1978). However, if adequate doses of heparin were given, AT III might effectively block the action of Factor Xa. Levels of protein C, a naturally occurring inhibitor of Factors V and VIII in plasma, were frequently reduced, especially when measured by bioassay rather than immunological methods. Protein C is activated by thrombin, factor Va and *V. russelli* venom itself. Protein C depletion will exacerbate the fall in Factors V and VIII, thereby potentiating the haemostatic defect. In the patients bitten by *V. russelli*, serum FDP levels were initially very high. Up to about 10 per cent of plasma FDP was in the form of D-dimer, but the fact that most was uncross-linked suggests that the mechanism involved either primary fibrinogenolysis or inhibition of Factor XIII-induced cross linking (Edgar *et al.*, unpublished). Activation of fibrinolysis was indicated by reduced levels of plasminogen and α_2-antiplasmin. Most of these observations can be explained by properties of Russell's viper venom which have been demonstrated by *in vitro* studies. The venom contains at least two procoagulants, one activating Factor X and the other Factor V (Schiffman, Theodor, and Rapaport 1969). Anticoagulants (Bowers and Hall 1958), an activator of fibrinolysis (Didisheim and Lewis 1956) and a platelet aggregating factor (Davey and Lüscher 1965) have also been described.

Disseminated intravascular coagulation with deposition of fibrin thrombi in important organs such as the kidney is an important pathological process in Russell's viper envenoming (see below). This is not the case with most other venoms that results in defibrination (e.g. *Echis carinatus*, *C. rhodostoma*, *T. albolabris*). Spontaneous systemic haemorrhage is another important cause of death following Russell's viper bite. During the acute phase of envenoming, patients may die from intracranial or massive gastrointestinal haemorrhage (Maung-Maung-Aye 1976; Hla-Myint *et al.* 1982). Spontaneous bleeding following snake bite is usually thought to be the result of discrete venom factors, haemorrhagins, which damage the vascular endothelium, leading to profuse bleeding because the blood is incoagulable and deficient in normally functioning platelets. The haemorrhagins of some venoms (e.g. habu, *Trimeresurus flavoviridis*) have been well characterized (Ohsaka 1979), but there has been no recent work on the haemorrhagins of *V. russelli* venom (Taylor and Mallick 1935). Severe late intracranial haemorrhage, especially involving the pituitary, is not explained by disseminated intravascular coagulation, as blood coagulability has been restored by this time. There is, however, evidence of a sustained increase in fibrinolytic activity and prolonged thrombocytopenia (Hutton *et al.*, unpublished; Myint-Lwin *et al.* 1985).

Mechanism of acute renal failure following V. r. siamensis bites   Russell's viper bite is an occasional cause of acute renal failure in northern India and Thailand, but in southern India (Matthai and Date 1981), Sri Lanka, and Burma it is the commonest cause of this medical emergency (Myint-Lwin *et al.* 1985). In Rangoon, Burma, 51 per cent of all cases treated with peritoneal dialysis are victims of *V. r. siamensis*. The mortality rate is 35 per cent (Hla-Mon, Maung-Maung-Khin, and Thet-Win 1981). The principal histological changes in the kidney are fibrin deposition in glomerular and peritubular vessels and acute tubular necrosis (Aung-Khin 1977). Prolonged hypotension as well as DIC could produce ischaemic damage, but a direct nephrotoxic action was suggested by morphological studies of human and animal material (Myint-Myint-Than 1978). The most convincing demonstration of the nephrotoxic factor was provided by studies using the isolated perfused rat kidney preparation (Ratcliffe, Pukrittayakamee, Ledingham, and Dunnill 1985). In the absence of coagulopathy and circulatory disturbances, venom concentrations in the range found in human victims produced dose-dependent disturbances of glomerular filtration rate and proximal tubular handling of sodium, which could be prevented by monospecific antivenom.

Since renal failure is the main cause of death following Russell's viper bite, it is very important that its mechanism should be understood. If by the time the patient is admitted to hospital there is irreversible tubular damage or diffuse obstruction of the renal microvasculature with fibrin deposits, antivenom will not prevent the development of acute renal failure. Ischaemia caused by DIC might, however, be reversed by using a thrombolytic agent, such as tissue plasminogen activator, although this could be dangerous in the presence of such a severe haemostatic disorder. Patients with established acute tubular necrosis can be salvaged with peritoneal dialysis (Hla-Mon *et al.* 1981), but it would be difficult to provide sufficient provincial centres capable of carrying out this demanding treatment. Another approach would be to attempt to protect high-risk communities, such as rice farmers, in Burma, Thailand, and Sri Lanka, by immunization with venom toxoids (Sawai 1979; Aung-Khin, Khin-Ohn-Lwin, and Thant-Zin 1980).

Antivenom

Antivenom remains the only specific treatment for snake venom poisoning that is of proved value. Until recently, antivenoms were the least researched and least developed of biological agents. Now, the development of new methods of immunization using stabilized liposomes (New, Theakston, Zumbuhl, Iddon and Friend 1984), improved methods of purifying IgG antibodies using affinity chromatography (Russell, Sullivan, Egen, Jeter, Markland, Wingert, and Bar-Or 1985) and the demonstration that, in some circumstances, monoclonal antibodies may reverse neuromuscular blockade by polypeptide toxins (Boulain and Menez 1982), makes possible a dramatic improvement in antivenom therapy. Even more neglected than the development of antivenoms is their clinical testing: very few randomized or controlled clinical trials have been attempted. Recently, in Thailand, three different monospecific antivenoms for *C. rhodostoma* were compared in a randomized clinical trial in patients with systemic envenoming, defined by their having incoagulable blood and in a parallel laboratory study carried out in Liverpool, using standardized venom assays in mice (Warrell,

Looareesuwan, Theakston, Phillips, Chanthavanich, Viravan, Supanaranond, Karbwang, Ho, Hutton, and Vejcho 1986). The results will indicate to the antivenom manufacturers specific ways in which their products should be improved.

Quantitative measurement of serum venom antigen and therapeutic antivenom concentrations using ELISA is producing valuable information about the kinetics of venom absorption, the speed of venom neutralization and the pharmacokinetics of antivenom (Khin-Ohn-Lwin, Aye-Aye-Mint, Tun-Pe, Theingie-Nwe, and Min-Naing 1984; Thein-Than, Kyi-Thein and Mg-Mg-Thwin 1985; Ho, Warrell, Looareesuwan, Phillips, Chanthavanich, Karbwang, Supanaranond, Hutton, and Vejcho 1986). Enzyme-refined antivenoms may be rapidly eliminated with a mean apparent plasma clearance time of 36 h (Thein-Than *et al.*, 1985). Venoms of some species such as *C. rhodostoma*, may continue to be absorbed from the injected 'depot' for several days despite effective initial neutralization of venom antigenaemia by antivenom. The combination of late antigenaemia and rapid antivenom clearance may result in recurrent severe envenoming several days after the bite (Ho *et al.* 1986). These observations should lead to modifications in antivenom treatment schedules and should encourage physicians to follow up their patients carefully even after signs of envenoming have been controlled initially by antivenom.

Antivenom reactions

Early (anaphylactic), pyrogenic, and late (serum sickness) reactions can occur after antivenom treatment. Reported incidence of early reactions following intravenous antivenom ranges from 3 to 5 per cent, depending partly on the dose and refinement of antivenom, but also on the quality of clinical observation during the critical 1–2 h after treatment. About 40 per cent of these reactions involve severe systemic anaphylaxis (bronchospasm, hypotension, or angioneurotic oedema). Very few fatal cases have been reported, but some anaphylactic deaths may have been misattributed to envenoming. Skin or conjunctival sensitivity tests have been widely practised, in the belief that early reactions were Type I immediate hypersensitivity reactions to equine serum proteins. Sutherland (1977) found that most commercial antivenoms were strongly anticomplementary *in vitro* and proposed the alternative hypothesis that antivenom reactions resulted from complement activation. In a clinical study carried out in Nigeria and Thailand (Malasit, Warrell, Chanthavanich, Viravan, Mongkolsapaya, Singhthong, and Supich 1986), 12 early reactions, two of them severe, were not predicted by hypersensitivity testing. It is therefore thought unjustifiable to delay antivenom treatment for the 20 or 30 min required to read the results of these tests. Most authorities have recommended that antivenom should be diluted in isotonic fluid and given by slow intravenous infusion.

Certainly, the rate of administration can be more easily controlled by this method, but in the rural tropics, setting up an infusion is more difficult and expensive than giving the antivenom by intravenous 'push' injection. A study of 33 patients in Thailand (Malasit *et al.* 1986) demonstrated no significant difference in the incidence or severity of early reactions whether the antivenom was given by push injection over 10 min or diluted and given as an infusion over 30 min. Doses of up to 50 ml of unrefined antivenom failed to produce detectable evidence of complement activation or immune complex formation in these patients, whether or not they developed early reactions. However, the anaphylactic reactions in hypogamma-globulinaemic patients caused by homologous serum are associated with marked complement depletion and immune complex formation (Day, Good and Wahn 1984) and it is possible that larger doses of equine anti-venom, comparable to the 200 mg kg^{-1} of homologous serum, might produce similar changes. Complement activation results from aggregation of Ig G molecules. Refinement of antivenoms should remove or prevent the formation of these aggregates.

Acknowledgements — I am grateful to my many colleagues in Thailand, Burma, Sri Lanka, and Britain, and especially to Drs M. J. Warrell, Sornchai Looareesuwan, R. E. Phillips, May Ho, R. D. G. Theakston, R. A. Hutton, and Chaisin Viravan. Professor Danai Bunnag and Professor Khunying Tranakchit Harinasuta (Bangkok), Dr Aung-Than-Batu (Rangoon) and Dr Dennis J. Aloysius (Colombo), in particular, have given me enormous support and encouragement.

The late Dr H. Alistair Reid was the inspiration for much of the work reviewed in this chapter.

References

Aung-Khin, M. (1977). Histological and ultrastructural changes of the kidney in renal failure after viper envenomation. *Toxicon* **16**, 71–5
—— (1980). The problem of snake bites in Burma. *Snake* **12**, 125–7.
——, Khin-Ohn-Lwin, and Thant-Zin (1980). Immunogenicity of the toxoid of Russell's viper venom. *Snake* **12**, 45–53.
Balozet, L. (1964). Le scorpionisme en Afrique de Nord. *Bull. Soc. Pathol. exot.* **57**, 37–38.
Bawaskar, H. S. (1982). Diagnostic cardiac premonitory signs and symptoms of red scorpion sting. *Lancet* **i**, 552–4.
Boulain, J. C. and Ménez, A. (1982). Neurotoxin-specific immunoglobulins accelerate dissociation of the neurotoxin-acetylcholine receptor complex. *Science* **217**, 732–3.

Bowers, E. F. and Hall, G. H. (1958). The separation and properties of anti-coagulant principle from Russell's viper venom (RVV). *Br. J. Haematol.* **4**, 220–7.

Bücherl, W. (1978). Venoms of Tityinae. In *Arthropod venoms* (ed. S. Bettini), *Handbook of experimental pharmacology* Vol. 48, pp. 371–9. Springer, Berlin.

Budzynski, A. Z., Pandya, B. V, Rubin, R. N., Brizuela, B. S., Soszka, T., and Stewart, G. J. (1984). Fibrinogenolytic afibrinogenemia after envenomation by Western diamondback rattlesnake (*Crotalus atrox*). *Blood* **63**, 1–14.

Burma Gazetteer (1959) Tharrawaddy District Volume A. Govt. Printing and Staty, Union of Burma, Rangoon, p. 21.

Chagnon, N. A. (1968). *Yanomamo — the fierce people*, p. 20. Holt, Rinehart and Winston, New York.

Dao, L. (1971). Emponzoñamiento ofidico en el estado lara. *Gaceta Medica de Caracas* **79**: 383–410.

Davey, M. G. and Lüscher, E. F. (1965). Actions of some coagulant snake venoms on blood platelets. *Nature* **207**: 730–2.

Day, N. K., Good, R. A. and Wahn, V. (1984). Adverse reactions in selected patients following intravenous infusion of gammaglobulin. *Am. J. Med.* **76** (3A), 25–32.

Deraniyagala, P. E. P. (1960–61). The taxonomy of the cobras of South Eastern Asia. *Spolia Zeylanica* **29**, 41–63, 205–32.

De Silva, A. (1981). Snakebites in Anuradhapura district *Snake* **13**: 117–30.

Didisheim, P. and Lewis, J. H. (1956). Fibrinolytic and coagulant activities of certain snake venoms and proteases. *Proc. Soc. Exp. Biol. Med.* **93**, 10–13.

Eapen, C. K., Chandy, N., Kochuvartey, K. L., Zacharia, P. K., Thomas, P. J., and Ipe, T. I. (1976). Unusual complications of snake bite: hypopituitarism after viper bites. In *Plant, animal and microbial toxins* (ed. A. Ohsaka, K. Hayashi, and Y. Sawai), Vol. II, pp. 467–73. Plenum Press, New York.

——, ——, and Joseph, J. K. (1984). A study of 1000 cases of snake envenomation. XIth International Congress of Tropical Medicine and Malaria, Calgary, Canada, 16–22 September.

Fayrer, J. (1982). Destruction of life in India by poisonous snakes. *Nature* **27**, 205–8.

Freiberg, M. and Walls, J. G. (1984). *The world of venomous animals* p. 162. T. F. H. Publications, Hong Kong.

Fulde, G. W. O. and Smith, F. (1984). Sea snake envenomation at Bondi. *Med. J. Austr.* **141**, 44–5.

Gajdusek, D. C. (1977). *Symposium on health and diseases in tribal societies* pp. 100–176. Ciba Foundation Symposium New Series, No. 49. Elsevier, New York.

Hla-Mon, Maung-Maung-Khin, and Thet-Whin (1981). Profile in acute renal failure. Proceedings: First Congress of Medical Specialities, Rangoon, Burma. 25–28, September pp. 1–7.

Hla-Myint, Hla-Mon, Maung-Maung-Khin, and Thet-Win (1982). Snake bite and envenomation. In *Textbook of internal medicine* (ed. Internal Medicine Section, Burma Medical Association), pp. 10–26. BMA, Rangoon.

Ho, M., Warrell, M. J., Warrell, D. A., Bidwell, D., and Voller, A. (1986). A critical reappraisal of the use of ELISA in the study of snake bite. *Toxicon* **24**, 211–21.

——, Warrell, D. A., Looareesuwam, S., Phillips, R. E., Chanthavanich, P., Karbwang, J., Supanaranond, W., Hutton, R. A., and Vejcho, S. (1986). Clinical significance of venom antigen levels in patients envenomed by the Malayan pit viper (*Calloselasma rhodostoma*). *Am. J. Trop. Med. Hyg.* **35**, 579–87.

Jeyarajah, R. (1984). Russell's viper bite in Sri Lanka. A study of 22 cases. *Am. J. trop. Med. Hyg.* **33**, 506–10.

Khin-Ohn-Lwin, Aye-Aye-Myint, Tun-Pe, Theingie-Nwe, and Min Naing (1984). Russell's viper venom levels in serum of snake bite victims in Burma. *Trans. R. Soc. trop. Med. Hyg* **78**, 165–8.

Kitchens, C. S. and Van Mierop, L. H. S. (1983). Mechanism of defibrination in humans after envenomation by the Eastern diamond back rattlesnake. *Am. J. Haemotol.* **14**, 345–53.

Klemmer, K. (1963). Liste der rezenten Giftschlangen. In *Die Giftschlangen der Erde* (ed. Behringwerk-Mitteilungen), pp. 255–464 (plate 37). N. G. Elwert, Marburg.

Kramer, E. (1977). Zur Schlangen fauna von Nepal. *Rev. Suisse Zool.* **84**, 721–61.

Kundert, F. (1974). *Fascination, Schlangen und Echsen* pp. 33, 144. F. Kundert, Spreitenbach.

McCarthy, N. J. (1984). Snake venom detection kit. *Med. J. Austr.* **140**, 140, 518.

Malasit, P., Warrell, D. A., Chanthavanich, P., Viravan, C., Mongkulsapaya, J., Singhthong, B., and Supich, C. (1985). Prediction, prevention and mechanism of early (anaphylactic) antivenom reactions in victims of snakebites. *Br. Med. J.* **292**, 17–20.

Marciniak, E. (1973). Factor-Xa inactivation by antithrombin III: evidence for biological stabilization of factor Xa by factor V-phospholipid complex. *Br. J. Haemotol.* **24**: 391–400.

Marshall, L. R. and Herrmann, R. P. (1984). Cross-reactivity of bardick snake venom with death adder antivenom *Med. J. Austr.* **140**, 541–2.

Matthai, T. P. and Date, A. (1981). Acute renal failure in children following snake bite. *Ann. trop. Paediat.* **1**, 73–6.

Maung-Maung-Aye (1972). Some experience in the management of snake bite. *Burma med. J.* **20**, 33–40.

—— (1976). Snakes of Burma with venomology and envenomation. M.Sc. (Zoology) Thesis, Arts and Science University, Rangoon.

—— (1984). The clinical features and management of Russell's viper bite. XIth International Congress of Tropical Medicine and Malaria, Calgary, Canada, 16–22 September.

Mazzotti, L. and Bravo-Becherelle, M. A. (1963). Scorpionism in the Mexican Republic. In *Venomous and poisonous animals and noxious plants of the Pacific Region* (ed. H. L. Keegan and W. V. Macfarlane), pp. 119–31. Pergamon Press, Oxford.

Miletich, J. P., Jackson, C. M., and Majerus, P. W. (1978). Properties of the Factor Xa binding site on human platelets. *J. biol. Chem.* **253**, 6908–16.

Mitrakul, C. (1973). Effects of green pit viper (*Trimeresurus erythrurus* and

Trimeresurus popeorum) venoms on blood coagulation, platelets and the fibrinolytic enzyme systems: studies *in vivo* and *in vitro*. *Am. J. clin. Pathol.* **60**, 654–62.

—— (1979). Effects of five Thai snake venoms on coagulation fibrinolysis and platelet aggregation. *S.E. Asian J. trop. Med. publ. Hlth* **10**, 266–75.

—— and Impun, C. (1973). The hemorrhagic phenomena associated with green pit viper (*Trimeresurus erythrurus* and *Trimeresurus popeorum*) bites in children. A report of studies to elucidate their pathogenesis. *Clin. Pediat.* **12**, 215–8.

Munasinghe, D. R. and Kulasinghe, P. (1965). Snake-bite — a case report. *Ceylon med. J.* **10**, 140–3.

Myint-Lwin, Warrell, D. A., Phillips, R. E., Tin-Nu-Swe, Tun-Pe, and Maung-Maung-Lay (1985). Bites by Russell's viper (*Vipera russelli siamensis*) in Burma: haemostatic, vascular and renal disturbances and response to treatment. *Lancet* ii, 1259–64.

Myint-Myint-Than (1978). Changes in the renal tubules in viper envenomation. M.Sc. (Zoology) Thesis, Arts and Science University, Rangoon.

New, R. C., Theakston, R. D. G., Zumbuhl, O., Iddon, D., and Friend, J. (1984). Immunization against snake venoms. *New Engl. J. Med.* **311**, 56–7.

Nimalasuriya, A. (1971). Anti-cholinesterases in the control of the neurological manifestations of Russell's viper bite. *J. Colombo gen. Hosp.* **2**, 186–8.

Nootpand, W. (1971). *Poisonous snakes of Thailand* pp. 47, 50. Mitraphadung, Bangkok.

Ohsaka, A. (1979). Hemorrhagic, necrotizing and edema-forming effects of snake venoms. In *Snake venoms* (ed. C.-Y. Lee). *Handbook of experimental pharmacology* Vol. 52, pp. 480–546. Springer, Berlin.

Peiris, O. A., Wimalaratne, K. D. P., and Nimalasuriya, A. (1969). Exchange transfusion in the treatment of Russell's viper bite. *Postgrad. med. J.* **45**, 627–9.

Pugh, R. N. H. and Theakston, R. D. G. (1980). Incidence and mortality of snake bite in savanna Nigeria. *Lancet* ii, 1181–3.

——, ——, Reid, H. A., and Bhar, I. S. (1980). Epidemiology of human encounters with the spitting cobra, *Naja nigricollis* in the Malumgashi area of Northern Nigeria. *Ann. trop. Med. Parasitol.* **74**, 523–30.

Ratcliffe, P. J., Pukrittayakamee, S., Ledingham, J. G. G., and Dunnill, M. S. (1985). Acute renal failure in the isolated perfused kidney, induced by Russell's viper venom. *Clin. Sci.* **68**, (suppl. 11), 39–40.

Regenass, U. and Kramer, E. (1981). Zur Systematik der grunen Grubenottern der Gattung *Trimeresurus* (Serpentes, Crotalidae). *Rev. Suisse Zool.* **88**, 163–205.

Regoeczi, E., Gergely, J., and McFarlane, A. S. (1966). *In vivo* effects of *Agkistrodon rhodostoma* venom: studies with fibrinogen [131]I. *J. clin. Invest.* **45**, 1202–12.

Reid, H. A. (1964). Cobra bites. *Br. med. J.* **2**, 540–5.

——, Chan, K. E., and Thean, P. C. (1963b). Prolonged coagulation defect (defibrination syndrome) in Malayan viper bite. *Lancet* i, 621–6.

—— and Lim, K. J. (1957). Sea-snake bite. A survey of fishing villages in north-west Malaya. *Br. med. J.* **2**, 1266–72.

——, Thean, P. C., Chan, K. E., and Baharom, A. R. (1963a). Clinical effects of bites by Malayan viper (*Ancistrodon rhodostoma*.) *Lancet* i, 617–21.

Russell, F. E., Sullivan, J. B., Egen, N. B., Jeter, W. S., Markland, F. S., Wingert, W. A., and Bar-Or, D. (1985). Preparation of a new antivenin by affinity chromatography. *Am. J. trop. Med. Hyg.* **34**, 141–50.

Sawai, Y. (1979). Vaccination against snake bite poisoning. In *Snake venoms* (ed. C. -Y. Lee). *Handbook of experimental pharmacology* Vol. 52, pp. 881–97. Springer, Berlin.

——, Toriba, M., Itokawa, H., de Silva, A., Perera, G. L. S., and Kottegoda, M. B. (1984). Study on deaths due to snakebite in Anuradhapura district, Sri Lanka. *Snake* **16**, 7–15.

Schiffman, S., Theodor, I., and Rapaport, S. I. (1969). Separation from Russell's viper venom of one fraction reacting with Factor X and another reacting with Factor V. *Biochemistry* **8**, 1397–406.

Sheehan, H. L. (1939). Simmonds's disease due to post-partum necrosis of the anterior pituitary. *Q. J. Med.* N.S. **32**, 277–309.

Smith, M. A. (1943). *The fauna of British India, Ceylon, and Burma. Reptiles and amphibians.* Vol. III *Serpentes.* Taylor and Francis, London.

Soderberg, P. (1973). On eleven Asian elapid snakes with specific reference to their occurrence in Thailand. *Nat. Hist. Bull. Siam. Soc.* **24**, 205–317.

Spaar, A. E. (1910). The bite of Russell's viper. *Spolia Zeylan.* **6**, 188–90.

Sutherland, S. K. (1977). Serum reactions: an analysis of commercial antivenoms and the possible role of anticomplementary activity in *de novo* reactions to antivenoms and antitoxins. *Med. J. Austr.* April 23, 613–5.

Swaroop, S. and Grab, B. (1954). Snakebite mortality in the world. *Bull. W.H.O.* **10**, 35–76.

Talalak, P. (1977). Action of *Trimeresurus erythrurus* and *Trimeresurus popeorum* venom on blood coagulation. *J. med. Ass. Thailand* **60**, 9–18.

Taylor, E. H. (1965). The serpents of Thailand and adjacent waters. *Univ. Kansas Sci. Bull.* **45**, 609–1096.

Taylor, J. and Mallick, S. M. K. (1935). Observations on the neutralization of the haemorrhagins of certain viper venoms by antivenene. *Ind. J. med. Res.* **23**, 121–30.

Theakston, R. D. G. (1983). The application of immunoassay techniques, including enzyme-linked immunosorbent assay (ELISA), to snake venom research. *Toxicon* **21**, 341–52.

——, Lloyd-Jones, M. J., and Reid, H. A. (1977). Micro-elisa for detecting and assaying snake venom and venom-antibody. *Lancet* **ii**, 639–41.

——, Pugh, R. N. H., and Reid, H. A. (1981a). Enzyme-linked immunosorbent assay of venom-antibodies in human victims of snake bite. *J. trop. Med. Hyg.* **84**, 109–113.

—— and Reid, H. A. (1983). The development of simple standard assay procedures for the characterization of snake venoms. *Bull. W.H.O.* **61**, 949–56.

——, Reid, H. A., Larrick, J. W., Kaplan, J., and Yost, S. A. (1981b). Snake venom antibodies in Ecuadorian Indians. *J. trop. Med. Hyg.* **84**, 199–202.

Thein-Than, Kyi-Thein, and Mg-Mg-Thwin (1985). Plasma clearance time of Russell's viper (*Viper russelli*) antivenom in human snake bite victims. *Trans. R. Soc. trop. Med. Hyg.* **79**, 262–3.

Tweedie, M. F. W. (1983). The snakes of Malaya (2nd ed.) p. 114. Singapore National Printers, Singapore.

Vidal, G. W. (1890). A list of the venomous snakes of Kanara. *J. Bombay nat. Hist. Soc.* **5**, 64–71.

Viravan, C., Veeravat, U., Warrell, M. J., Theakston, R. D. G., and Warrell, D. A. (1986). ELISA-confirmation of acute and post-envenoming by the monocellate Thai cobra (*Naja kaouthia*). *Am. J. trop. Med. Hyg.* **35**, 173–81.

Visudhiphan, S., Dumavibhat, B., and Trishnananda, M. (1981). Prolonged defibrination syndrome after green pit viper bite with persisting venom activity in patient's blood. *Am. J. clin. Pathol.* **75**, 65–9.

Visuvaratnam, M., Vinayagamoorthy, C., and Balakrishnan, S. (1970). Venomous snake bites in North Ceylon — a study of 15 cases. *J. trop. Hyg.* **73**, 9–14.

Wall, F. (1921). *Ophidia taprobanica or the snakes of Ceylon.* H. R. Cottle, Colombo.

Warrell, D. A. and Arnett, C. (1976). The importance of bites by the saw-scaled or carpet viper (*Echis carinatus*). *Acta trop.* **33**, 307–41.

——, Greenwood, B. M., Davidson, N. McD., Ormerod, L. D., and Prentice, C. R. M. (1976). Necrosis, haemorrhage and complement depletion following bites by the spitting cobra (*Naja nigricollis*). *Q. J. Med.* **45**, 1–22.

——, Looareesuwan, S., White, N. J., Theakston, R. D. G., Warrell, M. J., Kosakarn, W., and Reid, H. A. (1983). Severe neurotoxic envenoming by the Malayan krait, *Bungarus candidus* (Linnaeus): response to antivenom and anticholinesterase. *Br. med. J.* **286**, 678–80.

——,——, Theakston, R. D. G., Phillips, R. E., Chanthavanich, P., Viravan, C., Supanaranond, W., Karbwang, J., Ho, M., Hutton, R. A., and Vejcho, S. (1986). Randomized comparative trial of three monospecific antivenoms for bites by the Malayan pit viper (*Calloselasma rhodostoma*) in southern Thailand: clinical and laboratory correlations. *Am. J. Trop. Med. Hyg.* **35**, 1235–47

Waterman, J. A. (1950). Two cases of scorpion poisoning characterized by convulsions with electrocardiograms. *Caribbean med. J.* **12**, 127–9.

Wolff, H. (1958). Insuficiência hipofisária anterior por picada de ofidio. *Arq. bras. Endocrin. Metab.* **7**, 25–47.

World Health Organization (1981). Progress in the characterization of venoms and standardization of antivenoms. WHO Offset Publ. No. 58. WHO, Geneva.

3

Recent developments in ciguatera research

Manabu Nukina, Kazuo Tachibana, and
Paul J. Scheuer

Introduction

Ciguatera is a fish intoxication associated with tropical coral reefs. It has been documented in Western literature for well over 400 years, but the aetiology of ciguatera has begun to unfold only since 1977, when the organism causing the disease was discovered (Yasumoto, Nakajima, Bagnis, and Adachi, 1977). Each of the three major seafood intoxications — red tides, pufferfish poisoning, and ciguatera — has presented a unique set of constraints that have governed its research progress. A brief account of some of these parameters is in order. It must be borne in mind that spectacular advances in separation methods and analytical instrumentation have played significant roles in the rate of progress of marine toxin and all natural product research over the past 20 years.

In all natural product research the isolation of a pure product and the determination of its molecular structure are convenient and important benchmarks of research progress. Crystalline tetrodotoxin (TTX) (then called spheroidine) was first obtained in 1948 and its structure was elucidated in 1964. Although the determination of its structure was accomplished by classical methods, it must be remembered that the supply of toxin was never a serious problem. The Nagoya group (e.g. Goto, Kishi, Takahashi and Hirata 1965) published a procedure for the isolation of 1–2 g of crystalline tetrodotoxin from 100 kg of pufferfish ovaries (about 500 fish), which are commercially available. Yet it is sobering to reflect that even today — 20 years later — we are still puzzled by the occurrence of tetrodotoxin in diverse animal phyla, such as fishes, molluscs, and amphibians, and we do not know the path of tetrodotoxin biogenesis. In fact, the first analogues of tetrodotoxin, be they precursors or degradation products, have only recently come to light (Nakamura and Yasumoto 1985).

In marked contrast to our lack of knowledge of the synthetic pathways involved in the synthesis of TTX, the biogenetic link between red tides and paralytic shellfish poisons (PSP) is indicated even in the nomenclature. In the saxitoxin–gonyautoxin family of compounds, red tides caused by blooms of dinoflagellates (*Gonyaulax* spp.) are the visible indicators of shellfish toxicity. Also helpful to this research was the circumstance that the Alaska butter clam, *Saxidomus giganteus*, retains one of the most stable of the compounds, saxitoxin, in its syphon for long periods of time and in respectable quantities. Laboratory culture of the organisms, though difficult, has long been accomplished and has led to the recognition of a large (and still growing) family of related toxins. More importantly, it has permitted research on the biosynthesis of these toxins (Shimizu, Norte, Hori, Genenah, and Kobayashi 1984). The molecular structure of saxitoxin was determined by X-ray diffraction methods in 1974 (Schantz, Ghazarossian, Schnoes, Strong, Springer, Pezzanite, and Clardy 1975). This knowledge was essential for the study of the unstable and elusive members of this family of toxins.

The so-called Florida or Gulf of Mexico red-tide toxins bear little resemblance to the temperate zone (PSP) red tides. The Florida phenomenon also arises from a dinoflagellate, *Gymnodinium breve* (*Ptychodiscus brevis*), which manifests itself by red-coloured blooms. There the resemblance ends. Massive fish kills and relatively minor incidents of human intoxication are characteristically associated with the Florida red tides. *Gymnodinium breve* has been cultured, but the complexity of the toxin mixture, difficulties involved in the purification of the different fractions and the bewildering nomenclature given to both the dinoflagellate itself and the toxins it elaborates, have contributed to the problems associated with this research. The structure of one of the compounds, brevetoxin B, was determined in 1981 by X-ray crystallography (Lin, Risk, Ray, Van Engen, Clardy, Golik, James, and Nakanishi 1981). Unlike tetrodotoxin or the saxitoxin-gonyautoxins group of toxins, brevetoxin B contains no nitrogen and belongs to a class of compounds known as polyethers. These molecules are constructed from highly oxygenated long-chain polyketides which are coiled into complex cyclic ethers of various sizes. Some of the known polyether representatives are antibiotics and have ionophoric properties.

Ciguatera

Source of toxin

Ciguatera research has been beset with many difficulties. Outbreaks of ciguatera tend to take place in isolated island groups in the Pacific and the Caribbean. There are no tell-tale signs as in red tides, nor are there simple precautions as in pufferfish poisoning (removal of gonads and liver), which would help prevent human intoxication. In fact, human illness has been the only means of discovering an outbreak. In the usual pattern of events, the geographic limits of an outbreak will be rather narrow, but the spectrum of affected fish species will be broad. Screening of fish for toxicity is nearly impossible, as one either has to feed the fish to a susceptible animal (cat, mongoose), or inject an extract into a mouse or mosquito. In a documented toxic fish (human or animal bioassay) the concentration of toxin is only about 1×10^{-6} per cent which is fortunate for the consumer in that it means that ciguatera is rarely fatal, but unlucky for the researcher, who needs toxin. The concentration of toxin in the viscera is higher, often by one or two orders of magnitude, but in human cases of poisoning the viscera have normally been discarded by the time the first human symptoms appear. These various difficulties — the procurement of fish of questionable toxicity from remote locales and the purification of a trace constituent by a complex process of isolation which has to be monitored by a toxin-consuming bio-assay — have compounded to retard research progress. Little wonder, then, that Yasumoto's discovery (Yasumoto *et al.* 1977) of *Gambierdiscus toxicus* as a ciguatera-causing dinoflagellate led to the belief that the toxin would become readily available as soon as the dinoflagellate was cultured. This has not been the case. Unlike the red-tide dinoflagellates, which float on the surface, *G. toxicus* is a benthic organism that settles on macroalgae or on coral detritus —the very reason it had remained undetected for so long. The algal settling is highly specific (Shimizu, Shimizu, Scheuer, Hokama, Oyama, and Miyahara 1982) and the factors that determine it are unknown. *G. toxicus* cultured in different laboratories and under a variety of conditions (Yasumoto, Raj, and Bagnis 1984) have produced only trace amounts of ciguatoxin, the predominant toxin in carnivorous ciguateric fish. The principal toxin in laboratory cultures of *G. toxicus* is maitotoxin. This is a water-soluble toxin found in the viscera of herbivorous ciguateric fishes, which appears to bear little structural relationship to ciguatoxin (Yasumoto, Bagnis, and Vernoux 1976). The most favourable ratio in any culture of 'ciguatoxin-like' to 'maitotoxin-like' toxicity is 28:71 (Durand, Squiban, Viso, and Pesando 1985). Their success, not yet repeated elsewhere, appears to be derived from the selection of a ciguatoxin-producing strain. The preferential algal settling (Shimizu *et al.* 1982) suggest that unknown ecological factors have yet to be discovered. Until laboratory cultures can be manipulated for ciguatoxin production, toxic fish remain the sole source of toxin.

Toxin detection

Since neither the appearance of the toxic fish nor of the ocean indicate ciguatoxicity, a simple and rapid method of detection has long been an important goal of ciguatera research. The injection of a fish extract into mice has for many years been the only well-documented procedure (Banner,

Sasaki, Helfrich, Alender, and Scheuer 1961). Its drawbacks are numerous. It is complex and slow and it relies on the availability of suitable animals on which to perform the assay. While it is adequate as a research procedure, it is useless to the fisherman or the consumer who wonders about the wholesomeness of a reef fish which he is about to prepare for dinner. Even as a research tool bioassay involving mice is flawed, as it consumes far too much precious toxin. Chungue, Bagnis, and Parc (1984) have developed a bioassay using the mosquito in which fish extract is injected into the thorax of *Aedes aegypti*. Because of the small size of mosquitoes, this assay conserves toxin, but it is clearly unsuitable as a detection device in the market place.

Hokama and co-workers (Hokama, Osugi, Honda, and Matsuo 1985) have pioneered an immunological approach to ciguatoxin detection, which in its latest modification shows every indication that it will be successful. Initially, Hokama, Banner, and Boylan (1977) coupled ciguatoxin to human serum albumin and then isolated antiserum from sheep or rabbits that had been treated with the ciguatoxin conjugate. After purification the antiserum was labelled with radioiodine. This preparation was used effectively for the mass screening of fish samples (Amberjack, *Seriola dumerili*) to be marketed in Hawaii. In a subsequent improvement (Hokama, Abad, and Kimura 1983) the previously purified antiserum fraction was coupled to horseradish peroxidase. The resulting enzyme preparation was as satisfactory as the radio-labelled compound in distinguishing between (documented) ciguatoxic and nontoxic fish tissue, and it was also faster and simpler to use. Most recently Hokama, (1985) has used monoclonal antibodies raised against the toxin to develop a new more rapid and potentially inexpensive assay procedure. The new test (a stick test) is currently being evaluated in several independent laboratories. It is equally applicable to raw fish and fish extracts.

Toxin structure

To minimize problems that might arise from biological or geographical factors affecting the nature of the toxin, we have always attempted to isolate toxin from a single species of fish in one location. In our earliest work we utilized red snapper (*Lutjanus bohar*) from Palmyra island (162°W, 6°N). When the level of toxicity declined in the Line islands, we moved to Johnston atoll (165°W, 17°N), where we collected moray eels (*Gymnothorax ≡Lycodontis javanicus*) and sharks (*Carcharhinus menisorrah*). We soon abandoned shark livers as a source of toxin because of exceptionally difficult purification problems. We continued to concentrate on moray eels, although low toxicity levels at Johnston have forced us to procure the animals from Tarawa atoll (173°E, 1°30′N), Republic of Kiribati. Our early work (Scheuer, Takahashi, Tsutsumi, and Yoshida 1967) convinced us that in ciguateric carnivores a single lipid toxin was the causative toxic agent. We confidently named it ciguatoxin, although our early structural guesses were far off the mark. With the benefit of hindsight (Tachibana 1980) we now know that the 'toxin' we isolated in 1967 contained approximately 0.1 per cent ciguatoxin (CTX).

Isolation of a trace constituent (1×10^{-6} per cent) from a biological matrix is invariably difficult. Since CTX is u.v.-transparent > 215 nm, we had to monitor the progress of the purification by toxin-consuming mouse bioassay. Our isolation scheme, always a combination of solvent partition and chromatography, is continuously being evaluated, modified, and improved. Successive co-workers soon became convinced that the scheme must be made simpler. This factor, in conjunction with technological advances in separation science, has led to our present procedures, outlined in Figs 3.1 and 3.2. In a notable departure from our most recently published isolation scheme (Nukina, Koyanagi, and Scheuer 1984) we use countercurrent techniques prior to the final HPLC step. Specifically, we have employed an Ito multilayer coil separator–extractor (Ito, Sandlin, and Bowers 1982) (P.C. Inc., Potomac, MD) at a rapid flow rate of 240 ml h^{-1}. The four-component solvent system (hexane/ethyl acetate/methanol/water) had been used by Mandava and Ito (1982) for the purification of terrestrial plant hormones. It allows easy change of the distribution coefficient by manipulating the solvent ratio. Since 1981, when a toxin sample (0.45 μg kg^{-1} i.p.

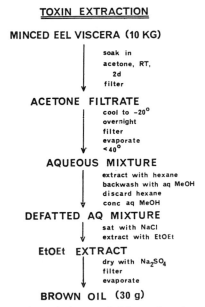

TOXIN EXTRACTION

MINCED EEL VISCERA (10 KG)

soak in
acetone, RT,
2d
filter

ACETONE FILTRATE

cool to –20°
overnight
filter
evaporate
<40°

AQUEOUS MIXTURE

extract with hexane
backwash with aq MeOH
discard hexane
conc aq MeOH

DEFATTED AQ MIXTURE

sat with NaCl
extract with EtOEt

EtOEt EXTRACT

dry with Na$_2$SO$_4$
filter
evaporate

BROWN OIL (30 g)

Fig. 3.1 Scheme for extraction of 'ciguatoxin' from the minced viscera of the Moray Eel.

TOXIN PURIFICATION

ETHER RESIDUES (41 g)

| partition between
| hexane/EtOAc/MeOH/H₂O
↓ 3 : 7 : 5 : 5

NON-AQUEOUS RESIDUE (149 mg)

| Sephadex LH-20
| CH₂Cl₂/MeOH
↓ 1 : 1

TOXIC FRACTIONS (46 mg)

| BondElut C₁₈
↓ MeOH/H₂O

TOXIC FRACTIONS (23 mg)

| CCC
| hexane/EtOAc/MeOH/H₂O
↓ 3 : 7 : 5 : 5

TOXIC FRACTIONS (1.1 mg)

| HPLC
| Lichrosorb RP-18
| MeOH/H₂O
↓ 4 : 1

CRYSTALLINE TOXIN (160 μg)

Fig. 3.2 Scheme for the purification of ciguatoxin. from the crude extract of the minced viscera of the Moray Eel.

mice) serendipitously crystallized in an NMR tube while en route to Hawaii from a mainland applications laboratory, our toxin samples crystallize spontaneously following the final HPLC step, which constitutes welcome evidence of toxin homogeneity.

Ciguatoxin (LD_{50} 0.45 μg kg^{-1} i.p. mice) is a colourless crystalline solid, soluble in methanol, ethanol, 2-propanol, and acetone. It is optically active with a molecular ellipticity of −620. The only functional groups which the infrared spectrum of CTX reveals unequivocally are hydroxyl and ether. None of the mass spectral techniques that were routinely available in the late 1970s (EI, CI) produced a molecular ion. ^{252}Cf plasma desorption mass spectrometry (Macfarlane and McNeil, personal communication) revealed a molecular ion corresponding to a weight of 1111.7 ± 0.3 dalton. High resolution mass data, which would permit conclusions regarding elemental composition of CTX are not yet in hand.

Virtually all of our structural information is derived from ^{1}H NMR studies at 300–600 MHz (Tachibana 1980). The toxin possesses five hydroxyl, four carbon–carbon double bonds and five methyl groups bonded to sp^3 carbons. As a likely number of oxygen atoms is 24, and as carbonyl-containing functions are not obvious, the number of ether linkages in the molecule is large. Our most important clue for the nature of the molecule came from a fortunate circumstance in Yasumoto's laboratory (Murakami, Oshima, and

Yasumoto 1982). A TLC examination of the toxic constituents of a marine dinoflagellate *Prorocentrum lima* revealed that one of the compounds exhibited chromatographic mobility indistinguishable from that of CTX. The identity of this constituent was, however, okadaic acid (Fig 3.3(a)), a compound that had been isolated from a sponge, *Halichondria okadai*, and whose structure had been determined by X-ray diffraction techniques (Tachibana, Scheuer, Tsukitani, Kikuchi, Van Engen, Clardy, Gopichand, and Schmitz 1981).

Although okadaic acid, $C_{44}H_{68}O_{13}$, m.w. 784 dalton, is a much smaller

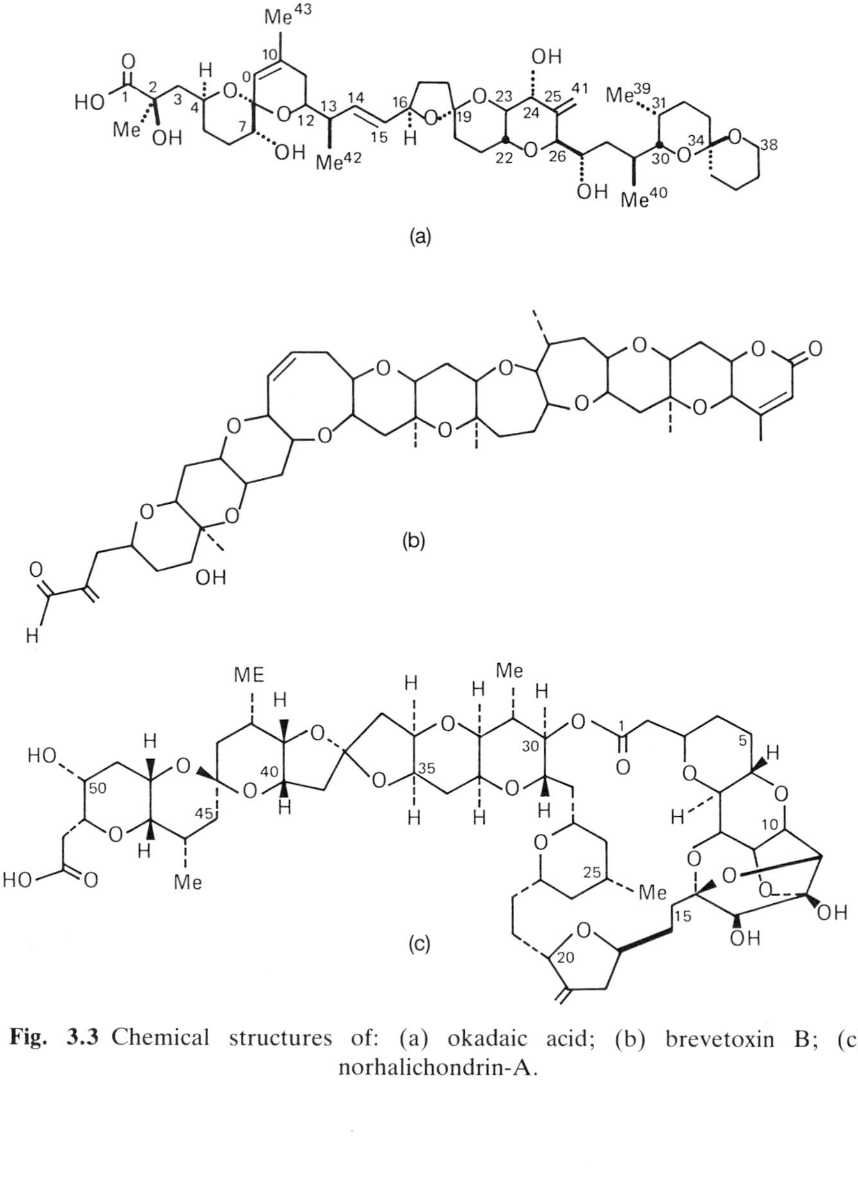

(a)

(b)

(c)

Fig. 3.3 Chemical structures of: (a) okadaic acid; (b) brevetoxin B; (c) norhalichondrin-A.

molecule than CTX, both compounds are polyethers, i.e. highly oxygenated long-chain fatty acids which exist as curls of cyclic ethers. As has been pointed out earlier, brevetoxin B (Fig 3.3(b)) is a notable representative of this class of compounds. Its composition of $C_{50}H_{70}O_{14}$ (M.W. 894 dalton), with only one hydroxyl group, makes this a less polar molecule than okadaic acid, which possesses four hydroxyls and a nonlactonized carboxyl group. Yet another polyether constituent, norhalichondrin-A (Fig 3.3(c)), which is close in molecular size to CTX and is of extraordinary structural complexity has recently been isolated from *Halichondria okadai*, the sponge that previously had produced okadaic acid (Uemura, Takahashi, Yamamoto, Katayama, Tanaka, Okumura and Hirata 1985).

The largest amount of CTX that we have had in hand was 1.3 mg. It was insufficient for a useful ^{13}C NMR spectrum, which is still a desirable goal in structural elucidation. Although CTX is a crystalline compound, the crystals are of a size and quality that are unsuitable for X-ray studies. Even if we can grow better crystals, it might not be possible to solve as large a structure as CTX without incorporation of a heavy atom. Our foremost goals, therefore, are the production of more pure CTX and the preparation of a crystalline heavy atom derivative.

Although we have adhered to our basic assumption (Scheuer *et al.* 1967) that CTX is a single entity, the question of multiple toxins is bound to arise in a research project that involves isolation of a trace constituent from a complex substrate. Even more suggestive of the presence of multiple toxins is the broad spectrum of often contradictory symptoms that have been described to physicians and others by patients poisoned by ciguatoxic fishes. We have thus been alert to the possibility that multiple toxins do exist, which give rise to the ciguatera syndrome.

Occasionally, we have observed (Tachibana 1980) that from samples of extracts that had been stored for some time, ciguatoxin would be eluted from a silica column with a less polar solvent mixture (chloroform/methanol 97:3) than is normally the case (the bulk of the toxin is normally eluted with a 9:1 chloroform/methanol solution). This phenomenon, the existence of a less polar form of ciguatoxin, can be demonstrated by chromatography on basic alumina of different activity grades. We showed (Nukina *et al.* 1984) that the two forms of ciguatoxin, while chromatographically distinct, are interconvertible. The two forms have [1]NMR spectra that differ only in minor details and elicit comparable symptoms in mice.

An epidemiological survey including detailed case studies in the Gambier islands, where ciguatera intoxication arises principally from eating parrot-fishes (Scaridae), led Bagnis, Loussan, and Thevenin (1974) to suggest that either a new toxin or multiple toxins were involved. In her follow-up study Chungue (1977) (Chungue, Bagnis, Fusetani, and Hashimoto 1977), isolated from the flesh of *Scarus gibbus* a toxic mixture that was separable by

DEAE cellulose chromatography into a toxin designated scaritoxin, and a more polar toxin, that strongly resembled ciguatoxin. Scaritoxin was reported to cause hind limb paralysis in mice, a symptom not normally observed with ciguatoxin.

Recently (Joh and Scheuer 1985) we had an opportunity to examine parrot-fishes (*Scarus sordidus*) from a toxic reef on Tarawa atoll, Republic of Kiribati. We also isolated two toxins separable on DEAE cellulose. However, by manipulation on basic alumina we were able to interconvert the two toxins. By TLC comparison we showed that scaritoxin and the less polar ciguatoxin (Nukina *et al.* 1984) are identical, though this finding remains to be confirmed by spectral comparison.

Acknowledgement — We thank the National Marine Fisheries Service through a subcontract with the Medical University of South Carolina for financial support.

References

Bagnis, R., Loussan, E., and Thevenin, S. (1974). Les intoxications par poissons perroquets aux iles Gambier. *Méd. trop.* **34**, 523–7.

Banner, A. H., Sasaki, S., Helfrich, P., Alender, C. B., and Scheuer, P. J. (1961). Bioassay of ciguatera toxin. *Nature* **189**, 229–30.

Chungue, E. (1977). Le complexe toxinique des poissons perroquets. Ph.D. Thesis, Academie de Montpelier, Université des sciences et techniques due Languedoc, Montpelier, France.

——, Bagnis, R., Fusetani, N., and Hashimoto, Y. (1977). Isolation of two toxins from a parrot-fish *Scarus gibbus*. *Toxicon* **15**, 89–93.

——, ——, and Parc, F. (1984) The use of mosquitoes *Aedes aegypti* to detect crude ciguatoxin in surgeon fishes *Ctenochaetus striatus*. *Toxicon* **22**, 161–4.

Durand, M., Squiban, A., Viso, A.-C., and Pesando, D. (1985). Production and toxicity of *Gambierdiscus toxicus*. Effects of its toxins (maitotoxin and ciguatoxin) on some marine organisms. *Proceedings of the Fifth International Coral Reef Congress*, Vol. 4, pp. 483–7. Papeete, Tahiti, Antenne Museum-ephe, Moorea, French Polynesia.

Goto, T., Kishi, Y., Takahashi, T., and Hirata, Y. (1965). Tetrodotoxin. *Tetrahedron* **21**, 2059–88.

Hokama, Y. (1985). A rapid simplified enzyme immunoassay stick test for the detection of ciguatoxin and related polyethers from fish tissues. *Toxicon* **23**, 939–46.

——, Abad, M. A., and Kimura, L. H. (1983). A rapid enzyme immunoassay for the detection of ciguatoxin in contaminated fish tissues. *Toxicon* **21**, 817–24.

——, Banner, A. H., and Boylan, D. B. (1977). A radio immunoassay for the detection of ciguatoxin. *Toxicon* **15**, 317–25.

——, Osugi, A. M. Honda, S. A. A., and Matsuo, M. K. (1985). Monoclonal antibodies in the detection of ciguatoxin and other toxic polyethers in fish tissues by a rapid poke stick test. *Proceedings of the Fifth International Coral Reef*

Symposium, Vol. 4, pp. 449–55. Papeete, Tahiti, Antenne Museum-ephe, Moorea, French Polynesia.

Ito, Y., Sandlin, J., and Bowers, W. G. (1982). High-speed preparative counter-current chromatography with a coil planet centrifuge. *J. Chromatogr.* **244**, 247–58.

Joh, Y.-G. and Scheuer, P. J. (1985). The chemical nature of scaritoxin. *Mar. Fish. Rev.* (In press.)

Lin, Y. Y., Risk, M., Ray, S. M., Van Engen, D., Clardy, J., Golik, J., James, J. C., and Nakanishi, K. (1981). Isolation and structure of brevetoxin B from the 'red tide' dinoflagellate *Ptychodiscus brevis* (*Gymnodinium breve*). *J. Am. chem. Soc.* **103**, 6773–5.

Mandava, N. B. and Ito, Y. (1982). Separation of plant hormones by counter-current chromatography. *J. Chromatogr.* **247**, 315–25.

Murakami, Y., Oshima, Y., and Yasumoto, T. (1982). Identification of okadaic acid as a toxic component of a marine dinoflagellate *Prorocentrum lima*. *Bull. Jap. Soc. Sci. Fish.* **48**, 69–72.

Nakamura, M. and Yasumoto, T. (1985). Tetrodotoxin derivatives in pufferfish. *Toxicon* **23**, 271–6.

Nukina, M., Koyanagi, L. M., and Scheuer, P. J. (1984). Two interchangeable forms of ciguatoxin. *Toxicon* **22**, 169–76.

Schantz, E. J., Ghazarossian, V. E., Schnoes, H. K., Strong, F. M., Springer, J. P., Pezzanite, J. O., and Clardy, J. (1975). The structure of saxitoxin. *J. Am. chem. Soc.* **97**, 1238–9.

Scheuer, P. J., Takahashi, W., Tsutsumi, J., and Yoshida, T. (1967). Ciguatoxin: isolation and chemical nature. *Science* **155**, 1267–8.

Shimizu, Y., Norte, M., Hori, A., Genenah, A., and Kobayashi, A. (1984). Bio-synthesis of saxitoxin analogues: the unexpected pathway. *J. Am. chem. Soc.* **106**, 6433–4.

——, Shimizu, H., Scheuer, P. J., Hokama, Y., Oyama, M., and Miyahara, J. T. (1982). *Gambierdiscus toxicus*, a ciguatera-causing dinoflagellate from Hawaii. *Bull. Jap. Soc. Fish.* **48**, 811–13.

Tachibana, K. (1980). Structural studies on marine toxins. Ph.D. Dissertation, University of Hawaii, Honolulu.

——, Scheuer, P. J., Tsukitani, Y., Kikuchi, H., Van Engen, D., Clardy, J., Gopichand, Y., and Schmitz, F. (1981). Okadaic acid, a cytotoxic polyether from two marine sponges of the genus *Halichondria*. *J. Am. chem. Soc.* **103**, 2469–71.

Uemura, D., Takahashi, T., Yamamoto, T., Katayama, C., Tanaka, J., Okumura, Y., and Hirata, Y. (1985). Norhalichondrin A: an antitumor polyl-ether macrolide from a marine sponge. *J. Am. chem. Soc.* **107**, 4796–8.

Yasumoto, T., Bagnis, R., and Vernoux, V. P. (1976). Toxicity of the surgeon-fishes. II. Properties of the principal water soluble toxin. *Bull. Jap. Soc. Sci. Fish.* **42**, 359–65.

——, Raj, U., and Bagnis, R. (1984). *Sea food poisonings in tropical regions*. Tohoku University, Sendai, Japan.

——, Nakajima, I., Bagnis, R., and Adachi, R. (1977). Finding of a dinoflagellate as likely culprit of ciguatera. *Bull. Jap. Soc. Sci. Fish.* **43**, 1021–6.

4

Toxicoses induced by ticks and reptiles in domestic animals

Bernard F. Stone

Introduction

For the purposes of this review, domestic animals are considered to comprise companion animals and livestock. The main aim is to report on tick toxicoses in these animals. Particular emphasis will be placed on tick paralysis and on research into this syndrome in Australia. The review by Stone and Wright (1981) of tick toxins and protective immunity will be updated where possible. An additional aim is to discuss envenomation of domestic animals by reptiles, as in Australia there are some similarities in symptomatology with tick paralysis.

A toxicosis is regarded as a pathological/physiological condition likely to have been induced in an animal by a toxin or, in the case of a reptile, by a venom. The view is taken that venoms are utilized for offence or defence and are complex mixtures often containing a number of individual toxins. Therefore envenomation by a reptile may result in one or a series of toxicoses. Tick toxins do not appear to be weapons but may be accidentally acquired by the victim when the parasite injects saliva. This fortuitous (or fateful) type of toxicosis is not uncommon (Sutherland 1983).

Gothe (1981) estimated that approximately 50 of the 800 described tick species are potentially capable of transferring toxins to their hosts. The pathophysiological changes produced by the ticks could not be attributed to infectious organisms and therefore must be regarded as being due to toxicoses. Not all of these ticks necessarily affect domestic animals, but 13 species possibly affect cattle.

During their period of attachment and feeding, ticks of most species 'cement' themselves to the host. All species then establish a feeding lesion, which receives tissue fluids and blood. The salivary secretions of the tick may contain attachment cement precursors, vasoactive agents to increase blood flow, enzymes, and other proteins that may be antigenic, often leading to the destruction of host tissue by the host's own immune reactions (Kemp, Stone, and Binnington 1983). Sometimes anticoagulants are present. One of the principal functions of the salivary secretions is to excrete surplus water and ions by returning them to the host during concentration of the blood meal. The role of a toxin in relation to these physiological processes is obscure.

Tick toxicoses other than tick paralysis

Six non-paralysing toxicoses of domestic animals have been reported. They may be categorized into four types, according to the vector.

Type 1 may logically include three apparently related toxicoses of cattle, sheep, and pigs in central, eastern, and southern Africa. These are 'sweating sickness', a fatal form, and 'Mhlosinga' and 'Magudu', which are milder forms (Neitz 1962). Certain strains of the small bontpoot tick, *Hyalomma truncatum*, have been incriminated. The symptoms are fever, profuse moist eczema, anorexia, and degeneration of condition. It is not possible to transfer the causal agent responsible via blood inoculations from affected animals, and removal of ticks results in an immediate clinical recovery. Thus, toxins are considered to be responsible. Despite attempts to demonstrate a sweating sickness toxin, none has yet been isolated; rickettsiae, which are almost always present in carrier strains, are a possible source of the toxin (Bezuidenhout and Malherbe 1981). There is some evidence of immunity (Neitz 1962; Dolan and Newson 1980). Sweating sickness may also occur in southern India and Sri Lanka (Neitz 1959).

Type 2 is caused by the sand tampan *Ornithodoros savignyi*, and affects young calves and sheep in the Kalahari region of north-west Cape Province, South Africa, and in Namibia (South-West Africa). Rapid death may occur, and a heat-stable, proteinaceous salivary toxin with an isoelectric point of pH 5 and a molecular weight of 15 400 dalton has been demonstrated in laboratory studies. This demonstration of the presence of a toxin probably refutes the popular belief that exsanguination is responsible for the condition (Howell 1966; Neitz, Howell, and Potgieter 1969; Howell, Neitz, and Potgieter 1975).

The last two types of toxicosis to be considered in this section appear to be induced only by massive infestations of ticks (Neitz 1962).

Type 3 is induced by the brown ear tick, *Rhipicephalus appendiculatus*, and affects cattle in southern Africa, causing pyrexia, anaemia, wasting, and necrosis of lymph nodes. It has been suggested that a leucocytotropic toxin casues a paralysis or dysfunction of the reticuloendothelial system or direct toxic damage to the bone marrow. Relapses resulting from latent blood infections such as babesiosis often follow. Immunity to the apparent toxicosis appears to be established and maintained by periodic reinfestation. In type 4, the cattle tick, *Boophilus microplus*, in Australia is reputed to have caused pyrexia, anorexia, and some direct interference with host metabolism, including possible liver dysfunction (O'Kelly and Seifert 1970). Although it has been reported that conditions were such that exsanguination or blood parasitaemia could not have been responsible, more evidence is needed on this apparent toxicosis.

Gothe (1981) is disinclined to accept that type 4 is a true toxicosis and only accepts type 3 with reservations.

Tick paralysis

Incidence and economic and social effects

Murnaghan and O'Rourke (1978) listed 35 species of ticks and Gothe, Kunze, and Hoogstraal (1979) listed 43 species that were possibly implicated in tick paralysis. Some species were not common to both lists, suggesting that at least 43 species may be involved, but not all indentifications for the individual species were fully documented. Additional paralysing species were reported by Dipeolu (1976), Magalhaes (1979), and Gothe, Bucheim, and Schrecke (1981); 25 species are recorded as paralysing domestic animals in 14 countries (Table 4.1).

The most troublesome species to domestic animals on three continents are: Africa — *I. rubicundus*, *R. evertsi evertsi*, and *A. (P.) walkerae*; Australia — *I. holocyclus*; North America — *D. andersoni*, *D. variabilis*, and *A. (P.) radiatus*. These ticks not only cause serious economic loss to the livestock industries on these continents but may be of social importance also for owners, who lose their pets.

Possibly the most consistently toxic tick in the world is the Australian paralysis tick *I. holocyclus* (Plate 4.1), which is present along the eastern coastal strip from Cairns in north Queensland to Lakes Entrance in Victoria. The Tasmanian paralysis tick *I. cornuatus* and Hirst's marsupial tick *I. hirsti* are capable of producing paralysis but are not so widely or abundantly distributed (Fig. 4.1).

A single tick may paralyse and kill even a large dog such as a German Shepherd or a Labrador. As a result of infestations by *I. holocyclus* there may be at least 20 000 domestic animals in Australia affected by tick paralysis each year and, of these, at least 10 000 may have been companion animals referred to veterinarians for treatment (B. F. Stone, unpublished data from a recent survey). However, livestock animals are also vulnerable and the deaths of calves in northern New South Wales alone have been estimated at about 10 000 per year (I. Lewis, personal communication); calves may be paralysed by as few as three to four ticks (Doube, Kemp, and Bird 1977; B. F. Stone, unpublished data). There are many other livestock

Table 4.1 World distribution of ticks reported to paralyse domestic animals

Species	Country	Additional references[a]
Ixodid ('hard') ticks		
Amblyomma maculatum	Uruguay	—
A. variegatum	Nigeria	Dipeoulu (1976)
Dermacentor andersoni	Canada	—
Dermacentor andersoni	USA	—
D. auratus	India	—
D. occidentalis	USA	—
D. variabilis	USA	—
Haemaphysalis punctata	Crete	—
Haemaphysalis punctata	Bulgaria (Macedonia)	—
Hyalomma truncatum	South Africa	—
Ixodes cornuatus	Australia	—
I. crenulatus	USSR (Moldavia, Transcarpathia, Ukraine)	—
I. hirsti	Australia	—
I. holocyclus	Australia	
I. ricinus	Crete	—
I. ricinus	USSR	—
I. ricinus	Turkey	—
I. ricinus	Yugoslavia	—
I. rubicundus	South Africa	—
I. scapularis	USA	—
Rhipicentor nuttalli	South Africa	—
Rhipicephalus evertsi evertsi	South Africa	—
R. sanguineus	USA	—
Argasid ('soft') ticks		
Argas (Argas) africolumbae	Upper Volta	Gothe *et al.* (1981)
A. (Persicargas) miniatus	Brazil	Magalhaes (1979)
A. persicus	South Africa	—
A. persicus	India	—
A. persicus	Upper Volta	Gothe *et al.* (1981)
A. persicus	USA	Brown and Cross (1941)
A. (P.) radiatus	USA	—
A. (P.) sanchezi	USA	—
A. (P.) walkerae	South Africa	—
Ornithodoros lahorensis	USSR	—

[a] Other than shown in Murnaghan and O'Rourke (1978) and in Gothe *et al.* (1979).

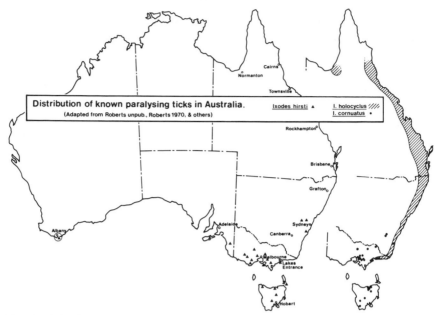

Distribution of known paralysing ticks in Australia.
(Adapted from Roberts unpub., Roberts 1970, & others)

Ixodes hirsti ▲   I. holocyclus ////
I. cornuatus •

Fig. 4.1 Distribution of the Australian paralysis tick *Ixodes holocyclus*, the Tasmanian paralysis tick *I. cornuatus*, and Hirsts's marsupial tick *I. hirsti*. Adapted from Roberts (1970), Roberts (unpublished), and others.

areas along the east coast of Australia where *I. holocyclus* occurs and adult cattle may also be affected by somewhat heavier infestations as are adult horses, sheep, goats, and deer (Seddon 1968; B. F. Stone, unpublished data). However, juveniles such as piglets, foals, kids, lambs, and fawns (raised as part of deer farming programmes), are at greatest risk. Therefore, it is estimated that each year in Australia 100 000 animals or more may be affected to some degree (B. F. Stone, unpublished data).

Paralysing toxins: separation and characterization

It is usually well accepted that toxins are responsible for tick paralysis, but so far a toxin has been unequivocally incriminated only for the syndrome induced by *I. holocyclus*. Since the work of Ross (1926), the paralysing ability of extracts of salivary glands of this tick has been repeatedly demonstrated. Stone and Wright (1981) reviewed the attempts made to demonstrate paralysing toxins in a number of ticks, in their eggs and in their salivary glands or saliva. Progress made in isolation, purification, and characterization of the paralysing toxin obtained from the salivary glands of *I. holocyclus* was also reviewed. More recently, it has been shown that a paralysing toxin with similar characteristics to that extracted from salivary glands, is secreted by these ticks when fed artificially and the medium collected (Stone, Commins, and Kemp 1983). This study provided verification, if it were needed, that the tick oral secretions contain the paralysing toxin. A method thus became available for the harvesting and comparison of secreted and extracted toxin. Sadly, yields by artificial feeding were no better than by extraction. Stone and Binnington (1986) discuss this and other developments in research into the nature of this toxin and the role of the salivary gland in its biosynthesis.

As a result of these recent studies of the salivary glands by electron microscopy (Stone and Binnington 1986) and a consideration of preliminary biochemical evidence (Stone 1979) it has been concluded that this toxin is probably an unusual Pronase-resistant protein originating in cell 'b' of the granular acinus II of the salivary gland. These latter results tended to confirm the light microscopical and toxinological studies of Binnington and Stone (1981) which showed that the peak of toxin content of salivary glands on the fifth day of feeding coincided closely with the peak of cell 'b' granular density and synthesizing activity. The other three candidate cells failed to show a correlation. Cell 'b' is rich in carbohydrates and proteins during toxin secretion but it is not known if the toxin is a glycoprotein. More direct evidence supporting the involvement of cell 'b' in the biosynthesis of the toxin may eventually be obtainable by the removal by micromanipulation of acinus II or cell 'b' material and verification by immunoassay of extractives using specific labelled antibodies to the toxin.

'Holocyclotoxin' was suggested by Stone and Wright (1981) as an appropriate name for the biologically active entity contained in the paralysing, secretory material obtained from *I. holocyclus*. It was clear that a pure chemical substance had not been obtained but the active extracts and fractions were regarded as containing holocyclotoxin. However, very recent work on the purification of this toxin has provided most encouraging results and it is possible that holocyclotoxin itself may have been isolated in size-homogeneous form by gel filtration on HPLC. The apparent molecular weight was approximately 50 000 (Aylward, Gauci, and Stone, unpublished data) which falls satisfactorily within the range of 40 000–60 000 obtained for the putative toxin contained in the Pronase-resistant fraction (Stone 1979) and verifies a more recent estimate of approximately 50 000 based on the original data (Stone, Neish, and Gauci, in manuscript).

Mode of action of paralysing toxins

Most of the in-depth physiological and pharmacological investigations of tick paralysis have been on *D. andersoni*-paralysed animals, and special attention will be paid to this unique, pioneering series of studies. The reviews of Gregson (1973), Murnaghan and O'Rourke (1978) and Gothe *et al.* (1979) have been drawn on heavily in compiling the following summary.

It was suggested that the condition is basically due to presynaptic blockage of conduction at neuromuscular junctions, but curare-like competitive blocking was eliminated by a number of findings, including the result that paralysed muscle responded normally to injection of acetylcholine (ACh); depolarizing blocking agents or anticholinesterases were not responsible for the condition, as their antagonists did not lessen paralysis. Tick paralysis due to *D. andersoni* was considered to be due to failure of release or synthesis of ACh, as the amount of ACh liberated from a perfused muscle preparation by nerve or muscle stimulation was either significantly less than for normal muscle or absent.

Failure in synthesis of ACh was eliminated as a cause of *D. andersoni* paralysis; the activity of the synthesizing enzyme, choline acetyltransferase, was similar in nerve preparations for normal and paralysed dogs, and the hemicholinium test for inadequate ACh synthesis was negative. No reduction of paralysis occurred when acetylcoenzyme A (jointly responsible with choline acetyltransferase for the final step of ACh synthesis) was added to perfused paralysed muscle preparations or injected into the intact animal. The stores of ACh were also adequate in the paralysed animal because a marked release of ACh occurred in perfusates of normal and paralysed muscles from reserpenized, paralysed dogs. Lack of calcium ions or excess magnesium ions, which interfere with release of ACh, appeared to be excluded as did absence of essential plasma-borne release factors in causing tick paralysis.

Blocking of motor and sensory nerve conduction was considered to be an important factor in *D. andersoni* paralysis but was only detectable in longer nerves probably because of the increasing likelihood of impulses meeting toxin-depressed nodes of Ranvier thought to be present in these nerves. The amplitude of nerve action potentials was reduced in long nerves tested *in situ*, and conduction velocity was also reduced particularly in the smaller diameter, slower acting fibres (Murnaghan and O'Rourke 1978). However, in *A. walkerae* paralysis of fowls, faster-conducting fibres were affected more than the slower ones (R. Gothe, personal communication). No changes from the normal pattern were found in nerve action potentials or in maximum nerve conduction velocities in *in situ* preparations for *I. holocyclus*-paralysed dogs (Cooper, Cooper, Ilkew, and Kelly 1976). Reduced muscle action potentials have been recorded from a child probably paralysed by *D. andersoni*, in fowls paralysed by *A. persicus* larvae (Murnaghan and O'Rourke 1978) and in dogs paralysed by *I. holocyclus* (Cooper *et al.* 1976).

Although it is clear that interference with peripheral motor nerve function is principally responsible for paralysis it has been stated that there is evidence of some central nervous system (CNS) involvement. Stretch reflexes were absent in *D. andersoni*-paralysed animals with only slight neuromuscular disturbance; human ataxia also has been reported with no accompanying muscular weakness. Undisturbed consciousness and mental alertness are features of *I. holocyclus* paralysis and therefore the CNS cortex is unaffected but the retention of sensation coupled with loss or modification of reflexes and normal contractions in paralysed muscle (on stimulating appropriate nerves) caused Ross (1926) to conclude that a toxin may be acting on the motor neurones of the CNS. However, Cooper and Spence (1976) considered that most aspects of motor paralysis may be explained on the basis of action at the neuromuscular junction. They also ruled out interference with conduction as there was no decline in amplitude of compound action potentials in phrenic nerves from hemidiaphragm preparations taken from mice paralysed by nymphal *I. holocyclus*.

Murnaghan and O'Rouke (1978) drew attention to the difficulty in detecting reduced amplitude of the action potential over the short stretch of nerve involved in such *in vitro* preparations. Cooper and Spence (1976) demonstrated a most interesting direct, temperature-dependent inhibition of transmitter release at neuromuscular junctions in these isolated, paralysed phrenic nerve-hemidiaphragm preparations; muscle contraction in response to nerve stimulation occurred much more readily at lower than higher temperatures. These authors proposed that holocyclotoxin inhibits transmitter release at neuromuscular junctions via some intermediate step between depolarization of the terminal membrane and release of ACh.

Symptomatology

The symptomatology of the syndromes due to *D. andersoni* and to *I. holocyclus* have been studied in the greatest detail and are somewhat similar with one notable difference, viz. that symptoms rapidly disappear following removal of the former ticks but usually worsen for some time after removal of the latter ticks. The symptoms are loss of appetite and voice, incoordination, ascending flaccid paralysis, ocular irritation, excessive salivation and vomiting, respiratory distress, asymmetric pupillary dilatation, and frequently death. Cardiovascular studies on *I. holocyclus*-paralysed dogs revealed an increase in blood pressure with a decrease in cardiac output indicating an intense vasoconstriction followed by a dramatic decrease in heart rate in terminal stages (Cooper *et al.* 1976). However, *D. andersoni*-paralysed dogs have normal blood pressure (Murnaghan and O'Rourke 1978).

Treatment

The early work of Ross (1935) and Oxer and Ricardo (1942) in Australia had shown that it was possible to stimulate high antitoxin titres in dogs (see p. 64) and this gave rise to a small veterinary antiserum industry that provided the means of treating tick paralysis. This antiserum is still the basic therapeutic treatment but must be administered intravenously at the first sign of paralysis, preferably before removal of the tick and after injection of a little anitserum around the tick attachment site(s) to neutralize localized toxin. The success rate is variable but may be quite high for cases treated in the early stages. Only recently have there been attempts to standardize the antiserum by means of a neutralization test (Stone, Cowie, Kerr, and Binnington 1982) and this has resulted in higher titre anitserum becoming available. An enzyme-linked immunosorbent assay (ELISA) for antitoxin has been developed (Morrison, Gauci, Stone, and Pearn, in manuscript), which should greatly assist in further standardization. Improvements have also been made to this serum, which is heterologous for non-canines, by reducing the serum albumin content (K. C. Curtin, personal communication). Improving the antitoxin is of undoubted value and is seen as a continuing need.

Hyperexcitability, hypertension, and emesis are counteracted by such drugs as acetylpromazine or phenoxybenzamine (an adrenergic alpha blocker — most effective in severe cases). Anaphylaxis is controlled by antihistamines, corticosteroids or adrenalin. The established clinical practice of cooling the patient may now have a scientific basis (Cooper and Spence 1976).

Development of immunity to tick paralysis

Stone and Wright (1980, 1981) and Stone, Neish and Wright (1983) discussed the development of immunity to tick paralysis resulting from natural and artificially regulated feeding of *I. holocyclus* on wildlife and domestic animals and reported on a study of the kinetics of this form of immunization of beagle dogs. Serum antibody titres increased to maximal values of about 50 antitoxin units per ml (ATU ml^{-1} after 40 weeks when beagles could tolerate 23 female ticks feeding simultaneously to repletion. Titres declined rapidly in the absence of feeding ticks but once immunity was firmly established, dogs retained it for at least one year. The carefully regulated injection of six doses of toxic tick salivary gland extracts into beagles produced maximal titres of about 40 ATU ml^{-1} in about 20 weeks and the dogs were immune to otherwise lethal doses of extracts and infestations of ticks (Wright, Stone, and Neish 1983); similar results had been obtained previously with rabbits except that higher titres were achieved (Stone, Neish, and Wright 1982). This information provided encouragement to proceed with investigations into the feasibility of a vaccine against tick paralysis in Australia.

Vaccine research

A non-toxic vaccine was clearly preferable to a toxic one and it was shown that glutaraldehyde treatment of holocyclotoxin contained in partially purified preparations from salivary glands detoxified and also enhanced the

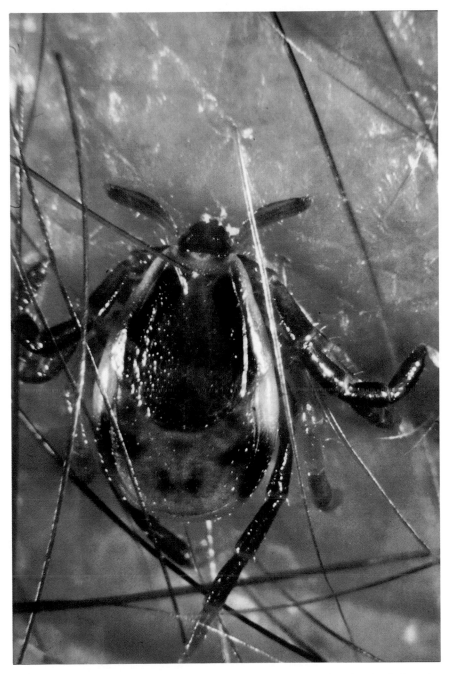

Plate 4.1 A recently-attached female Australian paralysis tick *Ixodes holocyclus* feeding on a host. (Photo: B. F. Stone).

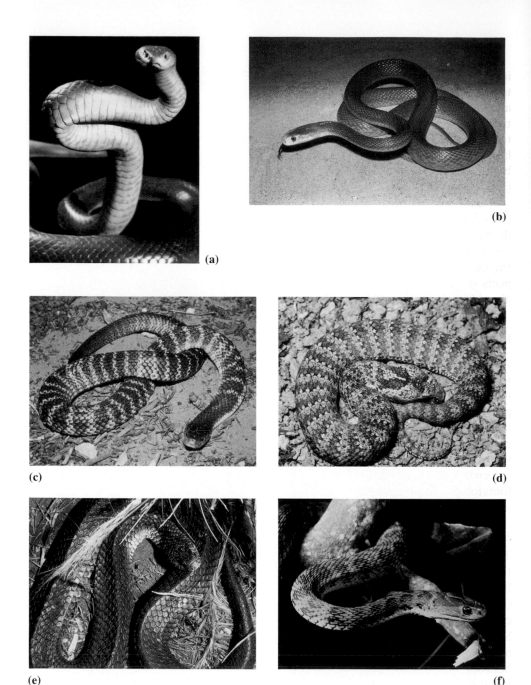

Plate 4.2 Some Australian snakes, dangerous to domestic animals.
(a) The common or eastern brown snake *Pseudonaja textilis*. (Photo: J. Pearn)
(b) The taipan *Oxyuranus scutellatus*. (Photo: J. White)
(c) The mainland or eastern tiger snake *Notechis scutatus*. (Photo: J. White)
(d) The death adder *Acanthopis antarcticus*. (Photo: Queensland Museum)
(e) The lowlands or proper copperhead *Austrelaps superbus*. (Photo: J. White)
(f) The Clarence River or rough-scaled snake *Tropidechis carinatus*. (Photo: G. Parker)

immunogenicity of an experimental vaccine (Stone and Neish 1984). When tested on rabbits, the toxoid vaccine produced antitoxin titres that were about 25 per cent higher and were achieved in 40 per cent of the previous time, using 50 per cent of the number of doses when compared with the toxin-based vaccine (Stone, *et al.* 1982; Stone and Binnington, 1986). Similarly encouraging results were obtained with dogs, titres of 60 ATU ml^{-1} being obtained in 11 weeks after three doses of the toxoid-based vaccine (Stone, Neish, Morrison and Uren, 1986; cf. p. 64).

It has been estimated that there may be a considerable demand in Australia for a vaccine because of the much greater preference of custodians of domestic animals for prophylaxis rather than therapeutics and because the cost of the latter approach is high. However, existing methods of harvesting the immunizing antigen are inadequate and it appears that the best prospects of commercialization are through genetic engineering. Research is about to commence on this aspect of the programme.

Reptile toxicoses in Australia

As in most other countries, the only reptiles in Australia known to be venomous to domestic animals are snakes, there being no Australian animals similar to the Gila monster *Heloderma suspectum suspectum*, the poisonous lizard of Arizona (Tinkham 1971). This is despite the not-undeserved reputation prevalent in other countries that Australia has the greatest variety of, as well as the most toxic, venomous creatures in the world, particularly terrestrial snakes, spiders, and marine animals.

Lewis (1978) and Sutherland (1983) reviewed the incidence, symptomatology, and treatment of snake bite in domestic animals in Australia, and data for this section have been largely taken from these references.

Incidence

There are about 20 species of venomous elapid snakes in Australia and 10 of these species are potentially lethal to animals (and humans). Eight of these latter snakes are listed in Table 4.2 in descending order of toxicity of venoms (Sutherland 1983). These snakes will be referred to by their abbreviated common names, e.g. 'fierce snake', and some are illustrated in Plate 4.2. Somewhat ironically but sadly for reptile conservation, an introduced amphibian (the cane toad, *Bufo marinus*) is apparently reducing the numbers of frog-eating snakes such as the brown snake, the death adder and the black snake (Covacevich and Archer 1975). The populations of mammal-eating snakes such as the taipan are unaffected (Shine and Covacevich 1983), and the toxic cane toad itself may be more of a threat to dogs, for example, than the snakes it displaced.

Approximately 350 cases of snake bite in domestic animals, mostly

Table 4.2 Some Australian snakes of importance in envenomation of domestic animals in descending order of toxicity of venoms (Sutherland 1983).

Species	Common name
Oxyuranus microlepidotus	Small scaled or 'fierce snake'
Pseudonaja textilis	Common or eastern 'brown snake'
Oxyuranus scutellatus	'Taipan'
Notechis scutatus	Mainland or eastern 'tiger snake'
Acanthopis antarcticus	'Death adder'
Austrelaps superbus	Lowlands or proper 'copperhead'
Tropidechis carinatus	Clarence River or 'rough scaled snake'
Pseudechis porphyriacus	Red-bellied or common 'black snake'

treated with antivenom, were reported to the Commonwealth Serum Laboratories over the period 1968–1977. Of these cases (peak period October to February), 49 per cent were from Victoria, 23 per cent from Queensland, 19 per cent from New South Wales and the balance presumably from the rest of Australia. Dogs accounted for 57 per cent of the cases and cats for 28 per cent. At least 2000 ampoules of brown snake antivenom, 700 ampoules of tiger snake antivenom and 40 ampoules of death adder antivenom are used annually for domestic animal treatment; therefore these three snakes will be the ones principally considered in this review. The cost of treatment with antivenom is such, combined with uncertain diagnosis in many instances, that these figures were thought to represent perhaps only 10 per cent of the real incidence.

More recently, Barr (1984) reported on the epidemiology of snake bite over a period of 10 years (1973–1983) for dogs and cats admitted to Melbourne University Veterinary Hospital in Victoria. Of the 240 animals treated, 52 per cent were dogs and in only 48 per cent of these cases was the snake actually seen. Tiger snakes were implicated in all cases except for one of brown snake bite.

Toxicity and symptomatology
The toxicity of venoms for domestic animals has not been determined with the same degree of accuracy as for laboratory animals such as mice because of the obvious difficulty and undesirability of using sufficiently large numbers of animals to ensure statistical significance. An LD_{50} is usually out of the question. For example, Sutherland (1983) has referred to the 'certain(ly) lethal dose' of tiger snake venom for the cat, dog, horse, sheep, and goat, which was 0.1, 0.045, 0.005, 0.01, and 0.018 mg kg^{-1}, respectively. These figures simply indicate that one or more animals were killed by the dose administered, the terminology and data being largely those of Kellaway (1929). It is not possible to draw conclusions concerning the comparative

susceptibility of these animals but there is other evidence that cats are less susceptible than dogs (Lewis 1978; Barr 1984).

Many Australian snake venoms contain combinations of neurotoxins, haemolysins, coagulants, and cytotoxins in various proportions. Thus, voluntary muscles may be paralysed or lysed (giving rise to myoglobinuria); blood may be affected in a number of ways including intravascular clotting, defibrination (followed by continuous bleeding at the site or elsewhere, haematemesis and haematuria), lysis of red cells (jaundice and haemoglobinuria); vascular endothelium may be damaged, resulting in haemorrhages in some tissues. The enzyme hyaluronidase, although not a direct toxin, is present in some snake venoms and is thought to assist their rapid entry into the circulation. This may account for the dramatic collapse of some animals soon after being bitten. Proteolytic enzymes, present in the venom of some snakes of other world areas and capable of producing severe local reactions at the bite site, appear to be absent in Australian snake venoms.

As neurotoxins are dominant in brown snake, tiger snake and death adder venoms, paralysis is the outstanding feature in all serious cases in domestic animals (Trinca 1959). Both brown and tiger snake venoms have presynaptic and postsynaptic action while death adder venom probably has only a postsynaptic action (Sutherland 1983). Characteristically the paralysis is ascending in nature, affecting the hind limbs first, resulting in ataxia, then proceeding to complete limb paralysis, and finally to respiratory distress and death. These symptoms are so similar to those caused by the Australian paralysis tick *Ixodes holocyclus* that it is understandable that diagnostic confusion may arise, in the absence of either tick or snake — the one having dropped off and the other having moved away. An early symptom in snake envenomation of domestic animals is pupillary dilatation and reduced light reflexes, possibly due to partial paralysis of intrinsic eye muscles. This may also occur in tick paralysis for the same reason.

The complexity of the effects of the coagulant factors in venoms has been described by Sutherland (1983) but the ultimate result is that blood often fails to clot or the clotting time is increased greatly. In the case of domestic animals a useful test can be made by checking a blood sample for clotting time above the usual 3 to 5 min.

Other symptoms include trembling, vomiting, and salivation. Severe muscle damage may occur in dogs receiving even low doses of brown snake venom, with rhabdomyolysis and elevated levels of creatine kinase (Lewis 1978) — c f. human tick paralysis due to *D. andersoni* (Boffey and Paterson 1973).

Treatment

Specific treatment depends on accurate diagnosis as some of the symptoms seen in snake bite may also be caused by other veterinary conditions such as poison baits and organophosphorus pesticides (salivation and vomiting), canine hepatitis or feline enteritis (prostration), leptospirosis (haemo-globinuria), botulism (paralysis), and of course tick paralysis (excessive salivation, vomiting, and ascending paralysis — see above). Knowledge of the identity of the snake is highly desirable as this allows the use of the specific monovalent antivenom (tiger snake, brown snake, death adder, or possibly taipan). In the absence of the offending snake itself, the ingenious venom detection kit (based on an enzyme-linked immunosorbent assay — Sutherland 1983), developed at the Commonwealth Serum Laboratories, may be used. Venom is detectable and identifiable in extracts of swabs from the bite site, in blood, or in urine samples at levels down to 5ng ml^{-1}. Although the cost of this procedure for veterinary application may well be prohibitive at present except for very valuable animals, this situation could change in the future.

Where no identification of the snake or venom is possible, regional distribution patterns may narrow down the likely number of species involved, so that a combination of monovalent antivenoms can be used for treatment with a reasonable chance of success. Thus the following antivenom combinations are recommended: brown snake + death adder (Queensland, north of Rock-hampton), tiger snake + brown snake + death adder (Queensland, south of Rockhampton; New South Wales, South Australia, West Australia and Northern Territory), tiger snake + brown snake (Victoria), and tiger snake only (Tasmania).

The survival rate for animals, mainly dogs and cats, treated with anti-venom was reported as 82 per cent and for untreated animals as less than 64 per cent (Lewis 1978). Surprisingly, 80 per cent of cases survived after treatment without identification of the snake, but using monovalent anti-venom. This may be compared with 84 per cent survival where a specific monovalent antivenom was used after identification of the snake or where a polyvalent antivenom was used, Polyvalent antivenom consists of a mixture of tiger snake, brown snake, death adder, black snake, and taipan anti-venoms, and may be indicated for particularly valuable animals in a region where the taipan or the fierce snake is found, However, Sutherland (1983) recommends taipan antivenom rather than polyvalent antivenom for taipan or fierce snake bite in humans and the same principle should apply for domestic animals. Apart from the advantage of a specific antivenom or one capable of cross-neutralization, large volume doses of polyvalent anti-venoms may be undesirable in dogs and cats. Anaphylactic-like reactions have been reported for animals treated with antivenoms, although there was no previous exposure to horse serum (Lewis 1978; Barr 1984). This effect is thought to be due to anticomplementary activity, necessitating dilution and slow infusion of the antivenom (Sutherland 1983).

Acknowledgements — The assistance of colleagues at CSIRO, Long Pocket

Laboratories, with the preparation of the manuscript is gratefully acknowledged; Mr Stan Fiske prepared Fig. 3.2 using data provided by Dr David Kemp and Mrs Jennifer Peters. Dr Struan Sutherland of the Commonwealth Serum Laboratories, Melbourne kindly reviewed the section on reptiles. Illustrations of snakes were made available by the Queensland Museum, Dr Julian White (Adelaide Children's Hospital, South Australia), Dr John Pearn and Mr John Morrison (Department of Child Health, University of Queensland), and Mr Greg Parker (Brisbane).

References

Barr, S. C. (1984). Clinical features, therapy and epidemiology of tiger snake bite in dogs and cats. *Austr. vet. J.* **61**, 208–12.

Bezuidenhout, J. D. and Malherbe, A. (1981). Sweating sickness: a comparative study of virulent and avirulent strains of *Hyalomma truncatum*. In: *Tick biology and control* (ed. G. B. Whitehead and J. D. Gibson), pp. 7–12. Tick Research Unit, Rhodes University, Grahamstown, South Africa.

Binnington, K. C. and Stone, B. F. (1981). Development changes in morphology and toxin content of the salivary gland of the paralysis tick *Ixodes holocyclus*. *Int. J. Parasitol.* **11**, 343–51.

Boffey, G. C. and Paterson, D. C. (1973). Creatine phosphokinase elevation in a case of tick paralysis *Can. med. Ass. J.* **108**, 866–68.

Brown, J. C. and Cross, J. C. (1941). A probable agent for the transmission of fowl paralysis. *Science* **93**, 528.

Cooper, B. J. and Spence, I. (1976). Temperature-dependent inhibition of evoked acetylcholine release in tick paralysis. *Nature, Lond.* **263**, 693–5.

——, Cooper, H. L., Ilkew, J. E., and Kelly, J. D. (1976). Tick paralysis. In Proceedings No. 30, pp. 57–61. Postgraduate Committee in Veterinary Science, University of Sydney.

Covacevich, J. and Archer, M. (1975). The distribution of the cane toad, *Bufo marinus*, in Australia and its effects on indigenous vertebrates. *Mem. Queensl. Mus.* **17**, 305–10.

Dipeolu, O. O. (1976). Tick paralysis in a sheep caused by nymphs of *Amblyomma variegatum*. A preliminary report. *Z. Parasitenkd* **49**, 293–5.

Dolan, T. T. and Newson, R. M. (1980). Sweating sickness in adult cattle. *Trop. Anim. Hlth Prod.* **12**, 119–24.

Doube, B. M., Kemp, D. H., and Bird, P. E. (1977). Paralysis of calves by the tick, *Ixodes holocyclus*. *Austr. vet. J.*. **53**, 39–43.

Gothe, R. (1981). Tick toxicoses of cattle. In: *Diseases of cattle in the tropics* (ed. M. Ristic and I. McIntyre), pp. 587–98. Martinus Nijhoff, The Hague.

——, Bucheim, C., and Schrecke, W. (1981). Zur paralyse-induzierenden kapazitat wildstammiger *Argas (Persicargas) persicus* — und *Argas (Argas) africolumbae* — populationen aus Ober Volta. *Berl. Münch. tierärztl. Wochenschr.* **94**, 299–302.

——, Kunze, K., and Hoogstraal, H. (1979). The mechanisms of pathogenicity in the tick paralyses. *J. med. Entomol.* **16**, 357–69.

Gregson, J. D. (1973). Tick paralysis: the appraisal of natural and experimental data. Canada Department of Agriculture, Monograph No. 9.

Howell, C. J. (1966). Collection of salivary gland secretion from the argasid *Ornithodoros savignyi* (Audouin, 1827) by use of a pharmacological stimulant. *J. S. A. vet. med. Ass.* **37**, 236–9.

Howell, C. J., Neitz A. W. H., and Potgieter, D. J. J. (1975). Some toxic, physical and chemical properties of the oral secretion of the sand tampan, *Ornithodoros savignyi* (Audouin, 1827). *Onderstepoort J. vet. Res.* **42**, 99–102.

Kellaway, C. H. (1929). The venom of *Notechis scutatus*. *Med. J. Austr.* **1**, 348–58.

Kemp, D. H., Stone B. F., and Binnington, K. C. (1983). Tick attachment and feeding: role of the mouthparts, feeding apparatus, salivary gland secretions and the host response. In *Physiology of ticks* (ed. F. D. Obenchain and R. Galun), pp. 119–68. Pergamon Press, Oxford.

Lewis, P. F. (1978). Snake bite in animals in Australia. In Proceedings No. 36, pp. 287–309. Postgraduate Committee in Veterinary Science, University of Sydney.

Magalhaes, F. E. P. (1979). Novos aspectos morfologicos, biologicos e toxicos de *Argas (Persicargas) miniatus* Kock, 1844 (Ixodoidea — Argasidae) no Estado do Rio de Janeiro. M.Sc. tese, Universidade Federal Rural do Rio de Janeiro.

Murnaghan, M. F. and O'Rourke, F. J. (1978). Tick paralysis. In: *Arthropod venoms* (ed. S. Bettini). *Handbook of Experimental Pharmacology* Vol. 48, pp. 419–64. Springer, Berlin.

Neitz, W. O. (1959). Sweating sickness: the present state of our knowledge. *Onderstepoort J. of vet. Res.* **28**, 3–38.

—— (1962). Tick toxicoses. Report on Second Meeting of the FAO/OIE Expert panel on Tick-Borne Diseases of Livestock, Cairo, UAR, pp. 6–8, 24. FAO Rome.

Neitz, A. W. H., Howell, C. J., and Potgieter, D. J. J. (1969). Purification of a toxic component in the oral secretion of the sand tampan, *Ornithodoros savignyi* (Audouin, 1827). *J. S. A. chem. Inst.* **22**, S142–9.

O'Kelly, J. C. and Seifert, G. W. (1970). The effect of the tick (*Boophilus microplus*) infestations on the blood composition of Shorthorn × Hereford cattle on high and low planes of nutrition. *Austr. J. biol. Sci.* **23**, 681–90.

Oxer, D. T. and Ricardo, C. L. (1942). Notes on the biology, toxicity and breeding of *Ixodes holocyclus* (Neumann). *Austr. Vet. J..* **18**, 194–199.

Roberts, F. H. S. (1970). *Australian Ticks*. CSIRO, Melbourne.

Ross, I. C. (1926). An experimental study of tick paralysis in Australia. *Parasitology* **18**, 410–29.

—— (1935). Tick paralysis: a fatal disease of dogs and other animals in eastern Australia. *J. Counc. sci. ind. Res.* **8**, 8–13.

Seddon, H. R. (1968). Dog paralysis tick (*I. holocyclus*). In: *Diseases of domestic animals in Australia* (2nd edn) (ed. H. E. Albiston), Part 3, pp. 68–80. Service Publications (Veterinary Hygiene) No. 7, Commonwealth of Australia, Department of Health, Canberra.

Shine, R. and Covacevich, J. (1983). Ecology of highly venomous snakes: the Australian genus *Oxyuranus* (Elapidae). *J. Herpet.* **17**, 60–69.

Stone, B. F. (1979). Chemical characterization studies on salivary gland toxins of the paralysis tick *Ixodes holocyclus*. In: *Neurotoxins: Fundamental and Clinical Advances* (ed. I. W. Chubb and L. B. Geffen), p. 273. Adelaide University Union Press, Adelaide.

—— and Binnington, K. C. (1986). The paralyzing toxin and other immunogens of the tick *I. holocyclus* and the role of the salivary gland in their biosyntheses. In: *Morphology, physiology and behavioral biology of ticks* (ed. J. R. Sauer and J. A. Hair), pp. 75–99. Ellis Horwood, Chichester, England.

——, Commins, M. A., and Kemp, D. H. (1983). Artificial feeding of the Australian paralysis tick *Ixodes holocyclus* and collection of paralyzing toxin. *Int. J. Parasitol.* **13**, 447–54.

——, Cowie, M. R., Kerr, J. D., and Binnington, K. C. (1982). Improved toxin/antitoxin assays for studies on the Australian paralysis tick *Ixodes holocyclus*. *Austr. J. exp. Biol. med. Sci.* **60**, 309–18.

—— and Neish, A. L. (1984). Tick-paralysis toxoid: an effective immunizing agent against the toxin of *Ixodes holocyclus*. *Austr. J. exp. Biol. med. Sci.* **62**, 189–91.

——, Neish, A. L., Morrison, J. J., and Uren, M. F. (1986). Toxoid stimulation in dogs of high titres of neutralizing antibodies against holocyclotoxin, the paralysing toxin of the Australian paralysis tick, *Ixodes holocyclus*. *Austr. vet. J.* **63**, 125–6.

——, ——, and Wright, I. G. (1982). Immunization of rabbits to produce high serum titres of neutralizing antibodies and immunity to the paralyzing toxin of *Ixodes holocyclus*. *Austr. J. exp. Biol. med. Sci.* **60**, 351–8.

——, ——, —— (1983). Tick (*Ixodes holocyclus*) paralysis in the dog — quantitative studies on immunity following artificial infestations with the tick. *Austr. vet. J.*. **60**, 65–8.

—— and Wright, I. G. (1980). Toxins of *Ixodes holocyclus* and immunity to paralysis. In: *Ticks and tick-borne diseases*, (ed. L. A. Y. Johnston and M. G. Cooper), pp. 75–8. Australian Veterinary Association, Sydney.

——, —— (1981). Tick toxins and protective immunity. In: *Tick biology and control* (ed. G. B. Whitehead and J. D. Gibson), pp. 1–5. Tick Research Unit, Rhodes University, Grahamstown, South Africa.

Sutherland, S. K. (1983). *Australian animal toxins*. Oxford University press, Melbourne.

Tinkham, E. R. (1971). The biology of the Gila monster. In: *Venomous animals and their venoms* (ed. W. Bucherl and E. E. Buckley), Vol. 2, pp. 387–413. Academic Press, New York.

Trinca, G. F. (1959). Snake bite as a veterinary problem. Australian Veterinary Association (Victorian Division) Proceedings, pp. 81–89.

Wright, I. G., Stone, B. F., and Neish, A. L. (1983). Tick (*Ixodes holocyclus*) paralysis in the dog — induction of immunity by injection of toxin. *Austr. vet. J.* **60**, 69–70.

5

The nutritional significance of naturally occurring toxins in plant foodstuffs

Irvin E. Liener

Introduction

If one accepts the Darwinian concept of natural selection, it follows that humans are at the pinnacle of the hierarchy of the animal kingdom because of their ability to utilize a wide variety of plants in the environment, either by direct consumption or indirectly by the feeding of animals when they are then used as a source of food. But plants did not evolve to serve humans or animals. The truth of the matter is that the primary concern of plants is to ensure their own survival. To this end, Nature has endowed them with the genetic capacity to synthesize substances that are toxic and thus serve to protect them from predators whether they be insects, fungi, animals, or humans. Being intelligent humans have learned which foods are safe to eat, or how such foods can be treated in order to eliminate their toxicity.

Although these substances are frequently referred to by such nondescript terms as 'toxins', 'toxicants', or 'toxic factors', these terms may be misleading. Strictly speaking, they imply that the substance in question is lethal beyond a certain level of intake, and the toxicologist may in fact assess its toxicity in terms of an LD_{50}, that is, that dose which causes the death of 50 per cent of the animals tested. Although some plants are known to produce an immediate and violent reaction, more subtle effects, produced only by prolonged ingestion, are more commonly observed. Such effects may include an interference with the bioavailability of nutrients, resulting in an inhibition of growth, or damage to specific organs such as the thyroid, pancreas, kidneys, or liver. A preferred term might be 'antinutritional', which may be liberally interpreted to mean nothing more or less than an adverse physiological response produced in humans or animals by a particular food or substance derived therefrom.

Although such toxic or antinutritional factors are widely distributed in the plant kingdom, only those foods that are eaten by a significant number of people on a fairly regular basis in some part of the world will be considered here. From a chemical point of view, it is convenient to classify these natural

Table 5.1 Examples of natural toxicants.

Toxicant	Food source	Toxic effect
Proteins		
Protease inhibitors	Legumes and cereals	Depressed growth/ Pancreatic hyperplasia
Lectins	Legumes and cereals	Depressed growth/death
Amino acid derivatives		
β-*N*-oxalyl-α,β-propionic acid	*Lathyrus sativus*	Lathyrism
Mimosine	*Leucaena*	Goitrogen/hair loss
Djenkolic acid	Djenkol bean	Kidney failure
Canavanine	Alfalfa seeds	Lupus erythematosus
Glycosides		
Glucosinolates	Cabbage family	Goitre
Cyanogen	Lima beans, cassava, fruit kernels	Respiratory failure/ goitre
Vicine/convicine	*Vicia faba*	Favism
Cycasin	Cycad nut	Carcinogen
Miscellaneous		
Alkaloids		
Pyrrolizidines	Tansy ragwort	Carcinogen
Swainosine	Locoweed	Locoism
Anagyrine	*Lupinus*	Crooked calf disease
Ptaquiloside	Bracken fern	Carcinogen
Tremetone	Snake root	Milk sickness
Solanine	Potatoes	Nervous paralysis
Gossypol	Cottonseed	Tissue damage

toxicants into the various categories shown in Table 5.1. No attempt will be made to present a detailed coverage of all of these natural toxicants, but rather specific examples from each of these categories will be presented.

Proteins

Protease inhibitors
Soya beans were originally introduced into the USA during the early part of this century primarily as a source of oil, with the extracted meal being utilized as a by-product that could provide animals with a rich source of protein. It was recognized quite early (Osborne and Mendel 1917) that it

was necessary to subject soya beans to heat treatment if they were to support
the growth of rats. The reason for the beneficial effect of heat treatment did
not become apparent until Kunitz (1945) isolated from raw soya beans a
protein that combines with trypsin to form an inactive complex. It is now
known that protease inhibitors in general are widely distributed throughout
the plant kingdom, particularly in legumes and, to a lesser extent, in cereal
grains and tubers, (Liener and Kakade, 1980).

Figure 5.1 shows the effect of heat treatment on the nutritive value of soya
beans and the concomitant inactivation of trypsin inhibitor activity. Proof
that the trypsin inhibitor itself is responsible for the poor growth on raw soya
flour comes from experiments showing that the purified inhibitor was
capable of producing a marked retardation of growth when incorporated
into the diet at a level equivalent to that present in raw soya beans (Liener,
Deuel, and Fevold 1949).

In addition to an inhibition of growth, one of the most characteristic
physiological responses of most animals to the trypsin inhibitor is an
enlargement of the pancreas (hypertrophy and hyperplasia) and an increase
in the secretory activity of the pancreas. The mechanism accounting for this
effect is only incompletely understood, but it is believed that pancreatic
secretion is controlled by a mechanism of negative feedback inhibition that
depends on the level of trypsin present at any given time in the small
intestine (Green and Lyman 1972). When the level of this enzyme falls
below a critical threshold value, the pancreas is induced to produce more
enzyme. The suppression of this negative feedback mechanism can thus
occur when trypsin is inactivated by the inhibitor. It is believed that the
mediating agent between trypsin and the pancreas is the hormone
cholecystokinin, which is released from the intestinal mucosa when the level

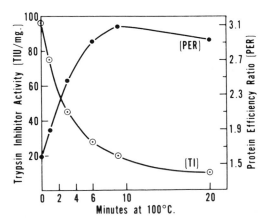

Fig. 5.1 Effect of heat on trypsin inhibitor activity (TI) and protein efficiency ratio
(PER) of soya bean. Taken from Rackis (1974).

of trypsin falls below its threshold level. These relationships are depicted in Fig. 5.2. Thus the depression of growth caused by trypsin inhibitor is believed to be a consequence of an endogenous loss of protein due to hypersecretion by the pancreas.

The stress on the pancreas produced by the prolonged feeding of raw soya flour to rats may eventually lead to the formation of adenomatous nodules on the pancreas (McGuiness, Morgan, Levison, Frape, Hopwood, and Wormsley 1980), and the incidence of tumours is positively associated with the level of trypsin inhibitor in the diet (Liener, Nitsan, Srisangnam, Rackis, and Gumbmann 1985).

There has been in recent years an upsurge of interest in the use of soya bean protein as a possible substitute for meat protein. This raises the question as to whether the trypsin inhibitor poses any risk in the human diet. Numerous feeding experiments with human subjects has failed to reveal any adverse physiological effects associated with the consumption of soya bean products that have been properly processed to inactivate the trypsin inhibitors (van Stratum and Rudrum 1979). Nevertheless there is the ever-present possibility that inadequately processed soya bean products may inadvertently find their way into the food chain and cause adverse reactions in those who consume such products (Gunn, Taylor, and Gangaros 1980).

Lectins

Another substance that is present in most legumes and cereals is a protein that has the unique property of being able to agglutinate the red blood cells of various species of animals — the so-called phytohaemagglutinins or lectins. This phenomenon involves the specific interaction of this protein with sugar residues such as are present in the glycoproteins of cell membranes (Liener 1976). It was recognized quite early that some of these lectins, such as ricin from the castor bean, are extremely toxic. Others, such as that present in the soya bean, however, appear to be relatively non-toxic, as evidenced by the fact that its removal from soya bean extracts by affinity chromatography did not serve to improve the nutritive value of the protein

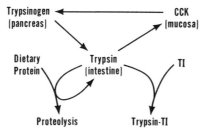

Fig. 5.2 Mode of action of soya bean trypsin inhibitors on pancreas. CCK = cholecystokinin. Taken from Anderson, Rackis, and Tallent (1979)

(Turner and Liener, 1975). On the other hand, lectins appear to be responsible to a large extent for the well-known fact that many other legumes, unless properly cooked, not only fail to support the growth of rats but may in fact lead to death (Honavar, Shih, and Liener 1962). Figure 5.3 shows the effect of adding lectins from two varieties of *Phaseolus vulgaris* (the black bean and the red kidney bean) to the diet of rats. Not only is there a marked depression in growth but at higher levels of lectin ($>$ 1 per cent) all of the animals died within 7 to 10 days, similar to the mortality observed with the raw bean.

The exact mechanism whereby lectins exhibit their toxic effects on animals upon ingestion is not known, but is most likely related to their ability to bind to the epithelial cells lining the intestinal tract. The *in vivo* binding of the kidney bean lectin can be demonstrated by an immunofluorescence technique which shows that the lectin ingested by the rat in the form of the raw bean becomes bound to the luminal surface of the microvilli in the proximal region of the small intestine (Fig. 5.4) and may cause actual disruption of the brush border (Fig. 5.5). As a consequence of this damage, there is a serious impairment in the absorption of nutrients through the intestinal barrier manifesting itself in an apparent decrease in the digestibility of the protein (Fig. 5.6). There is also evidence to indicate that bacteria and or bacterial toxins and the lectins themselves may enter the circulatory system to cause internal damage to the organs (Untawale, Pietraszek, and McGinnis 1978; Jayne-Williams, and Burgess 1974; King,

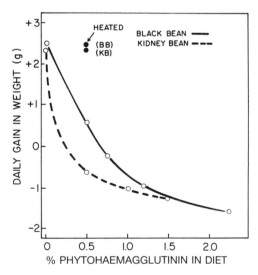

Fig. 5.3 Effect of feeding various levels of purified lectins from *Phaseolus vulgaris* on growth of rats. Based on data from Honavar *et al.* (1962).

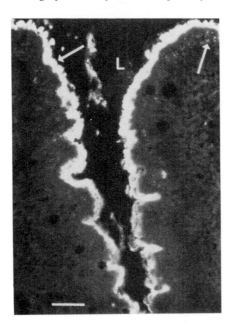

Fig. 5.4 Immunofluorescence micrograph of part of a transverse section through the duodenum of a rat fed on a diet containing kidney beans. Incubation with rabbit antilectin IgG shows immunofluoresence in brush border region and within apical cytoplasm of mature enterocytes (arrows). L = Lumen. Scale bar: 50 μm. Taken from King *et al.* (1980).

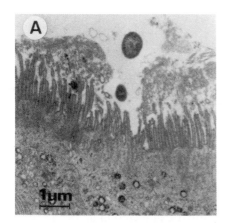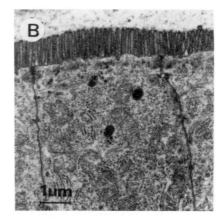

Fig. 5.5 Electron micrographs of sections through the apical regions from rats fed diets containing: (A), 5 per cent raw kidney beans and 5 per cent casein compared to (B), 10 per cent casein. Taken from Pusztai *et al.* (1979).

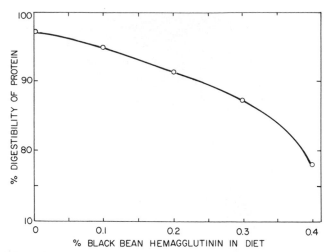

Fig. 5.6 Effect of increasing levels of black bean lectin on the apparent digestibility of dietary protein (casein). Based on data taken from Jaffé and Camejo (1961).

Pusztai, and Clarke 1980; Pusztai, Clarke, King, and Stewart 1979; Pusztai, Clarke, Grant, and King 1981).

Lectins are found in many other food items commonly consumed in the human diet including tomatoes, bean sprouts, raw vegetables, fruits, spices, dry cereals, and nuts (Nachbar and Oppenheim 1980). It is difficult, of course, to assess the significance of lectins in the human diet, but as long as sufficient heat treatment has been employed to insure their destruction, there need be little cause for concern. Nevertheless, there have been sporadic reports of cases of intoxication accompanying the ingestion of beans that have been inadequately cooked. For example, in 1948 a severe outbreak of gastroenteritis occurred among the population of West Berlin due to the consumption of partially cooked bean powder which had been airlifted into the city (Griebel 1950). In Africa, beans are frequently consumed as mixtures with maize, and such mixtures require a relatively short cooking time in order to prepare a palatable gruel for infant feeding. Such preparations have been found to retain significant levels of lectin and hence should be regarded as potentially harmful (Korte 1972). Similar problems can arise even in more affluent societies. A recent report from England (Bender and Reaidi 1982) has described several case histories of acute gastroenteritis, nausea, and diarrhoea following the consumption of raw kidney beans or beans in casseroles that had received inadequate heat treatment in a slow cooker. The presence of lectin could readily be detected in all of the bean samples implicated in cases of illness. Incidents such as this have prompted the placement of a warning label on packets of dry kidney beans now sold in retail food markets in the UK (Fig. 5.7).

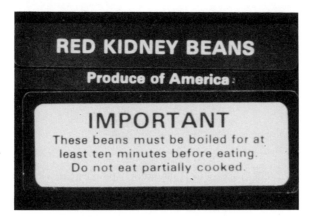

Fig. 5.7 Warning label that has been placed on packets of dry red kidney beans sold in the retail market in England.

Amino acids

Lathyrogens

Lathyrism, as it occurs in humans, is a paralytic disease associated with the consumption of the chickling pea or vetch, *Lathyrus sativus*. This disease is particularly prevalent in India, especially during periods of famine resulting from droughts when the crop fields become blighted, and, as an alternative crop, this particular legume is cultivated. We are not dealing here with an occasional case of poisoning but with a disease that can reach almost epidemic proportions. As recently as 1975 over 100 000 cases of lathyrism in men between the ages of 15 and 45 years was reported (Natarajan 1976). This disease seems to affect mostly young adults and is characterized by a nervous paralysis of the lower limbs that forces the victim to walk with short, jerky steps; death may result in extreme cases (Attal, Kulkarni, Chowbey, Palkar, and Deotale 1978).

Spencer and Schaumberg (1983) have described an outbreak of lathyrism that occurred during World War II among Romanian Jews confined to a forced labour camp on the Ukraine. For a period of four months their daily ration consisted of 400 g of *L. sativus* peas cooked in salt water plus 200 g of bread. The neurological symptoms of this disease remain even today among those survivors who now live in Israel.

The causative factor of lathyrism is believed to be an amino-acid derivative, β-*N*-oxalyl-α,β-diaminopropionic acid (Fig. 5.8). This compound when injected into rats, mice, chicks, and monkeys evokes neurological symptoms similar to those seen in humans (Padmanaban 1980). It is believed that this compound acts as a metabolic antagonist of glutamic acid,

STRUCTURE OF β-N-OXALYL-α,β-DIAMINO-
PROPIONIC ACID (ODPA) COMPARED WITH GLUTAMIC ACID

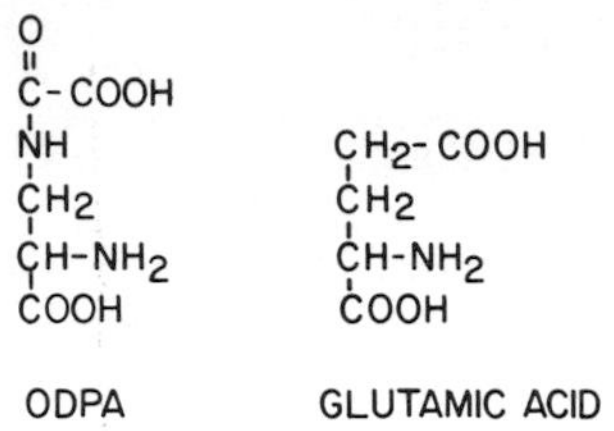

```
O
‖
C-COOH
|
NH                CH₂-COOH
|                 |
CH₂               CH₂
|                 |
CH-NH₂            CH-NH₂
|                 |
COOH              COOH

ODPA           GLUTAMIC ACID
```

Fig. 5.8 Structure of β-N-oxalyl-α,β-diaminopropionic acid, a compound believed to be a neurotoxin responsible for lathyrism by virtue of its structural similarity to glutamic acid.

which is involved in the transmission of nerve impulses in the brain (Lakshaman and Padmanaban 1974).

Mimosine

The National Academy of Sciences (1977) published a monograph that pointed out the potential value of the legume *Leucaena leucocephala* as a forage crop for livestock and human feeding. One of the principal factors limiting the use of this plant, however, is the fact that an unusual amino-acid, mimosine (Fig. 5.9), comprises 1–4 per cent of the dry weight of the protein. The adverse effect that this compound has on growth has been attributed to an underproduction of thyroxine, presumably due to the fact that rumen bacteria convert mimosine to 3,4-dihydroxypyridine, which acts as a goitrogen (Hegarty, Court, Christie, and Lee 1976). In non-ruminants such as the horse, pig, and rabbit, the goitrogenic effect is not very marked, but the animals nevertheless do very poorly on diets containing *leucaena*, one of the characteristic symptoms being a loss of hair (Owen 1958). In fact, it has even been suggested that mimosine might be used as a defleecing agent in sheep (Reis, Tunks, and Hegarty 1975). Certain segments of the human population, particularly in Indonesia, also display a loss of hair following the

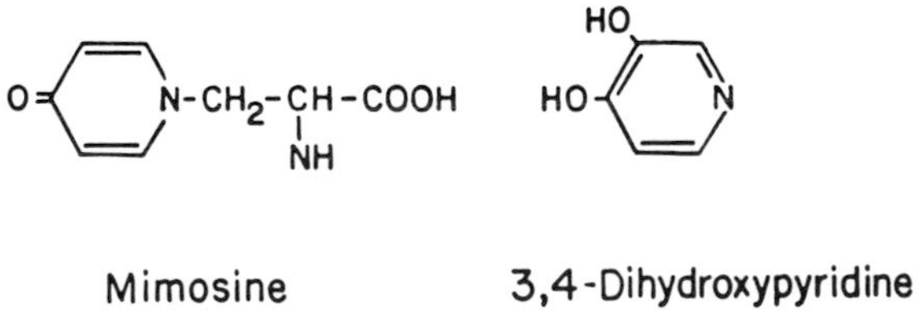

Mimosine   3,4-Dihydroxypyridine

Fig. 5.9 Structure of mimosine and its goitrogenic metabolite, 3,4-dihydroxypyridine.

consumption of the leaves, pods, and seeds of the *leucaena* in the form of a soup (van Veen 1973).

Although the goitrogenic effect of the mimosine in ruminants seems to be well established, the precise mechanism of toxicity in other animals remains obscure. The fact that it can act as an inhibitor of the enzymes crystathionine synthetase and cystathionase (Hylin 1969) may be of particular relevance to the symptomology accompanying the ingestion of mimosine, since an inhibition of the conversion of methionine to cysteine would account for hair loss. Mimosine may also exert a more direct effect on hair growth, since it has been reported that *leucaena* extracts destroyed the matrix of the cells of the hair follicles of mice (Montagna and Yun 1963).

Djenkolic acid

In certain parts of Sumatra, particularly in Java, the djenkol bean is a popular item of consumption (van Veen 1973). This bean is the seed of the leguminous tree, *Pithecolobium lobatum*, and resembles the horse chestnut in size and colour. Consumption of this seed sometimes leads to kidney failure, which is accompanied by the appearance of blood and white needle-like clusters in the urine. The latter substance has been identified as a sulphur-containing amino-acid known as djkenolic acid (Fig. 5.10), which is present to the extent of 1–4 per cent (van Veen and Latuassan 1949). Despite its structural resemblance to cystine, it cannot replace cystine in the diet of rats, although it can apparently be metabolized by the animal body. However, because of its relative insolubility, much of the djenkolic acid escapes metabolic degradation and tends to crystallize out in the kidney tubules and urine.

Glycosides

Goitrogens

Substances capable of causing goitre are present in those plants belonging to the cabbage family and include such common edible plants as cabbage itself,

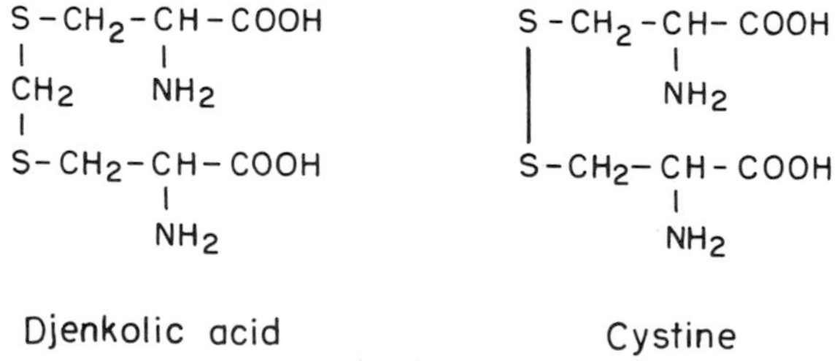

Djenkolic acid   Cystine

Fig. 5.10 The structure of djenkolic acid, an amino acid present in the djenkol bean, *Pithecolobium lobatum*, showing its structural relationship to cystine.

turnip, broccoli, cauliflower, brussel sprouts, and rutabega. They are also found in rape seed and mustard seed, the former being used as feed for livestock and the latter as a condiment. It has been estimated that approximately 4 per cent of the incidence of goitre in the world is due to antithyroid compounds present in many commonly consumed plants (Greer 1957). In most cases the chemical agents responsible for goitrogenicity have been identified as sulphur-containing glycosides, also referred to as glucosinolates (Tookey, van Etten, and Daxenbichler 1980). An example of such a compound is *progoitrin* (Fig. 5.11). The latter is non-toxic, and it is only after hydrolysis by an enzyme also present in the plant tissue that the goitrogenic agent, goitrin, is produced. This compound inhibits the uptake of iodine so that iodine supplementation is relatively ineffective as a therapeutic agent.

Cow's milk is believed to provide a vector for the transmission of goitrogens from cows fed kale and turnips, and may be responsible for endemic goitre in countries such as Australia (Tasmania) (Clements and Wishart 1956) and Finland (Peltola 1965).

Cyanogens

A number of plants are potentially toxic because they contain glycosides from which HCN may be released by enzymatic hydrolysis (Conn 1979). The most common plants eaten by humans are shown in Table 5.2, listed in order of their potential cyanide content. In the early years of the present century and again during World War I, lima beans imported from tropical

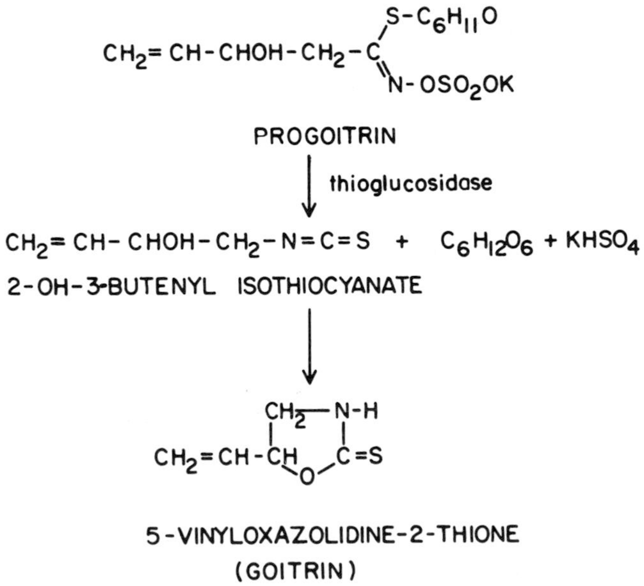

$$CH_2 = CH - CHOH - CH_2 - C\overset{\displaystyle S-C_6H_{11}O}{\underset{\displaystyle N-OSO_2OK}{}}$$

PROGOITRIN

thioglucosidase

$$CH_2 = CH - CHOH - CH_2 - N = C = S \quad + \quad C_6H_{12}O_6 + KHSO_4$$

2-OH-3-BUTENYL   ISOTHIOCYANATE

$$CH_2 = CH - CH \overset{\displaystyle CH_2 - N-H}{\underset{\displaystyle O}{\diagdown \diagup}} C = S$$

5-VINYLOXAZOLIDINE-2-THIONE
(GOITRIN)

Fig. 5.11 A goitrogenic factor in the cabbage family.

Table 5.2 Cyanide content of certain plants[a].

Plant	HCN yield, mg 100 g^{-1}
Lima bean (*Phaseolus lunatus*)	
Samples incriminated in fatal human poisoning	210.0–312.0
Normal levels	14.4–16.7
Sorghum	250.0
Cassava	113.0
Linseed meal	53.0
Black-eyed pea (*Vigna sinensis*)	2.1
Garden pea (*Pisum sativum*)	2.3
Kidney bean (*Phaseolus vulgaris*)	2.0
Bengal gram (*Cicer arietinum*)	0.8
Red gram (*Cajanus cajans*)	0.5

[a] Data taken from Montgomery (1980).

countries (Java, Burma, Puerto Rico, etc.) were responsible for serious outbreaks of cyanide poisoning, and even today cases of human intoxication are not uncommon in some of the tropical countries (Montgomery 1980). It is reassuring to note that most of the lima beans consumed in the USA and Europe are varieties which contain levels of cyanide well below the levels implicated in fatal cases of poisoning.

The poisonous nature of improperly prepared cassava has been recognized for hundreds of years by the African natives who consume large quantities of this plant in their daily diet. A neuropathological condition known as ataxic neuropathy in such countries as Nigeria and Tanzania has been attributed to the chronic ingestion of cassava from which the cyanide has been completely eliminated. A high incidence of goitre in these countries has also been attributed to the thiocyanate, which is one of the products of cyanide metabolism (Ekpechi 1973).

The principal cyanogenic glycoside present in cassava and lima beans is phaseolunatin (also known as linamarin) (Fig. 5.12). The enzymatic release of HCN can occur by the sequential action of two enzymes, a β-glucosidase and oxynitrilase. These enzymes are present in the plant tissue and can release HCN when the tissue is macerated either mechanically or during mastication. The natives have learned by experience that the toxicity of cassava can be considerably reduced by removal of the peel, by washing with running water to remove much of the cyanogen, followed by cooking and fermentation to inactivate the enzymes and to volatilize the HCN.

Favism-inducing factors
The field or broad bean (*Vicia faba*) is extensively used as a source of good quality protein for feeding livestock and poultry. Though widely consumed

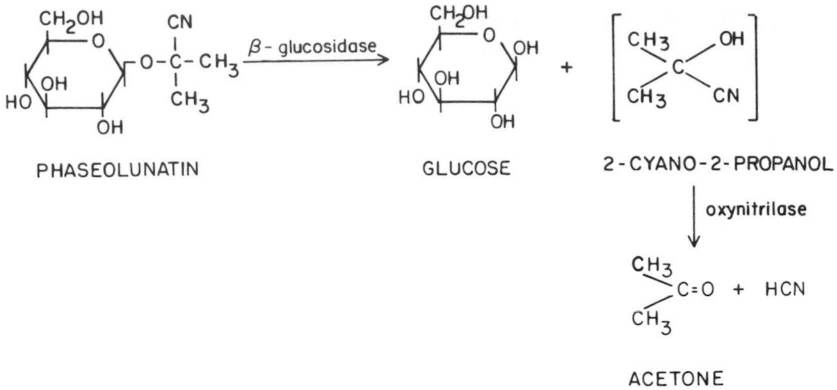

Fig. 5.12 Enzymatic hydrolysis of phaseolunatin, the cyanogenic glycoside of lima beans.

as a human food as well, its consumption frequently precipitates a condition known as favism, which is characterized by an anaemia due to the haemolysis of the red blood cells (Mager, Chevion, and Glaser 1980). This disease is confined largely to the inhabitants of the countries surrounding the Mediterranean basin (Italy, Sicily, Israel, Lebanon, North Africa, etc.), although individuals of the same ethnic background residing in other countries frequently suffer from favism.

From extensive clinical and biochemical studies on individuals with favism, one common feature has emerged, namely a genetic deficiency of glucose-6-phosphate dehydrogenase (G6PD) and low levels of reduced glutathione (GSH) in the red blood cells. GSH is essential for maintaining the structural integrity of the cell membrane. The role of G6PD is to generate NADPH via the pentose phosphate shunt, and GSH is produced from oxidized GSH (GS-SG) through the NADPH-mediated role of GSH-reductase. It follows that any metabolic challenge that leads to a decrease in GSH might be expected to render the blood cells more vulnerable to haemolysis. Such a challenge is provided by divicine and isouramil (Fig. 5.13), pyrimidine derivatives that occur in *V. faba* as β-glucosides (vicine and convicine, respectively) to the extent of about 0.5% of the bean seeds. As shown in Fig. 5.14, both of these aglycones are potent reducing agents, which in the presence of molecular oxygen, lead to the formation of H_2O_2. The latter, in turn, oxidizes GSH to GS-SG through the action of the enzyme GSH-peroxidase. Normally red blood cells can cope with such a challenge by increasing the activity of G6PD, which serves to maintain levels of GSH sufficient to protect the cell membrane from haemolysis. In the absence of G6PD, however, such as in favism-sensitive individuals, an insufficient supply of NADPH no longer permits the generation of protective levels of GSH, and thus the haemolytic crisis is precipitated.

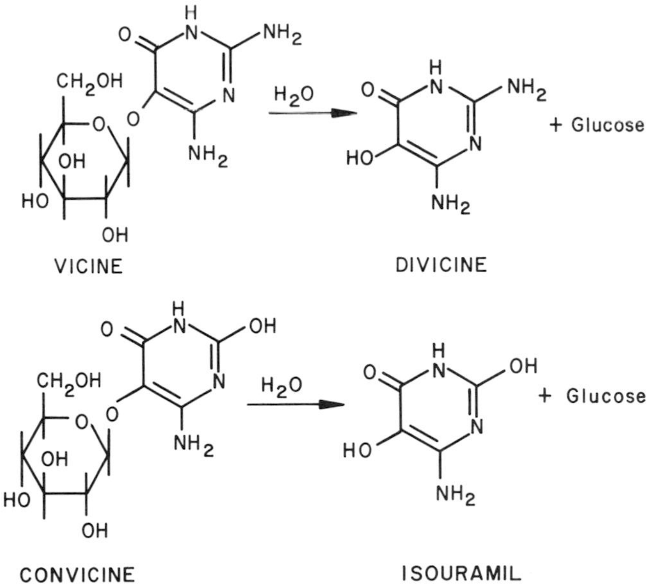

Fig. 5.13 Structures of vicine and convicine. Their active aglycones, divicine and isouramil respectively, arise from the removal of their sugar moiety (glucose) by a β-glucosidase.

Cycasin

Cycad seeds or nuts are obtained from *Cycad circinalis*, a palm-like tree that grows throughout the tropics and subtropics, and is sometimes used as a source of starch. The seeds, unless thoroughly washed, are extremely toxic and have not only produced tumours of the liver and kidneys in experimental animals, but have also been implicated in cases of human poisoning (see review by Matsumoto 1983). The toxic principle of the cycad is methylazoxymethanol (MAM), the aglycone of cycasin (Fig. 5.15). The latter is non-toxic but MAM is released on hydrolysis by intestinal bacteria. MAM can pass into the milk of lactating rats causing tumours in the offspring of such animals (Mickelsen, Campbell, Yang, Mugera, and Whitehair 1964). Whether this observation is of any significance as a health hazard to the human population in general is questionable, but would, in any event, affect only the small segment of the world's population that includes cycads in their diet.

Miscellaneous

The chemical structure of many of the toxic components in plant materials is so diverse that no common category is appropriate. To be considered here are several examples that illustrate this diversity.

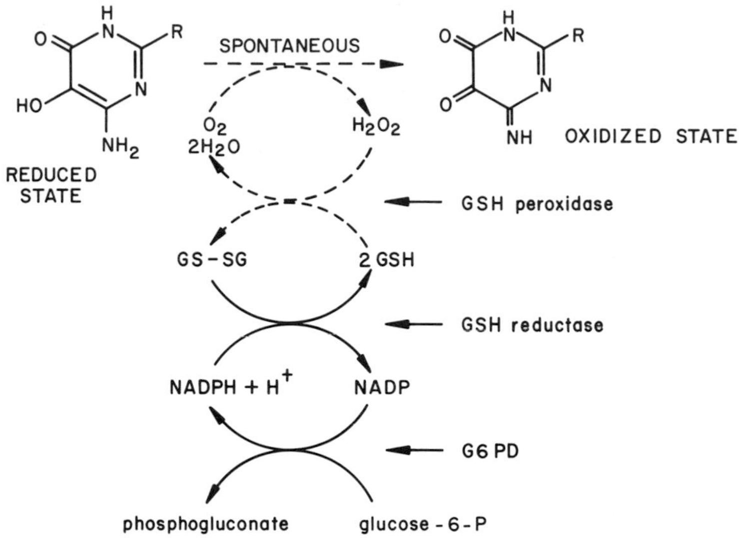

Fig. 5.14 The proposed mechanism for the pathogenesis of favism. Solid arrows denote pathway for the generation of reduced glutathione (GSH) which depends on the activity of glucose-6-phosphate dehydrogenase (G6PD) whereby the spontaneous oxidation of reduced isouramil (R=OH) or divicine (R=NH$_2$) leads to a depletion of GSH through the formation of oxidized glutathione (GS–SG). The latter pathway is favored in individuals who are deficient in G6PD. Based on mechanism proposed by Chevion, Navok, Glaser, and Mager (1982).

Alkaloids

Pyrrolizidine derivatives   Pyrrolizidine alkaloids (PA) are found in a wide variety of plant species which have been responsible for huge livestock losses throughout the world. Their principal effect is that of a hepatotoxin causing tumours and chronic liver damage. The toxic principle belongs to a class of compounds that are derivatives of pyrrolizidine (Fig. 5.16), over 150 of such derivatives have been identified and their structures elucidated (Bull, Culvenor, and Dick 1968). Since large numbers of people have been

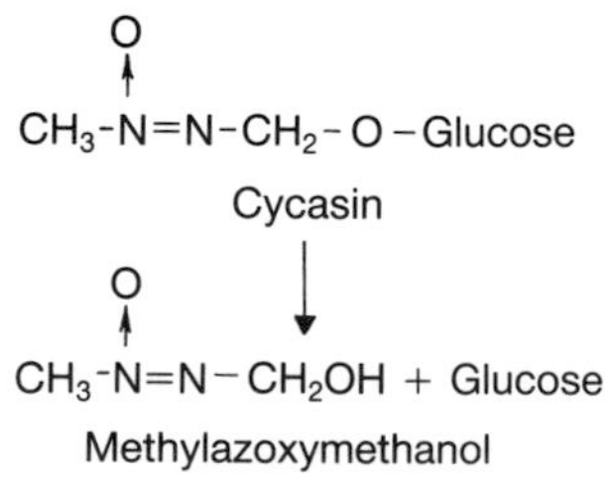

Fig. 5.15 Structure of cycasin and its toxic metabolite, methylazoxymethanol.

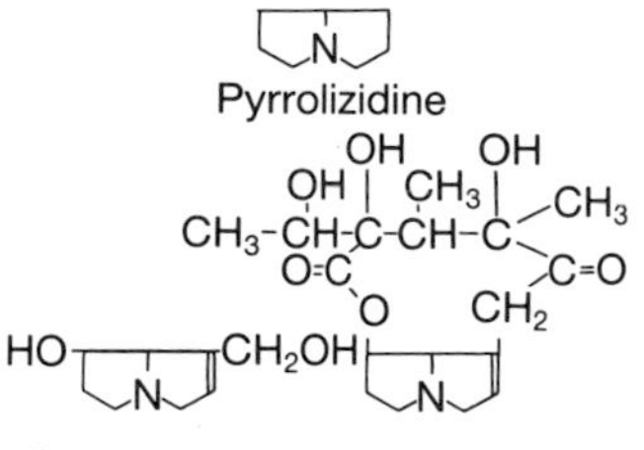

Fig. 5.16 Pyrrolizidine alkaloids in tansy ragwort (*Senecio jacobaea*).

poisoned through consumption of harvested cereal and grain crops contaminated with PA-containing plants (Mohabbat, Merzad, Srivastava, Sediq, and Aram 1976), there is obvious concern that the milk from animals grazing on pastures containing such plants could act as a vector for the transmission of PA. In the western part of the USA one such plant, the tansy ragwort (*Senecio jacobaea*), is readily consumed by cattle, and the milk from such animals was found to contain significant levels of a pyrrolizidine derivative that was identified as jacoline (Dickinson, Cooke, King, and Mohammed 1976). Similar results have been reported with goat's milk (Deinzer, Arbogast, Buhler, and Cheeke 1982) except that the PA were hydrolysed to retronecine prior to analysis so that the positive identification of the original pyrrolizidine in the milk was not possible. The final link in the chain of evidence implicating milk as a vector for the transmission of PA was the finding that rats fed milk from goats dosed with tansy ragwort developed biliary hyperplasia and hepatic lesions (Goeger, Cheeke, Schmitz, and Buhler 1982).

Swainosine The ingestion by range animals of certain species of *Astragalus* (locoweed) results in a chronic neurological disease known as locoism. The factor responsible for locoism has been identified as the indolizidine alkaloid known as swainosine (Molyneux and James 1982) (Fig. 5.17). The mechanism of toxicity appears to reside in the fact that this compound is a potent inhibitor of Golgi α-D-mannosidase II (Dorling, Huxtable, and Colegate 1980) and a consequent accumulation of mannose-rich oligosaccharides in the brain (Tulsiani, Broquist, James and Touster 1984). In this respect locoism in animals resembles the hereditary lysosomal disease, mannosidosis, in humans.

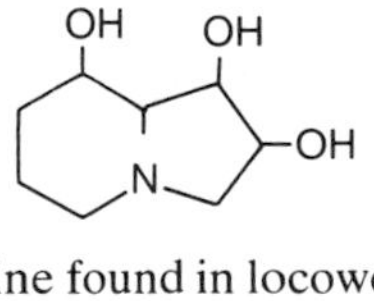

Fig. 5.17 Structure of swainosine found in locoweed and which is the toxic principle responsible for 'locoism'.

Lupin alkaloid In 1980 a baby was born in the back country of north western California with severe bone deformities of his arms and hands. (Kilgore, Crosby, Craigmill, and Poppen 1981). On questioning the mother it was learned that her goats has also given birth to deformed kids and that puppies born to a dog fed the goats' milk during pregnancy were likewise deformed. More significant was the fact that the mother herself had consumed the same goats' milk during her pregnancy. The symptoms in all cases bore a striking similarity to 'crooked calf disease', which had been previously reported to occur in calves born to cows that had consumed a plant belonging to the genus *Lupinus* during pregnancy (Shupe, Binns, James, and Keeler 1967). The specific compound responsible for crooked calf disease was subsequently identified as the quinolizidine alkaloid, anagyrine (Fig. 5.18) (Keeler 1976).

A survey of the area where the goats had browsed early in the mother's pregnancy revealed the principal forage plant to be *Lupinus latifolius* which was shown to contain anagyrine. When this plant was fed to lactating goats anagyrine could be detected in the milk. Thus the evidence seems to point to goat's milk as being the manner in which anagyrine was transferred to the mother and that the embryo was exposed to this compound at a critical time for limb formation. This particular incident, which might easily have escaped detection, illustrates the ease with which a teratogenic alkaloid could pass into the milk and thus provide an important route for prenatal exposure to toxins previously overlooked.

Bracken fern

Bracken fern (*Pteridium aquilinum*) is a forage contaminant which is responsible for a high rate of bladder cancer and intestinal tumours in grazing or experimental animals (see review by Pamukcu, Esturk, Yaleiner, Milli, and Bryan 1978). Identification of this carcinogen, however, has proved elusive. Among the diverse substances purported to be the active carcinogen of bracken fern are, a furan derivative with the molecular formula $C_7H_8O_4$ (Leach, Barber, Evans, and Evans 1971), shikimic acid (Evans and Osman 1974), an indanone derivative (Saito, Umeda, Enemoto, Natanaka, Natai, Yoshihira, Kukuoto, and Kuroyanagi 1975), condensed tannins (Wang, Chiu, Pamukcu, and Bryan 1976), and, more recently,

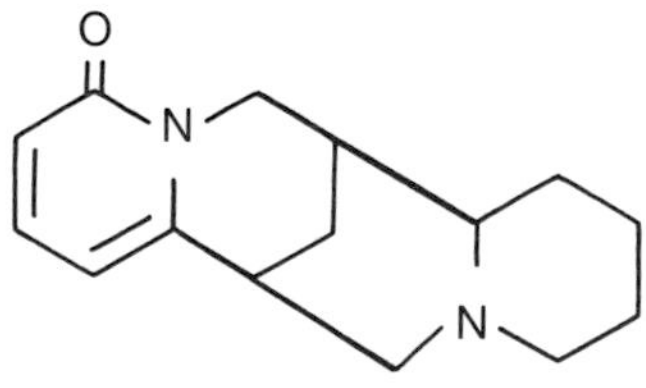

Fig. 5.18 Structure of anagyrine, a lupin alkaloid.

ptaquiloside, a novel norsesquiterpene glucoside of the illudane type (Hirono, Aiso, Yamaji, Mori, Yamada, Niva, Ojika, Wakamatsu, and Kigoshi 1984).

Bracken is also commonly used as a human food in Japan, where it is prepared by immersing fresh bracken in boiling water containing wood ash or sodium bicarbonate and seasoning. Bracken prepared in this manner has considerably reduced carcinogenic activity (Hirono, Shibuya, Shimizu, and Fushimi 1972).

Milk sickness

A disease known as 'milk sickness', characterized by weakness, nausea and prostration, has occasionally reached epidemic proportions in certain parts of the USA (Kingsbury 1964; Christensen 1965). This disease has been known to occur in grazing animals such as cows, sheep, and horses. The name was derived from the fact that this disease was associated with the consumption of milk from cows that were themselves ill with a disease characterized by muscle tremors known as 'trembles'. It is often stated that this disease was responsible for the death of Abraham Lincoln's mother.

After many years of investigation the cause of this disease was traced to the consumption by cattle of a plant known as snakeroot (*Eupatorium rugosum*). The causative principle was at one time thought to be a heat-stable unsaturated alcohol of unknown structure whose analysis suggested the formula $C_{16}H_{22}O_3$ and which was given the name 'tremetol' (Couch, 1929). A more recent review (Cooper-Driver 1983) attributes milk sickness to a sesquiterpene which is referred to as 'tremetone' (Fig. 5.19).

Conclusion

It should be apparent that, although there are numerous examples of minor constituents in plant materials that may be considered toxic or at least antinutritional in their action, plants have nevertheless provided humans and animals with a valuable source of protein. This can be attributed in part at least to the fact that people have learned how to destroy or eliminate these

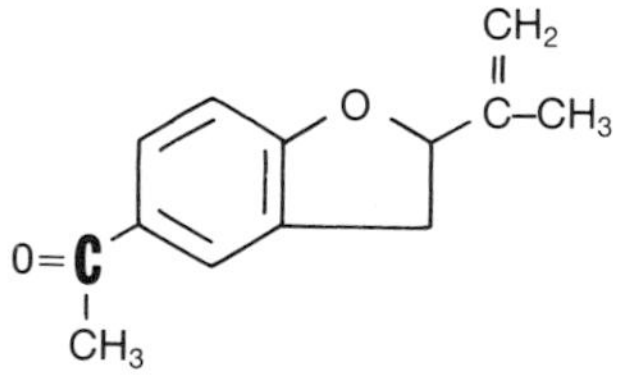

Fig. 5.19 Structure of tremetone found in snake root and believed to be causative agent of 'milk sickness'.

toxic or antinutritional factors by suitable modes of treatment. Neverthe-less, there is the ever present possibility that the prolonged consumption of a particular plant material can cause huge economic losses in livestock and may even endanger the health of humans. As the shortage of plant protein becomes more acute due to climatic changes or simply due to the pressure of a burgeoning population, the world may be faced with a more limited selection of sources of plant protein, many of which could be potential carriers of toxic constituents, both known and perhaps yet to be identified. The animal scientist, nutritionist, plant breeder, and certainly toxicologists should at least be cognizant of such a possibility and be prepared to apply their knowledge and skill to meeting this challenge should the occasion arise.

References

Attal, H. C., Kulkarni, S. W., Chowbey, B. S., Palkar, N. D., and Deotale, P. G. (1978). A field study of lathyrism — some clinical aspects. *Ind. J. med. Res.* **67**, 608–15.

Anderson, R. L., Rackis, J. J., and Tallent, W. H. (1979). Biologically active substances in soy products. In *Soy protein and human nutrition* (ed. H. L. Wilcke, D. T. Hopkins, and D. H. Waggle), pp. 209–33. Academic Press, New York.

Bender, A. E. and Reaidi, G. B. (1982) Toxicity of kidney beans (*Phaseolus vulgaris*) with particular reference to plant lectins. *J. Plant Foods* **4**, 15–22.

Bull, L. B., Culvenor, C. C. J., and Dick, A. T. (1968). *Pyrrolizidine alkaloids.* North-Holland, Amsterdam.

Chevion, M., Navok, T., Glaser, G., and Mager, J. (1982). The chemistry of favism-inducing compounds. The properties of isouramil and divicine and their reaction with glutathione. *Eur. J. Biochem.* **127**, 405–9.

Christensen, W. I. (1965). Milk sickness; a review of the literature. *Econ. Bot.* **19**, 293–300.

Clements, F. W. and Wishart, J. W. (1956). A thyroid-blocking agent in the etiology of endemic goiter. *Metab. clin. Exp.* **5**, 623–39.

Conn, E. E. (1979). Cyanogenic glycosides. In *Biochemistry of nutrition* (eds. A. Neuberger and T. H. Jukes), Vol. 1, pp. 21–43. University Park Press. Baltimore.

Cooper-Driver, G. A. (1983). Chemical substances in plants toxic to animals. In *CRC Handbook of naturally occurring food toxicants* (ed. M. Recheigl, Jr.), pp. 213–40. CRC Press, Boca Raton, Florida.

Couch, J. F. (1929). Tremetol, the compound that produces 'trembles' (milk-sickness). *J. Am. chem. Soc.* **51**, 3617–19.

Deinzer, M. L., Arbogast, B. L., Buhler, D. R., and Cheeke, D. R. (1982). Gas chromatographic determination of pyrrolizidine alkaloids in goat's milk. *Anal. Chem.* **54**, 1811–14.

Dickinson, J. O., Cooke, M. P., King, R. R., and Mohammed, P. A. (1976). Milk transfer of pyrrolizidine alkaloids in cattle. *J. Am. vet. med. Ass.* **169**, 1192–6.

Dorling, P. R., Huxtable, C. R., and Colegate, S. M. (1980). Inhibition of α-mannosidase by swainosine, an indolizidine alkaloid isolated from *Swainosa canescens*. *Biochem. J.* **191**, 649–51.

Ekpechi, O. L. (1973). Endemic goiter and high cassava diets in Eastern Nigeria. In *Chronic cyanide toxicity* (ed. B. Hestel and R. McIntyre), pp. 139–45. International Development Research Centre, Ottawa.

Evans, I. A. and Osman, M. A. (1974). Carcinogenicity of bracken and shikimic acid. *Nature* **250**, 348–9.

Goeger, D. E., Cheeke, P. R., Schmitz, J. A., and Buhler, D. R. (1982). Effect of feeding milk from goats fed tansy ragwort (*Senecio jacobaea*) to rats and calves. *Am. J. vet. Res.* **43**, 1631–3.

Green, G. M. and Lyman, R. L. (1972). Feedback regulation of pancreatic enzyme secretion as a mechanism for trypsin-induced hypersecretion in rats. *Proc. Soc. exp. biol. Med.* **140**, 6–12.

Greer, M. A. (1957). Goitrogenic substances in food. *Am. J. clin. Nut.* **5**, 440–62.

Griebel, C. (1950). Erkrankungen durch Bohnenflochen (*Phaseolus vulgaris L.*) und Plattererbsen (*Lathyrus tingitanus L.*). *Z. Lebensm. Unters. Forsch.* **90**, 191–7.

Gunn, R. A., Taylor, P. R., and Gangaros, E. J. (1980). Gastrointestinal illness associated with the consumption of a soybean protein extender. *J. food Protect.* **43**, 525–7.

Hegarty, M. P., Court, R. D., Christie, G. S., and Lee, C. P. (1976). Mimosine in *Leucaena leucocephala* is metabolized to a goitrogen in ruminants. *Aust. vet. J.* **52**, 490.

Hirono, I., Aiso, S., Yamaji, T., Mori, H., Yamada, K., Niva, H., Ojika, M., Wakamatsu, K., and Kigoshi, H. (1984). Carcinogenicity in rats of ptaquiloside isolated from bracken. *Gann* **75**, 833–6.

——, Shibuya, C., Shimizu, M., and Fushimi, K. (1972). Carcinogenic activity of processed bracken used as human food. *J. nat. Cancer Inst.* **48**, 1245–50.

Honavar, P. M., Shih, C. C., and Liener, I. E. (1962). Inhibition of the growth of rats by purified hemagglutinin fractions isolated from *Phaseolus vulgaris*. *J. Nut.* **77**, 109–14.

Hylin, J. W. (1969). Toxic peptides and amino acids in foods and feeds. *J. agric. food Chem.* **17**, 492–6.

Jaffé, W. G. and Camejo, G. (1961). The action of a toxic protein from the black bean (*Phaseolus vulgaris*) on intestinal absorption in rats. *Acta cient. venez.* **12**, 59–61.

Jayne-Williams, D. J. and Burgess, C. D. (1974). Further observations on the toxicity of navy beans (*Phaseolus vulgaris*) for Japanese quail (*Coturnix coturnix japonica*). *J. appl. Bacteriol.* **37**, 149–69.

Keeler, R. F. (1976). Lupin alkaloids from teratogenic and non-teratogenic plants. III. Identification of anagyrine as a possible teratogen by feeding trials. *J. Toxicol. environ. Hlth* **1**, 887–98.

Kilgore, W. W., Crosby, D. G., Craigmill, A. L., and Poppen, N. K. (1981). Toxic plants as possible teratogens. *Cal. Agric.* November–December, p. 6.

King, T. P., Pusztai, A., and Clarke, E. M. W. (1980). Immunocytochemical localization of ingested kidney bean (*Phaseolus vulgaris*) lectins in the rat gut. *Histochem. J.* **12**, 201–8.

Kingsbury, J. M. (1964). *Poisonous plants in the United States and Canada*. Prentice-Hall, Englewood Cliffs, New Jersey.

Korte, R. (1972). Heat resistance of phytohemagglutinins in weaning food mixtures containing beans (*Phaseolus vulgaris*). *Ecol. Food Nutr.* **1**, 303–7.

Kunitz, M. (1945). Crystallization of a trypsin inhibitor from soybeans. *Science* **101**, 688–9.

Lakshaman, J. and Padmanaban, G. (1974). Effect of β-*N*-oxalyl-L-α,β-diaminopropionic acid on glutamate uptake by synaptosomes. *Nature* **249**, 469–70.

Leach, H., Barber, G. D., Evans, I. A., and Evans, W. C. (1971). Isolation of an active principle from the bracken fern that is mutagenic, carcinogenic, and lethal to mice on intraperitoneal injection. *Proc. biochem. Soc.* **124**, 13–14.

Liener, I. E. (1976). Phytohemagglutinins. *A. Rev. plant Physiol.* **27**, 291–319.

——, and Kakade, M. L. (1980). Protease inhibitors. In *Toxic constituents of plant foodstuffs* (ed. I. E. Liener), pp. 7–71. Academic Press, New York.

——, Deuel, H. J. Jr., and Fevold, H. L. (1949). The effect of supplemental methionine on the nutritive value of diets containing concentrates of the soybean trypsin inhibitor. *J. Nutr.* **39**, 325–39.

——, Nitsan, Z., Srisangnam, C., Rackis, J. J., and Gumbmann, M. R. (1985). The USDA trypsin inhibitor study. II. Time related biochemical changes in the pancreas of rats. *Qualitas Plantarum. Plant Foods Hum. Nutr.* **35**, 259–74.

Mager, J., Chevion, M. and Glaser, G. (1980). Favism. In *Toxic constituents of plant foodstuffs* (ed. I. E. Liener), pp. 266–94. Academic Press, New York.

Matsumoto, H. (1983). Cycasin. In *Handbook of naturally occurring toxicants* (ed. M. Recheigl, Jr.), pp. 43–61. CRC Press, Boca Raton, Florida.

McGuiness, M. E., Morgan, R. G. H., Levison, D. L., Frape, G., Hopwood, G., and Wormsley, K. G. (1980). The effects of long-term feeding of soya flour on the rat pancreas. *Scan. J. Gastroenterol.* **15**, 497–502.

Mickelson, O., Campbell, M. E., Yang, M., Mugera, G. M., and Whitehair, C. K. (1964). Studies with cycad. *Fed. Proc. Fedn. Am. Socs. exp. Biol.* **23**, 1363–5.

Mohabbat, O., Merzad, A. A., Srivastava, R. N., Sediq, G. G., and Aram, G. N. (1976). An outbreak of hepatic veno-occlusive disease in north-western Afghanistan. *Lancet* **ii**, 269–71.

Molyneux, R. J. and James, J. F. (1982). Loco intoxication indolizidine alkaloids of spotted locoweed (*Astragalus lentiginosia*). *Science* **216**, 190–1.

Montagna, W. and Yun, J. S. (1963). The effects of the seeds of *Leucaena glauca* on the hair follicles of the mouse. *J. invest. Dermatol.* **40**, 325–30.

Montgomery, R. D. (1980). Cyanogens. In *Toxic constituents of plant foodstuffs* (ed. I. E. Liener), pp. 143–60. Academic Press, New York.

Nachbar, M. S. and Oppenheim, J. O. (1980). Lectins in the US diet: a survey of lectins in commonly consumed foods and a review of the literature. *Am. J. clin. Nutr.* **33**, 2338–45.

Natarajan, K. R. (1976). India's poison peas. *Chemistry* **49**, 12–13. National Academy of Sciences (1977). *Leucaena*, promising forage and tree crop for the tropics. Washington, D.C.

Osborne, T. B. and Mendel, L. B. (1917). The use of soybean as food. *J. biol. Chem.* **32**, 369–87.

Owen, L. N. (1958). Hair loss and other toxic effects of *Leucaena glauca*. *Vet. Rec.* **70**, 454–6.

Padmanaban, G. (1980). Lathyrogens. In *Toxic constituents of plant foodstuffs* (ed. I. E. Liener), pp. 239–63. Academic Press, New York

Pamukcu, A. M., Esturk, E., Yaleiner, S., Milli, U., and Bryan, G. T. (1978). Carcinogenic and mutagenic activities of milk from cows fed bracken fern (*Pteridium aquilinum*). *Cancer Res.* **38**, 1556–60.

Peltola, P. (1965). The role of L-5-vinyl-2-thiooxazolidone in the genesis of endemic goiter in Finland. In *Current topics in thyroid research* (eds. C. Cassano and M. Andreoli), pp. 872–6. Academic Press, New York.

Pusztai, A., Clarke, E. M. W., Grant, G., and King, T. P. (1981). The toxicity of *Phaseolus vulgaris* lectins. Nitrogen balance and immunochemical studies. *J. Sci. Food Agric.* **32**, 1037–46.

——, ——, King, T. P., and Stewart, J. C. (1979). Nutritional evaluation of kidney beans (*Phaseolus vulgaris*): chemical composition, lectin content and nutritional evaluation of selected cultivars. *J. Sci. Food Agric.* **30**, 843–8.

Rackis, J. J. (1974). Biological and physiological factors in soybeans. *J. Am. Oil Chem. Soc.* **51**, 161A–74A.

Reis, P. J., Tunks, D. A., and Hegarty, M. P. (1975). Fate of mimosine administered orally to sheep and its effectiveness as a defleecing agent. *Aust. J. Biol. Sci.* **28**, 495–8.

Saito, M., Umeda, M., Enemoto, M., Natanaka, Y., Natai, S., Yoshihira, K., Kukuoto, M., and Kuroyanagi, M. (1975). Cytotoxicity and carcinogenicity of pterosins and pterosides, 1-indanone derivatives from bracken (*Pteridium aquilinum*). *Experientia* **31**, 829–31.

Shupe, J. L., Binns, W., James, L. F., and Keeler, R. F. (1967). Lupin, a cause of crooked calf disease. *J. Am. vet. med. Ass.* **151**, 198–203.

Spencer, P. S. and Schaumberg, H. H. (1983). Lathyrism: a neurotoxic disease. *Neurobehav. Toxicol. Teratol.* **5**, 625–9.

Stratum, P. G. van and Rudrum, M. J. (1979). Effects of consumption of processed soy proteins on minerals and digestion in man. *J. Am. Oil. Chem. Soc.* **56**, 130.

Tookey, H. L., van Etten, C. H., and Daxenbichler, M. E. (1980). Glucosinolates. In *Toxic constituents of plant foodstuffs* (ed. I. E. Liener), pp. 103–42. Academic Press, New York.

Tulsiani, D. R. P., Broquist, H. P., James, J. F., and Touster, O. (1984). The similar effects of swainosine and locoweed on tissue glycosidases and oligosaccharides of the pig indicate that the alkaloid is the principal toxin responsible for the induction of locoism. *Arch. Biochem. Biophys.* **232**, 76–85.

Turner, R. H. and Liener, I. E. (1975). The effect of the selective removal of hemagglutinins on the nutritive value of soybeans. *J. Agric. food Chem.* **23**, 484–7.

Untawale, G. G., Pietraszek, A., and McGinnis, J. (1978). Effect of diet on adhesion and invasion of microflora in the intestinal mucosa of chicks. *Proc. Soc. exp. Biol. Med.* **159**, 276–80.

Veen, A. G. van (1973). Toxic properties of certain unusual foods. In *Toxicants occurring naturally in foods*, pp. 474–6. National Academy of Sciences, Washington, D. C.

——, and Latuassan, H. E. (1949). The state of djenkolic acid in the djenkol bean. *Chron. nat.* **105**, 288–90.

Wang, C. Y., Chiu, C. W., Pamukcu, A. M., and Bryan, G. T. (1976). Identification of carcinogenic tannin from bracken fern (*Pteridium aquilinum*). *J. nat. Cancer Inst.* **56**, 33–6.

Part III

Biochemical studies on the metabolism of natural toxins

6

Naturally occurring carcinogens: metabolism and biochemical effects in mammals

J. Lüthy

Introduction

Studies in cancer epidemiology in the past three decades have provided strong evidence for the importance of environmental factors in the aetiology of human cancer. It is particularly the role of diet that has been suspected to have an influence on some type of tumours, such as cancer of the gastrointestinal tract (Barna-Lloyd 1978; Wynder and Gori 1977; Doll and Peto 1981; Mirvish 1983). However, since causal dependencies cannot be proven by epidemiological studies because of the methods used, results derived from toxicological experiments as well as chemico analytical methods applied are of decisive importance for the interpretation of epidemiological correlations. A great effort has therefore been made in recent years to investigate the mechanisms by which chemical carcinogens act on living organisms. Additionally, it has become evident that modifying factors in carcinogenesis such as cocarcinogens, promotors, inhibitors, or suppressing agents also present in food can greatly influence the whole process of carcinogenesis and may be of even greater practical importance than the class of naturally occurring initiators, which are the subject of the present short review.

Structural characteristics of carcinogens and methods for their detection in the environment

Many of the strong carcinogens known today belong to a number of different chemical classes, all of which have been shown to be metabolized *in vivo* via electrophilic (i.e. chemically reactive) intermediates (Miller 1970). The covalent binding to DNA of such reactive intermediates seems to be an important early event in the chemical induction of a tumour (Lutz 1979). This binding to a biological macromolecule can lead to heritable cellular damage. If such DNA damage is not properly repaired before the cell divides, a mutation can be produced and forms the basis for a cell transformation and possible development into a tumour.

In addition to the effort that has gone into trying to predict the carcinogenicity of organic compounds on the basis of critical structural elements (Cramer, Ford, and Hall 1978; Lutz 1984), a wide variety of short-term test systems using different genetic endpoints have been developed in recent years. They include systems measuring gene mutations directly, or measuring other criteria of genetic damage such as sister-strand crossover, chromosomal abnormality, or unscheduled DNA synthesis. The most successful application of these methods has been in identifying compounds (synthetic or naturally occurring) that are mutagens and therefore suspected of being carcinogens. One of the most exciting discoveries in food toxicology in this respect was the detection of protein-pyrolysate derived mutagens in fried meat and other food rich in protein (Kawachi, Nagao, and Yahagi 1979). A more recent example — mutagens in larger fungi — is discussed in the following section.

Mutagens in mushrooms

Mushrooms are not only well known for the great variety in their appearance, they also often contain organic compounds of unusual structure. Therefore, they may represent an interesting pool for the detection of yet unknown carcinogens. Indeed, the screening of 48 species of larger fungi for mutagenic activity in the *Salmonella*/mammalian microsome assay (Ames, McCann, and Yamasaki 1975) gave positive results in almost 80 per cent of cases (Sterner, Bergman, Kesler, Magunssen, Nilsson, Wickberg, Zimerson, and Zeltberg 1982; von Wright, Knuutinen, Lindroth, Pelliner, Widen, and Seppa 1982). Although some mushrooms contain high amounts of free histidine, which can mimic the induction of revertants in the Ames test, at least in some species the mutagenicity can be attributed to certain individual compounds (von Wright and Suortti 1983). Preliminary results of our own investigations with mushrooms collected or commercially available in Switzerland using a histidine-independent bacterial mutagenicity test system with *S. typhimurium* TM 677 indicated mutagenicity in 38 per cent of the tested species (unpublished results). Surprisingly, the highest mutation factor was found with the juice or the alcoholic extract from the common cultivated *Agaricus bisporus*. This widely eaten mushroom contains relatively large amounts of agaritine (Fig. 6.1(a)) and further hydrazine derivatives in trace amounts (Levenberg 1961; Ross, Nagel, and Toth 1982; Fischer, Lüthy, and Schlatter 1984).

When testing the isolated or synthesized phenylhydrazine derivatives occurring in *Agaricus bisporus* (Table 6.1) it becomes clear that agaritine is only a weak mutagen. However, by addition of the mammalian enzyme

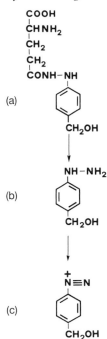

Fig. 6.1 Enzymatically catalysed conversion of agaritine (*a*) into *p*-hydroxy-methylphenyl-hydrazine (*b*) and *p*-hydroxymethylbenzene-diazonium ion (*c*) in *Agaricus bisporus*.

Table 6.1 Comparative direct mutagenicity in *Salmonella typhimurium* TA100 and TA1537 of agaritine and further hydrazine derivatives occurring in the commercial mushroom *Agaricus bisporus*.

| | Number of induced revertants per μMol | |
Compound	TA100	TA1537
p-hydrazino-benzoic acid	11	1.4
Agaritine	0	3.6
Agaritine + γGT	326	314
p-hydroxymethylphenyl-hydrazine	2.3	39
Hydroxymethyl-benzene diazonium ion	3072	918

Data from Fischer (1986).

γ-glutamyltransferase (γ-GT) to the incubation mixture the number of revertants is increased dramatically. The highest mutagenicity was found with hydroxymethylbenzene-diazonium ion (Fig. 6.1(c)), the suspected proximate or ultimate mutagen of agaritine.

Hydroxymethylbenzene-diazonium ion is a potent stomach carcinogen in mice (Toth, Nagel, and Ross 1982), acting via binding to DNA as shown by Fischer (1986; Table 6.3).

A further carcinogenic hydrazine, gyromitrin, detected in dried false morels (*Gyromitra esculenta*) at the p.p.m. levels, needs metabolic activation (Meier-Bratschi, Carden, Lüthy, Lutz, and Schlatter 1983).

Activation of genotoxic compounds and binding to DNA in mammals

One would expect that the now available methods for the detection of genotoxic compounds will lead to the discovery of new classes of mutagens in the near future. Nevertheless, most of the important classes of naturally occurring carcinogens listed in Fig. 6.2 have been found relatively early and their biological activity investigated first by classical long-term studies with mammals. This is certainly true for the pyrrolizidine alkaloids and the propenyl benzene derivatives (such as safrol, estragol, and others), two classes of carcinogenic secondary plant constituents of an extensive distribution among the botanical families, and the potent hepatocarcinogen aflatoxin B_1, as the most prominent representative of carcinogenic mycotoxins.

The metabolism to electrophilic intermediates of some naturally occurring carcinogens is shown in Fig. 6.2. Cycasin (methylazoxymethanol-β-glucoside), which occurs in the palm-like cycad trees, is highly carcinogenic for the liver and kidneys of rats. The compound is hydrolysed by β-glucosidase from the intestinal bacteria. The resulting product (methylazoxymethanol) decomposes spontaneously to an electrophilic methylating species similar to or identical with that formed in the metabolic activation of the better studied dimethylnitrosamine.

About 30 derivates of allyl- and propenylbenzene occur in many essential oils, herbs, and spices. Safrole, estragole, methyleugenol, and β-asarone have been shown to possess a rather weak carcinogenic activity. Evidence that these type of compounds are metabolically activated through the formation of 1'-hydroxy derivatives has accumulated. The ultimately carcinogenic species capable of binding to DNA *in vivo* appears to be the 1'-esters; in the case of safrol the corresponding sulphuric ester has been identified as the ultimate carcinogenic form of 1'-hydroxy-safrol in mouse liver (Boberg, Miller, Miller, Poland, and Liem 1983).

The carcinogenic potency of an initiating carcinogen can be estimated by the determination of the covalent binding to DNA. Lutz (1979) has defined a 'covalent binding index' (CBI) which generally expresses the ratio of a

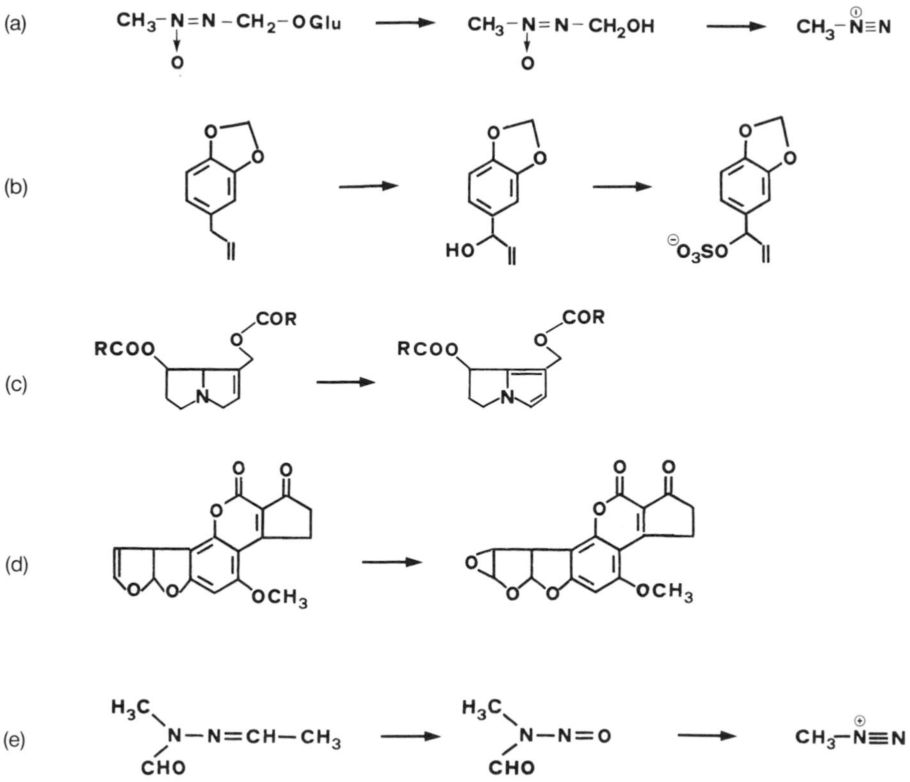

(a) CH$_3$–N=N–CH$_2$–OGlu   ⟶   CH$_3$–N=N–CH$_2$OH   ⟶   CH$_3$–N≡N

(b)

(c)

(d)

(e)

Fig. 6.2 Metabolism of naturally occurring carcinogens to electrophilic intermediates in mammals: cycasine (*a*), safrol (*b*), pyrrolizidine alkaloids (*c*), aflatoxin B$_1$ (*d*), gyromitrin (*e*).

DNA-damage (measured as radioactivity attached to DNA) per applied labelled substance administered to the corresponding animal.

A comparison of CBI for liver DNA with hepatocarcinogenic potency reveals a surprisingly good quantitative correlation for a set of standard carcinogens (Lutz 1982). Randerath, Haglund, Phillips, and Reyy (1984) studied the binding of a series of naturally occurring alkenylbenzenes to mouse liver DNA using the newly developed ^{32}P post-labelling assay, which allows testing also of non-radioactive chemicals. The results are summarized in Table 6.2. The known hepatocarcinogens safrole, estragole, and methyl-eugenol exhibited the strongest binding to the DNA while several related compounds, which have not been shown thus far to be carcinogenic in rodent bioassays (Miller, Swanson, Phillips, Fletcher, Liem, and Miller 1983), bounds to DNA at much lower levels. Comparing the CBI values of alkenylbenzenes with those of the highly potent carcinogens aflatoxin B$_1$ and

Table 6.2 *In vivo* binding to DNA of some naturally occurring alkenylbenzenes in mouse liver (Randerath 1984).

Compound	Covalent binding index[a]
Methyleugenol	31
Estragol	30
Safrol	29
Myristicin	11
Dill apiol	8
Parsley apiol	3
Elemicin	2
Isosafrol	1
Anethole	0.2

[a] Defined by Lutz (1979).

aflatoxin M_1 (Table 6.3) the data are in good correlation with the corresponding TD_{50} values (Gold *et al.* 1984).

The pyrrolizidine alkaloids from the *Senecio*, *Crotalaria*, and from some Boraginaceae genera have long been known to include a number of highly hepatotoxic members (Bull, Culvenor, and Dick 1968; Huxtable 1979). Several pyrrolizidine alkaloids are reported to be mutagenic as well as carcinogenic (Schimmer 1983). Humans can be exposed to low levels of pyrrolizidine alkaloids by the ingestion of contaminated milk, honey, or grains. Additionally, some medical herbs traditionally used in various countries have been found to contain pyrrolizidine alkaloids (Huxtable 1980; Lüthy, Zweifel, Schmid, and Schlatter 1983b; Lüthy, Brauchli, Zweifel, Schmid, and Schlatter 1984; Röder 1984). An allylic ester structure appears to be essential for both the hepatocarcinogenicity and hepatotoxicity. This type of unsaturated alkaloid is converted *in vivo* by a mixed function oxidase system to pyrrolic metabolites, which act as strong electrophilic reactants, mainly in liver and lung (Mattocks 1968). Beside the formation of pyrroles, two further principal metabolic reactions are involved: *N*-oxidation catalyzed by microsomal oxidases, and hydrolysis catalysed by esterases. The first is activating, the other two are detoxifying. Mattocks and Bird (Mattocks 1982; Mattocks and Bird 1983) have reported measurements relating to all three reactions in an attempt to correlate structure and toxicity in this chemically diverse group of plant toxins. Data on binding to DNA for a few pyrrolizidine alkaloids have been reported (Table 6.3) and indicate a low or moderate hepatocarcinogenicity.

Table 6.3 *In vivo* binding to DNA of some naturally occurring carcinogens, expressed in the units of covalent binding indices (CBI).

Compound	Species	Route	Organ	CBI[a]	Reference
Seneciphylline	rat (fem)	oral	liver	70	Candrian *et al.* (1985)
Senecionine	rat (fem)	oral	liver	200	Candrian *et al.* (1985)
Senecionine	rat (male)	oral	liver	50	Candrian *et al.* (1985)
Lasiocarpine	rat	i.p.	liver	40	Culvenor *et al.* (1969)
Aflatoxin B_1	rat	oral	liver	10 000	Lutz *et al.* (1980)
Aflatoxin B_1	mouse	oral	liver	240	Lutz *et al.* (1980)
Aflatoxin M_1	rat	oral	liver	2000	Lutz *et al.* (1980)
Aflatoxin D_1	rat	oral	liver	<70	Schröder *et al.* (1985)
Aflatoxin G_1	rat	i.p.	liver	700	Lijinski *et al.* (1970)
Gyromitrin	rat	oral	liver	15	Meier-Bratschi (1983)
4-(hydroxymethyl) benzenediazonium tetrafluoroborate	rat	oral	stomach	13	Fischer (1986)

[a] Defined by Lutz (1979).

Transfer of carcinogens in milk

The excretion of xenobiotica in mammalian milk has been extensively investigated for drugs and residues of pesticides. The fundamental principles have been described and used to construct a pharmacokinetic approach (Wilson *et al.* 1980). The two most important factors are the time-dependent plasma levels of a foreign compound and its distribution across the membrane between plasma and milk. Both factors are influenced by the lipophily of the compound and the degree of ionization at physiological pH.

Highest feed–milk transfer rates were found with pesticides of the organochlorine type (dieldrin, hexachlorbenzene, hexachlorcyclohexane, etc.): 10–30 per cent of the ingested amounts of such compounds are excreted with the milk of lactating dairy cows (van den Hoeck, Salverda, and Tuinstra 1975). Much less (about 1–2 per cent) aflatoxin B_1 ingested each day by a cow appears in the milk as aflatoxin M_1 (Patterson, Glancy, and Roberts 1980; Kiermeier 1973). This means an aflatoxin B_1 level of 300 $\mu g\ kg^{-1}$ in the feed could result in a *c.* 1 $\mu g\ l^{-1}$ of aflatoxin M_1 in the milk.

Considering the low analytical detection limit of c. 10 ng l^{-1} and the potential contamination of some dairy ration ingredients with aflatoxins, it should be no surprise that when surveys were carried out, aflatoxin M was found in commercial dairy products in a number of countries (Stoloff 1980).

The feed–milk transfer of the pyrrolizidine alkaloid seneciphylline has recently been determined as 0.1 per cent, using radiolabelled compound (Lüthy, Heim, and Schlatter, 1983a; Lüthy, Candrian, and Schlatter 1986). Considering further experimental data of Dickinson (1980) and Johnson (1979), the highest possible concentration of macrocyclic unsaturated pyrrolyzidine alkaloids like seneciphylline in the milk of unaffected cows can hardly exceed 10–20 μg l^{-1}. The analytical detection limit of pyrrolizidine alkaloids with the presently available methods is in about the same range.

References

Ames, B. N., McCann, J., and Yamasaki, F. (1975). Methods for detecting carcinogens and mutagens with the *Salmonella*/mammalian microsome mutagenicity test. *Mutat. Res.* **31**, 347–64.

Barna-Lloyd, G. (1978). 'Environmentally' caused cancers. *Science* **202**, 469.

Boberg, E. W., Miller, F. C., Miller, J. A., Poland, A., and Liem, A. (1983). Strong evidence from studies with brachymorphic mice and pentachlorophenol that 1'-sulfoöxysafrole is the major ultimate electrophilic and carcinogenic metabolite of 1'-hydroxysafrole in mouse liver. *Cancer Res.* **43**, 5163–73.

Bull, L. B., Culvenor, C. C. J., and Dick, A. T. (1968). *The pyrrolizidine alkaloids*. North Holland, Amsterdam.

Candrian, U., Lüthy, J., and Schlatter, Ch. (1985). *In vivo* covalent binding of retronecine-labelled (^{3}H)-seneciphylline and (^{3}H)-senecionine to DNA of rat liver, lung, and kidney. *Chem. biol. Interact.* **54**, 57–69.

Cramer, G. M., Ford, R. A., and Hall, R. L. (1978). Estimation of toxic hazard — a decision-tree approach. *Food cosmet. Toxicol.* **16**, 255–76.

Culvenor, C. C. J., Downing, D. T., and Edgar, J. A. (1969). Pyrrolizidine alkaloids as alkylating and antimitotic agents. *Ann. N.Y. Acad. Sci.* **163**, 837–47.

Dickinson, J. O. (1980). Release of pyrrolizidine alkaloids into milk. *Proc. west. Pharmacol. Soc.* **23**, 377–9.

Doll, R. and Peto, R. (1981). The causes of cancer: quantitative estimates of avoidable risks of cancer in the United States today. *J. Nat. Cancer Inst.* **66**, 1192.

Fischer, B. (1986). Genotoxicity of hydrazine derivatives in *Agaricus bisporus*. Thesis, ETH Zürich (in preparation).

——, Lüthy, J., and Schlatter, Ch. (1984). HPLC determination of agaritine in the commercial mushroom Agaricus bisporus. *Z. Lebensmittel. Forsch.* **179**, 218–3.

Gold, L. S., Sawyer, Ch. B., Magaw, R., Bachman, G. M., de Veciana, M., Levinson, R., Hooper, N. K., Havender, W. R., Bernstein, L., Peto, R., Pike, M. C., and Ames, B. N. (1984). A carcinogenic potency database of the standarized results of animal bioassays. *Env. Hlth. Perspect.* **58**, 9–319.

Hoek, J. van den., Salverda, M. H., and Tuinstra, L. G. M. Th. (1975). The excretion of six organochlorine pesticides into the milk of the dairy cows after oral administration. *Neth. Milk Dairy J.* **29**, 66–78.

Huxtable, R. J. (1979). New aspects of the toxicology and pharmacology of pyrrolizidine alkaloids. *Gen. Pharmacol.* **10**, 159–67.

—— (1980). Herbal teas and toxins: novel aspects of pyrrolizidine poisoning in the United States. *Perspect. Biol. Med.* **24**, 1–14.

Johnson, A. F. (1979). Toxicity of tansy ragwort. In *Symposium on pyrrolizidine (Senecio) alkaloids: toxicity, metabolism, and poisonous plant control measures* (ed. P. R. Cheeke). Nutrition Research Institutes, Oregon State University.

Kawachi, T., Nagao, M., and Yahagi, T. (1979). Mutagens and carcinogens in food. In *Advances in medical oncology, research and education Vol. 1: Carcinogenesis* (ed. G. P. Margison), pp. 192–206. Pergamon Press, Oxford.

Kiermeier, F. (1973). Ueber die Aflatoxin-M-Ausscheidung in Kuhmilch in Abhängigkeit von der aufgenommenen Aflatoxin-B$_1$-Menge. *Milchwissenschaft* **28**, 683–5.

Levenberg, B. (1961). Structure and enzymatic cleavage of agaritine, a phenylhydrazide of L-glutamic acid isolated from Agaricaceae. *J. Am. Chem. Soc.* **83**, 503–4.

Lijinski, W., Lee, K. Y., and Gallagher, C. H. (1970). Interaction of aflatoxins B$_1$ and G$_1$ with tissues of the rat. *Cancer Res.* **30**, 2280–3.

Lüthy, J., Candrian, U., and Schlatter, Ch. (1986). The transfer of the pyrrolizidine alkaloid seneciphylline into cow's milk. (in preparation).

——, Brauchli, J., Zweifel, U., Schmid, P., and Schlatter, Ch. (1984). Pyrrolizidin-Alkaloide in Arzneipflanzen der Boraginaceen: *Borago officinalis* I und *Pulmonaria officinalis* L. *Pharm. acta helvet.* **59**, 242–6.

——, Heim, Th., and Schlatter, Ch. (1983a). Transfer of (^{3}H)pyrrolizidine alkaloids from *Senecio vulgaris* L. and metabolites into rat milk and tissues. *Toxicol. Lett.* **17**, 283–8.

——, Zweifel, U., Schmid, P., and Schlatter, Ch. (1983b). Pyrrolizidin-Alkaloide in *Petasites hybridus* L. und *P. albus* L. *Pharm. acta helvet.* **58**, 97–128.

Lutz, W. K. (1979). *In vivo* covalent binding of organic chemicals to DNA as a quantitative indicator in the process of chemical carcinogenesis. *Mutat. Res.* **65**, 289–356.

—— (1982). Constitutive and carcinogen-derived DNA binding as a basis for the assessment of potency of chemical carcinogens. In *Biological reactive intermediates* (eds. R. Snider, D. V. Parke, J. J. Kocsis, D. J. Jollow, C. G. Gibson, and Ch. H. Willmer), Vol. II, Part B, pp. 1349–65. Plenum, New York.

—— (1984). Structural characteristics of compounds that can be activated to chemically reactive metabolites: use for a prediction of a carcinogenic potention. *Arch. Toxicol.* Suppl. **7**, 194–207.

——, Jaggi, W., Lüthy, J., Sagelsdorff, P., and Schlatter, Ch. (1980). *In vivo* covalent binding of aflatoxin B$_1$ and aflatoxin M$_1$ to liver DNA of rat, mouse and pig. *Chem. Biol. Interact.* **32**, 249–56.

Mattocks, A. R. (1968). Toxicity of pyrrolizidine alkaloids. *Nature* **217**, 723–8.

——(1982). Hydrolysis and hepatotoxicity of retronecine diesters. *Toxicol. Lett.* **14**, 111–16.

—— and Bird, I. (1983). Pyrrolic and *N*-oxide metabolites formed from pyrrolizidine alkaloids by hepatic microsomes *in vitro*: relevance to *in vivo* hepatotoxicity. *Chem. Biol. Interact.* **43**, 209–22.

Meier-Bratschi, A., Carden, B. M., Lüthy, J., Lutz, W. K., and Schlatter, Ch. (1983). Methylation of deoxyribonucleic acid in the rat by the mushroom poison Gyromitrin. *J. Agric. food Chem.* **31**, 1117–20.

Miller, E. C., Swanson, A. B., Phillips, D. H., Fletcher, T. L., Liem, A., and Miller, J. A. (1983). Structure–activity studies of the carcinogenicities in the mouse and rat of some naturally occurring and synthetic alkenylbenzene derivatives related to safrole and estragole. *Cancer Res.* **43**, 1124–34.

Miller, J. A. (1970). Carcinogenesis by chemicals: an overview — G. H. A. Clowes memorial lecture. *Cancer Res.* **30**, 559–76.

Mirvish, S. S. (1983). Intragastric nitrosamide formation and other theories. *J. nat. Cancer Inst.* **71**, 631–47.

Patterson, D. S. P., Glancy, E. M., and Roberts, B. A. (1980). The 'carry-over' of aflatoxin M_1 into the milk of cows fed rations containing a low concentration of aflatoxin B_1. *Food cosmet. Toxicol.* **18**, 35–7.

Randerath, K., Haglund, R. E., Phillips, D. H., and Reddy, M. V. (1984). ^{32}P-post-labelling analysis of DNA adducts formed in the livers of animals treated with safrole, estragole, and other naturally-occurring alkenylbenzenes. I. Adult female CD-1 mice. *Carcinogenesis* **5**, 1613–22.

Röder, E. (1984). Wie verbreitet und wie gefährlich sind Pyrrolizidinalkaloide? *Pharm. uns. Zeit* **13**, 33–38.

Ross, A. F., Nagel, D. L., and Toth, B. (1982). Evidence for the occurrence and formation of diazonium ions in the *Agaricus bisporus* mushroom and its extracts. *J. agric. food Chem.* **30**, 521–5.

Schimmer, O. (1983). Genotoxizität von Pyrrolizidinalkaloiden. *Dtsch. Apoth. Z.* **123**, 1361–5.

Schröder, T., Zweifel, U., Sagelsdorff, P., Friederich, U., Lüthy, J., and Schlatter, Ch. (1965). Ammoniation of aflatoxin-containing corn: distribution, *in vivo* covalent deoxyribonucleic acid binding, and mutagenicity of reaction products. *J. agric. food Chem* **33**, 311–16.

Sterner, O., Bergman, R., Kesler, F., Magunsson, G., Nilsson, L., Wickberg, B., Zimerson, F., and Zeltberg, G. (1982). Mutagens in larger fungi. I. Forty-eight species screened for mutagenic activity in the Salmonella/microsome assay. *Mutat. Res.* **101**, 269–81.

Stoloff, L. (1980). Aflatoxin M in perspective. *J. food Protect.* **43**, 226–30.

Toth, B., Nagel, D., and Ross, A. (1982). Gastric tumorigenesis by a single dose of 4-(hydroxymethyl)benzenediazonium ion of *Agaricus bisporus*. *Br. J. Cancer* **46**, 417–22.

Wilson, J. T., Brown, R. D., Cherek, D. R., Dailey, J. W., Hilman, B., Jobe, P. C., Manno, B. R., Manno, J. F., Redelzki, H. M., and Stewart, J. J. (1980). Drug excretion in human breast milk: principles, pharmacokinetics and projected consequences. *Clin. Pharmacokinet.* **5**, 1–66.

Wright, A. von, and Suortti, T. (1983). Preliminary characterisation of the mutagenic properties of 'necatorin', a strongly mutagenic compound of the mushroom *Lactarius necator*. *Mutat. Res.* **121**, 103–106.

——, Knuutinen, J., Lindroth, S., Pellinen, M., Widen, K.-G., and Seppa, E.-L. (1982). The mutagenicity of some edible mushrooms in the Ames test. *Food chem. Toxicol.* **20**, 265–7.

Wynder, E. L. and Gori, G. B. (1977). Contribution of the environment to cancer incidence: an epidemiologic exercise. *J. Nat. Cancer Inst.* **58**, 825–32.

7

Chemical aspects of livestock poisoning in South America

G. G. Habermehl and L. Busam

Introduction

Toxic plants have been known for centuries. They have been extensively used by all primitive cultures for medicinal purposes, as arrow and dart poisons, and as agents for ritual torture. As a result of this activity, many toxic plants are now well known, and numerous guides are available to inform the user of the potential dangers of a given plant. Despite this, unintentional intoxications still occur in both humans and animals as a result of the accidental ingestion of poisonous plants and the misuse of plants of medicinal value. Some of the plants most commonly implicated in poisonings of this kind are the foxgloves, *Digitalis* spp., the bulbs of *Tulipa* spp., which are often mistaken for edible onions, and the plants and corms of *Colchicum* spp, and *Anemonia* spp.

The isolation of the toxic factors from poisonous plants became a serious occupation around the turn of the century, and interest in this field of toxicology has continued to grow. It has become clear that poisoning by plants is not always as straightforward as is commonly supposed and recent investigations into a number of plants responsible for the large-scale poisoning of livestock have produced a number of unexpected results. In this chapter, some observations on the syndromes 'calcinosis' and 'sudden-death' are described. This is followed by a more detailed discussion of *Baccharis* poisoning in cattle.

Calcinosis

This syndrome is characterized by the calcification of various organs such as lungs, kidneys, and heart. It is a widespread chronic disease of cattle and it has been established that many different plants may be involved in precipitation of the problem. In South America, for example, the most important plant is *Solanum malacoxylon*; in the United States of America, several *Cestrum* spp. are involved and in the Alpine region of central Europe,

Trisetum flavescens has been implicated (Rosenberger 1970; Wasserman, Caradino, Krook, Hughes, and Haussler 1976).

These plants are not, of course, closely related to each other, but it seems that in each case the substance responsible for poisoning is 1,25-dihydroxy-cholecalciferol or 1,25-dihydroxyvitamin D_3 (the active form of vitamin D_3). In mammals this active form is synthesized from vitamin D_3 by hydroxylation at C-25 in the liver and subsequent hydroxylation at C-1 in the kidney. Excessive levels of 1,25–dihydroxyvitamin D_3 leads to hypercalcaemia, largely as a result of the mobilization of calcium from bone. The deposition of calcium salts in soft tissues is a natural outcome of prolonged hypercalcaemia.

It is most striking that plants of diverse families produce the same toxic compound. It is not clear whether the compound has a role in the metabolism of the plant or whether it is produced by the same synthetic route in the different families.

'Sudden death'

The syndrome 'sudden death' is seen in cattle that have consumed the plant *Polygala klotzschi*. The plant is endemic to Mato Grosso do Sul, Brazil (Fig. 7.1(a)). It is extremely poisonous, and the consumption of only 10 g of fresh plant per kg body weight may be fatal. The poisoned animals become ill within one hour after the ingestion of the plant. The animals fall, showing symmetrical but uncontrolled movements of the head. After 2–3 h, diarrhoea develops and breathing becomes irregular and accelerated. Recovery has rarely been observed. Post mortem findings include petechiae of the mucosa of the intestines, necrosis of the lymph tissues in spleen, lymph nodes and Peyer's patches as well as haemorrhages in the CNS (Tokarnia, Dobereiner, and Canella 1976).

Habermehl, Busam, Heydel, Mebs, Tokarnia, Dobereiner, and Spraul (1985) attempted the isolation of toxic material from fresh plants collected near Campo Grande, Mato Grosso do Sul, Brazil. Eight saponins were identified. All of them were based on 16α-medicagenic acid (the aglycone), but they were differentiated on the basis of the identity of the sugars that were released from the steroids following acid hydrolysis, and the site from which the sugars were released (Fig. 7.2).

The saponins were found to be toxic, causing haemolysis and damage to the kidneys and liver, but they were relatively slow to act.

A ninth compound 5-methoxypodophyllotoxin (Fig. 7.3) was also isolated. This compound caused haemolysis, haemorrhage in the endocardium and damage to the kidneys and liver, and was more rapidly acting than the saponins. No detailed information exists in the acute toxicity of this compound.

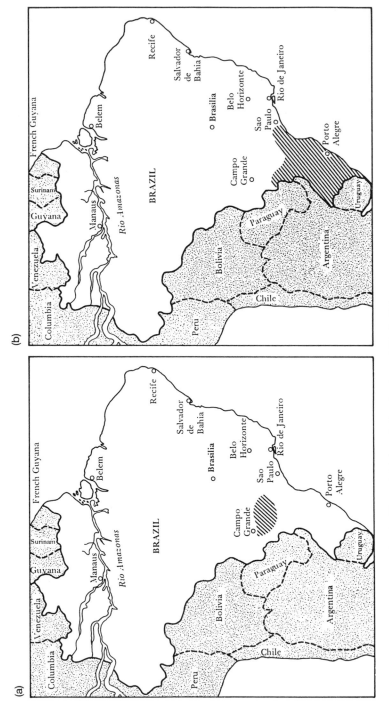

Fig. 7.1 Distribution of *Polygala klotzschi* (a) and *Baccharis coridifolia* (b).

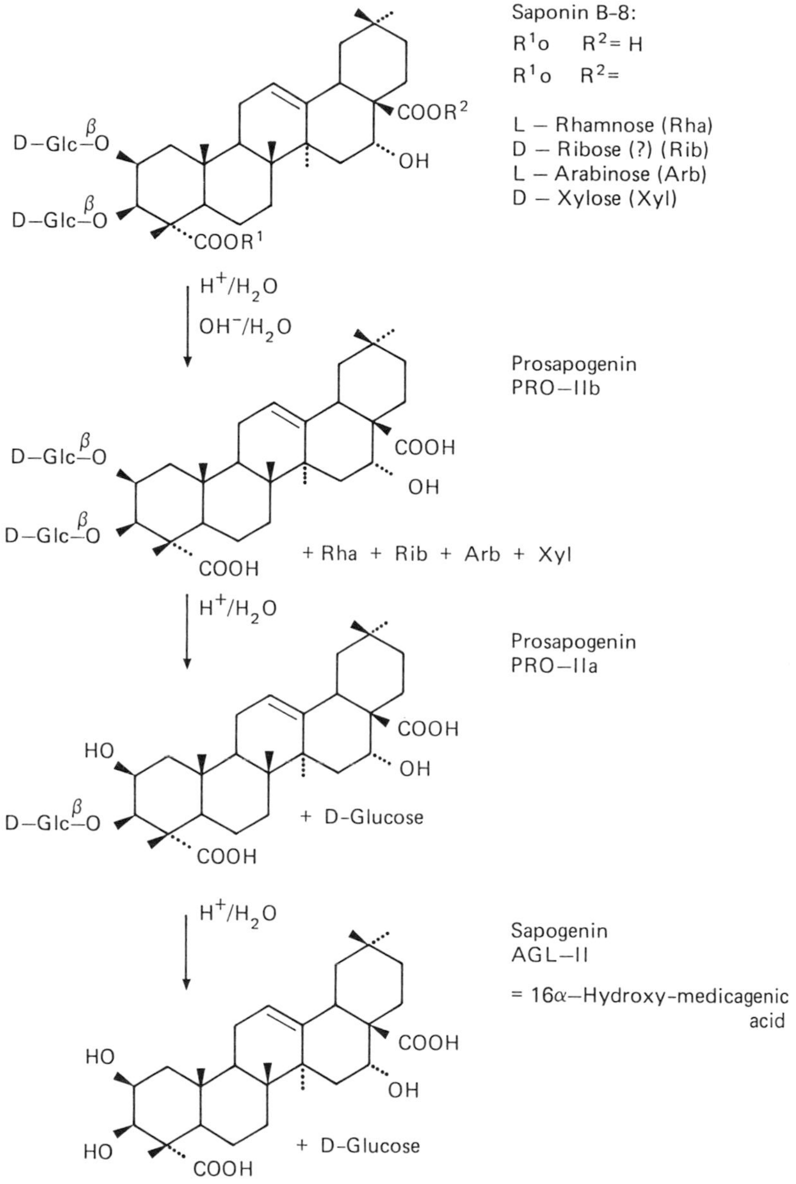

Fig. 7.2 Hydrolysis of saponin.

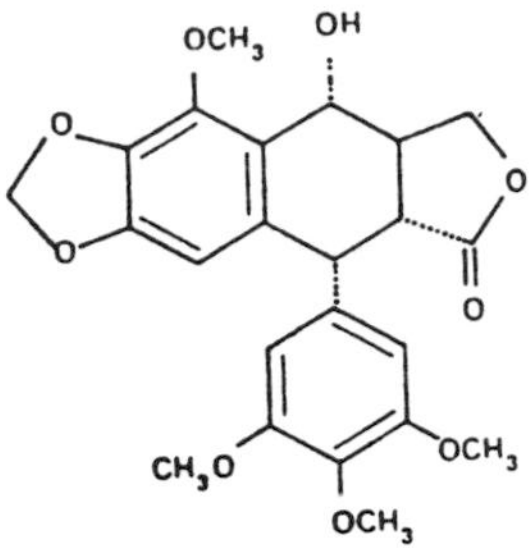

Fig. 7.3 5-Methoxypodophyllotoxin.

Baccharis poisoning

One of the most important plants responsible for the poisoning of cattle in South America is *Baccharis coridifolia*, a herbaceous shrub that is a characteristic representative of the savannah vegetation of Southern Brazil, Argentine, Paraguay, and Uruguay (Fig. 7.1(b)). Although the plant has been known to be toxic since the beginning of this century no experimental work was formally published before 1975 (Tokarnia and Dobereiner 1975; 1976; Dobereiner, Rezende, and Tokarnia 1976). All parts of the plant are toxic, but the flowers, seeds and leaves are particularly dangerous. Death occurs between 4 h and 34 h following the ingestion of a lethal amount of the plant (approximately 0.35 g kg^{-1} of the flowering plant in a young animal). More than 50 000 animals die in Brazil per year following the consumption of the plant (Dobereiner, personal communication).

Post-mortem findings include congestion of the mucosa and oedema of the wall of rumen and reticulum, and congestion and petechiae in the abomasum and small intestine. The liver is pale and haemorrhages occur in the epi- and endocardium. The main histopathological findings are epithelial necrosis and oedema of the mucosa of rumen and reticulum as well as oedema in the liver.

Extraction of the plant with chloroform, followed by chromatographic separation, yielded eight macrocyclic trichothecenes, as well as di-*O*-acetyl-verucarol and a metabolite thereof. All these compounds were isolated in pure form, and the structures elucidated by means of mass spectrometry, and two-dimensional n.m.r. spectroscopy. Two of the macrocyclic trichothecenes, roridin E and roridin A, were well known to toxicologists because they are metabolites of *Fungi imperfecti*. Five of the compounds were novel (although they were closely related to the roridins) and they were named miotoxins A, B, C, D, and iso-D, after the native name of the plant mio-mio. Two more of the trichothecenes, miophytocenes A and B, were non-toxic (Fig 7.4).

The toxic compounds possess an intact oxirane system (three-membered ring with one oxygen atom). In the non-toxic miophytocenes, this oxirane

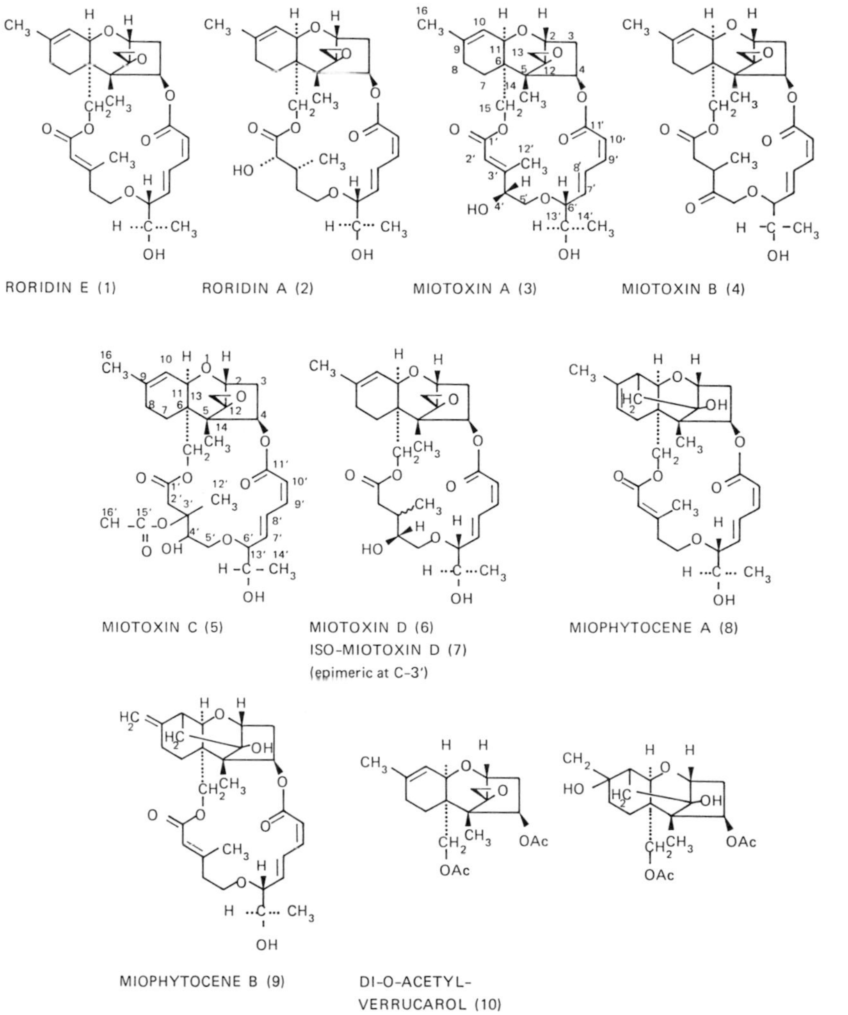

RORIDIN E (1) RORIDIN A (2) MIOTOXIN A (3) MIOTOXIN B (4)

MIOTOXIN C (5) MIOTOXIN D (6) MIOPHYTOCENE A (8)

ISO-MIOTOXIN D (7)
(epimeric at C-3')

MIOPHYTOCENE B (9) DI-O-ACETYL-
VERRUCAROL (10)

Fig. 7.4 The macrocyclic trichothecenes isolated from chloroform extracts of *Baccharis coridifolia*.

ring has been opened. Since it is well known that oxiranes are highly reactive chemical groups, it seems likely that an intact oxirane ring is essential and directly responsible for the toxicity of the tricothesanes.

The fact that trichothecenes such as roridins A and E as well as acetyl–verrucarol have been known for a long time as metabolites of *Fungi imperfecti*, and that such compounds are well known to be phytotoxins, led to the assumption that the compounds isolated from the plant material are not original products of *Baccharis coridifolia*. Further studies led to the finding that the roridins isolated from *B. coridifolia* are in fact produced by a soil fungus, *Myrothecium verrucaria*, which could be isolated from the surface of the roots as well as from the soil around the plants. It is possible that trichothecenes from *Myrothecium verrucaria* are taken up from the roots and then metabolized within the plant in part, to the non-toxic miophytocenes. A similar mechanism was suggested by Kupchan, Streelman, Jarvis, Dailey, and Sneden (1977), who isolated antileukaemic trichothecenes from *Bacharis megapotamica*.

Another plant of the same genus, *Baccharis dracunculifolia*, has been considered toxic in some cases, but not in others (Dobereiner, personal communication). We have checked this plant without finding any evidence of toxicity. No trichothecenes could be isolated from it. Earlier reports of the toxicity may be due to improper classification of the plant and confusing it for *B. coridifolia*.

Two questions still remain open. Why do some species from this genus appear to have established a kind of symbiosis with a fungus while others have not? And what is the reason that *B. coridifolia* is able to store and metabolize large amounts of trichothecenes which are otherwise able to kill plants in amounts of a few parts per million?

References

Dobereiner J., Rezende A. M. L., and Tokarnia C. H. (1976). Intoxicacao experimental por *Baccharis coridifolia* em coelhos. *Pesq. agropec. Bras. Ser. Vet.* **11**, 27–35.

Habermehl, G. G., Busam, L., Heydel, D., Mebs, D., Tokarnia, C. H., Dobereiner, J., and Spraul, M. (1985). Macrocyclic Trichothecenes: cause of livestock poisoning by the Brazilian plant *Baccharis coridifolia*. *Toxicon* **23**, 731–45.

Kupchan, S. M., Streelman, D. R., Jarvis, B. B., Dailey, R. G., and Sneden, A. T. (1977). Isolation of potent new antileukemic trichothecenes from *B. megapotamica*. *J. org. Chem.* **42**, 4221–5.

Rosenberger, G. (1970) *Krankheiten des Rindes*, Paul Parey, Berlin, Hamburg.

Tokarnia, C. H., and Dobereiner, J. (1975). Intoxicacao experimental em bovinos por mio-mio, *Baccharis coridifolia*. *Pesq. agropec. Bras. Ser. Vet.* **10**, 79–97.

—— and —— (1976). Intoxicacao experimental em bovinos por mio-mio, *Baccharis cordifolia*. *Pesq. agropec. Bras. Ser. Vet.* **11**, 19–26.

——, ——, and Canella, C. F. C. (1976). Intoxicacao experimental em bovinos por *Polygala klotzschii*. *Pesq. agropec. Bras. Ser. Vet.* **11**, 73–86.

Wasserman, R. H., Corradino, R. A., Krook, L., Hughes, M. R., and Haussler, M. R. (1976). Studies on the 1, 25-dihydroxycalciferol-like activity in a calcinogenic plant, *Cestrum diurnum*, in the chick. *J. Nutr.* **106**: 457–65.

8

Biosynthesis and biotransformation of marine invertebrate toxins

Yuzuru Shimizu

Introduction

A great number of marine invertebrates are known to contain toxic substances (Halstead 1978; Hashimoto 1979). Many of the compounds with unique structures and pharmacological actions are frequently discussed in terms of self-defence mechanisms, as the invertebrates are often dangerously exposed to attacks by predators. Aside from such teleological interpretations however, it has gradually become understood that more often than not the animals do not themselves biosythesize the toxins. Rather, they acquire the toxins from other organisms and then sometimes modify the structures. The purpose of this article is to focus on the generation of marine invertebrate toxins and their pathways with the intention of broadening our general understanding of the complexities of the formation of secondary metabolites in marine environments.

Paralytic shellfish poisoning (PSP) toxins

For about two decades after its discovery (Schantz, Mold, Stanger, Shavel, Reil, Bowden, Lynch, Wyler, Reigel, and Sommer 1957), saxitoxin was considered to be the sole toxin involved in paralytic shellfish poisonings. In 1975 a group of new toxins, named gonyautoxins and neosaxitoxin, was isolated from the US east coast red tide organism, *Gonyaulax tamarensis* (Shimizu, Alam, Oshima, and Fallon 1975; Oshima, Buckley, Alam, and Shimizu 1977). Since then additional toxins have been reported from various sources. To date, more than a dozen PSP toxins have been isolated and their structures elucidated (Fig. 8.1) (Shimizu 1984).

Biosynthesis of PSP toxins

Although a number of suggestions had been made regarding the molecular origin of saxitoxin analogues and the possible significance of the toxin

115

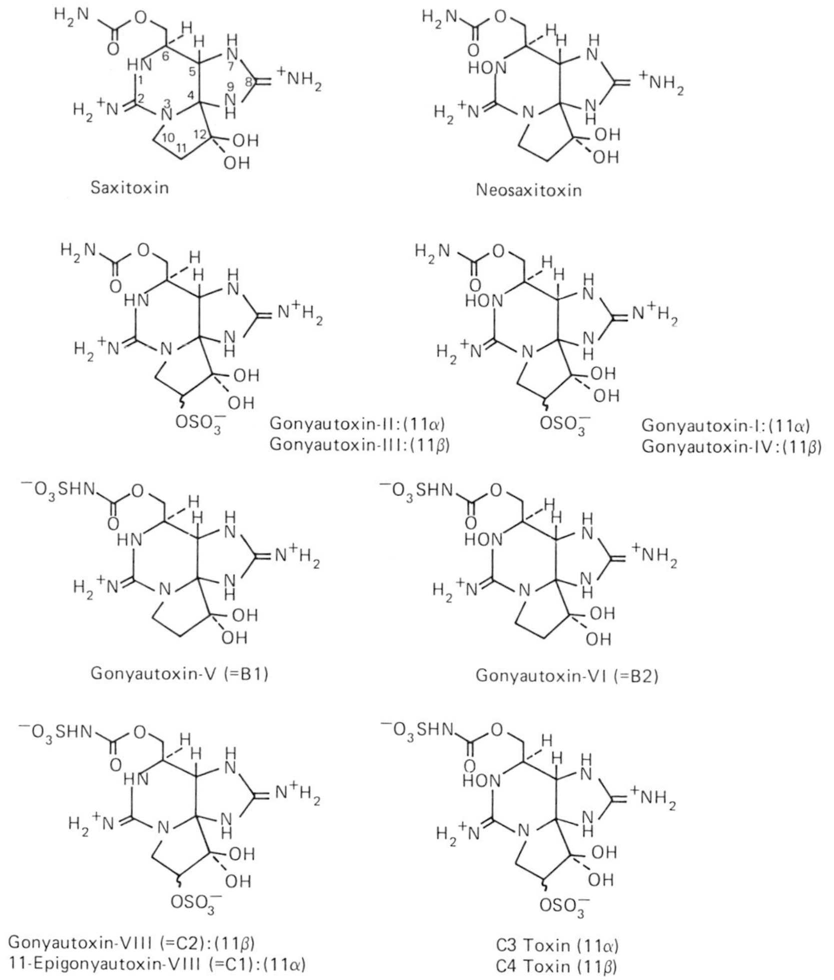

Fig. 8.1 Structures of paralytic shellfish toxins.

biosynthesis to the toxin-producing organisms, there were no experimentally proven pathways given to the PSP toxins until very recently.

By feeding various isotopically labelled precursors to cultures of *Gonyaulax tamarensis*, it was shown that α-ketoglutarate can be incorporated into the toxin molecule probably via arginine (Shimizu 1982, Shimizu, Kobayashi, Genenah, Ichihara 1984a). After several twists, it was finally proved, by feeding ^{13}C-labelled precursors to cultures of *Aphanizomenon flos-aquae*, that the condensed perhydropurine ring system is formed by the condensation of arginine and an acetate unit with the decarboxylation of arginine C-1 carbon (Shimizu, Norte, Hori, Genenah, and Kabayashi

1984b). The pathway was quite unexpected. More recently it has also been established that the extra carbon (C-13) on the ring is derived from methionine via *S*-adenosylmethionine (Shimizu *et al.*, unpublished). The complete biosynthetic pathway of the saxitoxin analogues is summarized in Fig. 8.2.

Acquisition of PSP toxins by marine invertebrates

Sommer and Meyer's finding that the paralytic shellfish poison saxitoxin is produced by the dinoflagellate *Gonyaulax catenella* in blooms and then accumulated by the filter-feeding shellfish, was the first to record the presence of such metabolite transfers through the food chain (Sommer and Meyer 1937). This original scenario, however, held some unanswered questions. Already in 1964 it was pointed out that high contents of saxitoxin were found in association with the siphons of Alaska butter clam, *Saxidomus*

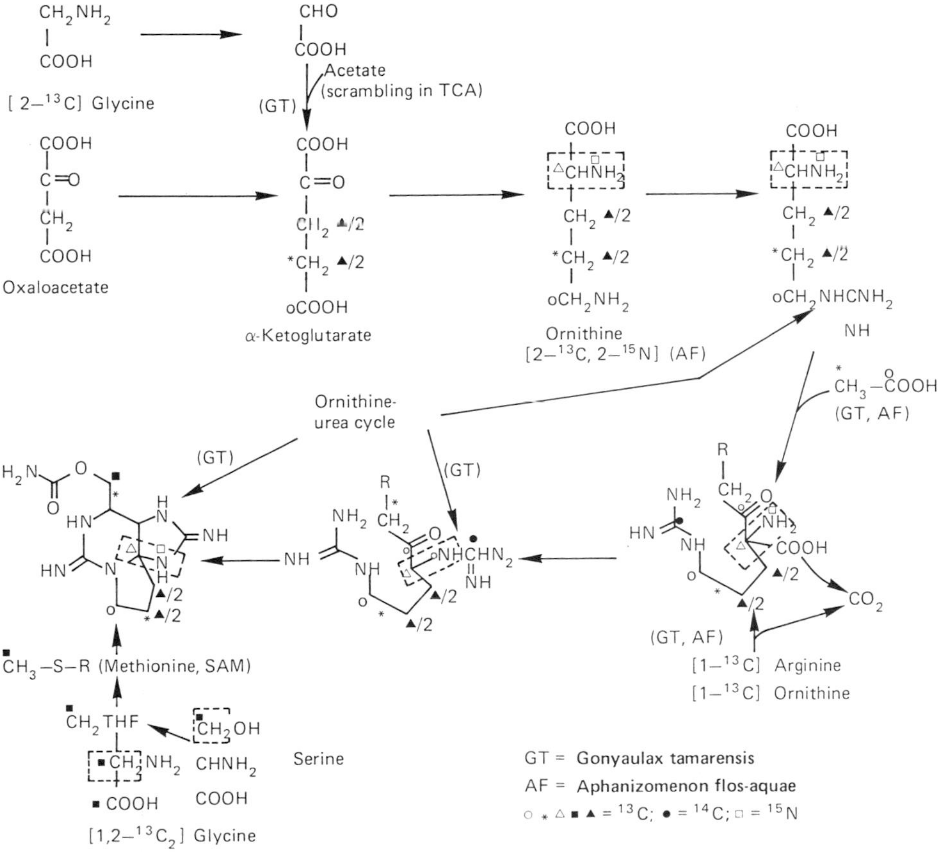

Fig. 8.2 Biosynthetic scheme for paralytic shellfish toxins proved by isotope feeding studies using *Gonyaulax tamarensis* and *Aphanizomenon flos-aquae*.

giganteus, although no visible bloom of the toxin-producing organism was present in the proximate water (Schantz and Magnusson 1964). Several speculations were made about the origin of the toxin; the clam siphon has a high affinity to saxitoxin and is able to accumulate the toxin even in high dilutions; a symbiotic organism is producing the toxins; the toxin is derived from the toxic cysts found in the sediments, etc. Equally puzzling is the origin of neosaxitoxin and saxitoxin found in various crabs in tropical waters (Yasumoto, Oshima, and Konta 1981; Koyama, Noguchi, and Ueda 1981). The discovery of the dinoflagellate *Pyrodium bahamense* var. *compressa* as a PSP causative organism in tropical waters does not settle the question, because no such dinoflagellate was found in the vicinity of the crab habitats. The rather astonishing finding that the macro red algae, *Jania* spp., contain PSP toxins and are often found among the contents of crab stomachs (Kotaki, Tajiri, Oshima, and Yasumoto 1983) does not explain the total toxin contents, which are very high compared to rather low concentrations of PSP toxins in the algae. PSP toxins are also found in other non-filter feeding invertebrates such as marine snails (Kotaki, Oshima, and Yasumoto 1981). The secondary metabolite transfer may explain the acquisition of the toxins by carnivorous snails, but not herbivorous ones.

Filter-feeding zooplankton have been found to receive toxins from dino-flagellates, as might be expected. For example filter-feeding crustaceae are known to become toxic during *Gonyaulax catenella* blooms, and mixed zooplankton (mostly copepods) were the suspected intermediaries in fish kills in the bay of Fundy (White 1977).

Metabolism of PSP toxins in invertebrates

The PSP toxins introduced into bivalves are mostly accumulated in the hepatopancreas. The accumulation rate is proportional to the number of the dinoflagellate in the water. The depuration rate of the toxins may vary from several weeks to months. The precise kinetics of uptake and depuration has not been established.

Since the shellfish hepatopancreas is known to be rich in enzymes such as sulphatase, the bioconversion of toxins was anticipated. However, attempts to hydrolyse the O-sulphated toxins with the homogenates of hepato-pancreas or crystalline stylus from various shellfishes failed (Ichihara and Shimizu, unpublished). In fact the short-term toxin profiles in most shellfish closely reflect those of the causative dinoflagellates. However, the reductive cleavage of 11-*O*-sulphate and/or *N*-1-hydroxyl groups of PSP toxins takes place in other tissues of the shellfish. Thus Shimizu and Yoshioka (1980) reported that the homogenates of adductor muscle of the scallop, *Placopecten magellanicus* can convert gonyautoxins to saxitoxin, and neo-saxitoxin to saxitoxin. The pathways are summarized in Fig. 8.3. Further studies using ^{14}C-labelled gonyautoxins showed that the reductive cleavage

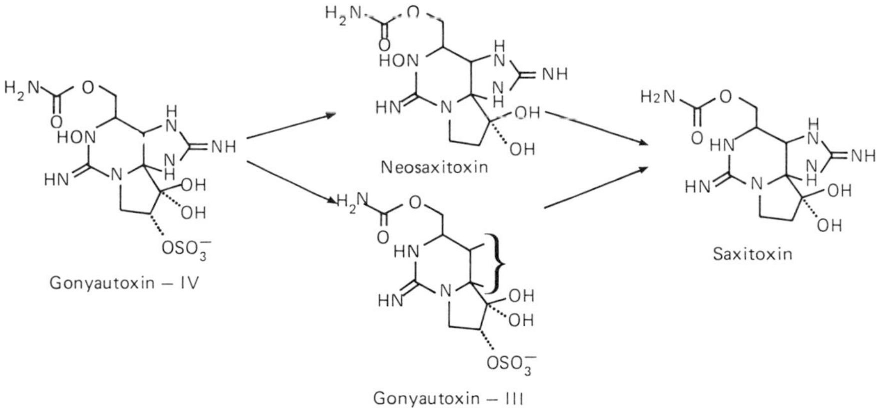

Fig. 8.3 Bioconversions of paralytic shellfish toxins in the scallops, *Placopecten magellanicus*.

could also occur non-enzymatically, probably with an involvement of –SH groups under anaerobic conditions (Shimizu *et al.* 1984; Ichihara and Shimizu, unpublished). Interestingly, certain bacteria such as *Pseudomonas* spp. or *Vibio* spp., which are common in marine invertebrates can carry out the same conversions (Kotaki, Oshima, and Yasumoto 1985). In 1980 the author's group analysed the toxin profiles in the mussels contaminated by a red tide in northern California. Initially, neosaxitoxin was the dominant toxin in the hepatopancras, but within two months it was mostly converted to saxitoxin (Shimizu, *et al.* 1984a). It is not certain if the observed conversion was due to a hepatopancreatic enzyme or to the symbiotic microorganisms.

Certain species of shellfish seem to affect particular biochemical conversions more than the others. Sullivan, Iwaoka, and Liston (1983) observed in their HPLC study of PSP toxins in several marine animals that the little-neck clam *Protothaca Staminea* can hydrolyse carbamoyl groups to form decarbamoylsaxitoxin and decarbamoyl gonyautoxins (Fig. 8.4). In

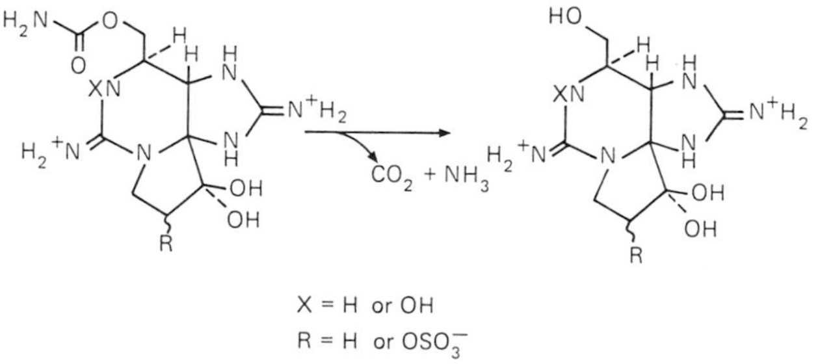

X = H or OH
R = H or OSO_3^-

Fig. 8.4 Decarbamoylation of paralytic shellfish toxins observed in the littleneck clam, *Protothaca staminea*, and the scallop, *Placopecten magellanicus*.

1979 the author's group reported the isolation of gonyautoxin-VII as an unidentified toxin in the scallop, *Placopecten magellanicus* (Hsu, Marchand, Shimizu, and Sims 1979). It is now believed that the compound was decarbamoylneosaxitoxin, probably formed by a similar biochemical process.

Only sketchy information is available on the metabolism of PSP toxins in marine invertebrates other than molluscs. Hayashi, Shimizu, and White (1982) compared the toxin profiles in copepods and *Gonyaulax tamarensis* in the same water. The result showed no significant biochemical conversions in the crustaceae organisms, at least in the short term. Thus the absence of gonyautoxins in tropical crab samples may reflect the toxin composition in the original toxin source or a result of the bioconversion of gonyautoxins over a long period of time.

Diarrhoeic shellfish poisoning (DSP) toxins and their origins

This new type of toxins was first discovered in Japanese shellfish by Yasumoto and his co-workers (Yasumoto, Oshima, and Yamauchi 1978; Yasumoto, Oshima, Sugawara, Fukuyo, Oguri, Igarashi, and Fujita, 1980). Later, DSP toxins were reported in various shellfish samples from many locations in both northern and southern hemispheres. The major toxins are okadaic acid and its derivatives with polyether structures. The toxin-producing organisms are the dinoflagellates, *Dinophysis fortii*, *Dinophysis acuminata*, and possibly other *Dinophysis* species (Yasumoto, Murata, Oshima, Matsumoto and Clardy 1984). Although not directly associated with DSP, the tropical dinoflagellate, *Prorocentrum lima* is also known to produce okadaic acid.

Yasumoto *et al.* (1984) also reported another group of toxins (pectenotoxins) in Japanese scallops, but their origins are not known.

Biosynthesis of DSP toxins

No experimentally supported biosynthetic pathway is reported in the literature. However, in view of a close analogy seen in the biosythesis of polyether-type antibiotics, the compounds are very likely formed from polyunsaturated fatty acids by epoxidation and concomitant opening of the resulting epoxide.

Acquisition and fate of DSP toxins in marine invertebrates

A parallel relationship seen between the population of *Dinophysis* spp. and the toxicity of shellfish (Yasumoto *et al.* 1980) indicates that the toxins are directly transferred to the shellfish, mostly in the hepatopancreas, as a result of filter-feeding. Toxins esterified with various fatty acids may result from modification by the shellfish. This conjugation with fatty acids has particular significance because toxins exterified with saturated fatty acids are apparently devoid of toxicity (Yasumoto, private communication). The toxicity in shellfish normally disappears in a few months, but the nature of the detoxification process is not known.

Polyether-type toxins seem to be widely distributed in various marine invertebrates. Okadaic acid was found in sponges (Tachibana, Sheuer, Tsukitani, Kikuchi, Van Eugen, Clardy, Copichand, and Schmitz 1981; Schmitz, Prasad, Gopichand, Hossain, Van der Heim, and Schmit 1981), and other types of compound in soft corals. It is an intriguing question how these organisms acquire the toxins or what is actually making the toxins. A similar question is also valid with toxins such as palytoxin, which is also considered to be an oxidized derivative of polyunsaturated alkene.

Neurotoxic shellfish poisoning (NSP) toxins

This general term is actually used only for those toxins derived from the naked dinoflagellate, *Gymnodinium breve (=Ptychodiscus brevis)*. The organism is mostly confined to the Gulf of Mexico.

The structures of several toxins are now conclusively identified (Fig. 8.5), although the structure of the most toxic component, brevetoxin A (=GB-1 toxin) is still unsolved, but see note added in proof, p. 122.

Fate of NSP Toxins

Although the toxins incorporated into the shellfish are known to cause neurological disorders as well as gastrointestinal troubles, surprisingly no

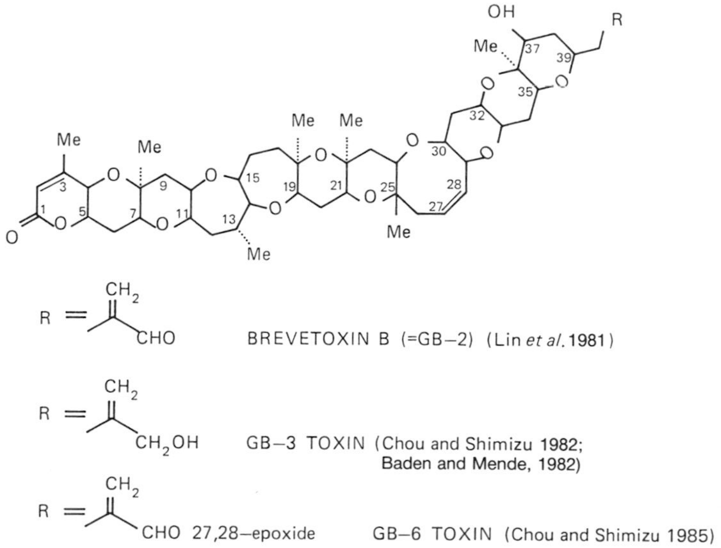

R = (CH$_2$)CHO BREVETOXIN B (=GB−2) (Lin *et al.* 1981)

R = (CH$_2$)CH$_2$OH GB−3 TOXIN (Chou and Shimizu 1982; Baden and Mende, 1982)

R = (CH$_2$)CHO 27,28−epoxide GB−6 TOXIN (Chou and Shimizu 1985)

Fig. 8.5 Examples of NSP toxins found in the dinoflagellate *Gymnodinium breve*.

one has isolated pure toxins from the toxic shellfish. Therefore it is not known if the toxins in shellfish are intact forms or are chemically modified. There is also some speculation that the toxins are transferred to other marine organisms, including fin fish.

Biosynthesis of NSP toxins

Like DSP toxins, the NSP toxins are also considered to be derived from polyunsaturated fatty acids, probably through concomitant openings of epoxide rings (see Fig. 8.6).

Conclusion

Despite the remarkable progress made in marine toxin research in recent years, there are still many unanswered questions regarding the toxigenesis mechanism and the metabolic fate of many important compounds. For example the actual origin of tetrodotoxin, which occurs in marine invertebrates such as octopus, crabs, and marine snails as well as in puffers, remains obscure (Mosher and Fuhrman 1984). The roles of blue-green algae (cyanobacteria) as possible sources of various toxic peptides and alkyl compounds found in marine invertebrates has been speculated upon for some time. However, only confirmed example is aplysiatoxin found in *Aplysia* sp., which is now known to come from the blue-green alga *Lyngbya majuscula* as the debromo derivative, which is then brominated in the *Aplysia* body (Mynderse, Moore, Kashiwagi, and Norton 1977).

The toxigenesis mechanism of toxic dinoflagellates themselves is also a mystery. The rather whimsical occurrence of the same toxins in remote taxa and variations of toxin production in an identical species make one suspect the existence of a transferable factor that contributes to the toxigenicity of the organism. Research on this subject is lacking but at least we can say that secondary metabolites found in marine environments do not seem to be formed by a single species but only through interactions of different organisms.

Acknowledgement — The author wish to thank Mr Ken Shimizu for the preparation of this manuscript. Some of the work described was carried out with grant support from the National Institutes of Health (GM 28754 and GM 24425), which is greatly appreciated.

Note added in proof — The structure of brevetoxin A has been elucidated (see Shimizu, Y., Chou, H-N., Bando, H., van Dyne, G. and Clardy, J. C. (1986)) Structure of brevetoxin A (GB-I Toxin), the most potent toxin in the Florida red-tide toxin, *Gymnodinium breve* (*Ptychodiscus brevis*). *J. Am. Chem. Soc.* **108**, 514–15.

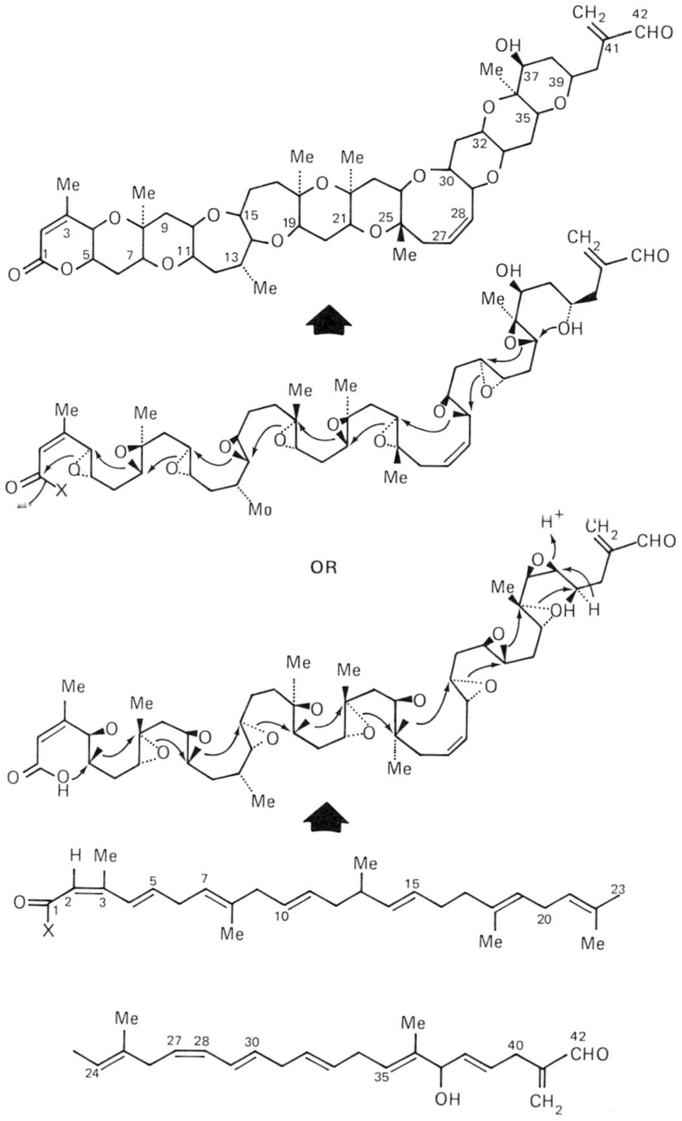

Fig. 8.6 Hypothetical biosynthetic pathway for *Gymnodinium breve* toxins.

References

Baden, D. G. and Mende, T. J. (1982). Toxicity of two toxins from the Florida red tide marine dinoflagellate *Ptychodiscus brevis*. *Toxicon* **20**, 457–461.

Chou, H.-N. and Shimizu, Y. (1982). A new polyether toxin from *Gymnodimium breve* Davis. *Tetrahedron Lett.* **23**, 5521–4.

—— and —— (1985). Isolation and structures of two new polycyclic ethers from *Gymnobinium breve* Davis (=*Ptychodiscus brevis*). *Tetrahedron Lett.* **26**, 2865–8.

Halstead, B. W. (1978). *Poisonous and venomous marine animals of the world.* Darwin, Princeton, New Jersey.

Hashimoto, Y. (1979). *Marine toxins and other bioactive marine metabolites.* Japan Scientific Societies Press, Tokyo.

Hayashi, T., Shimizu, Y., and White, A. W. (1982). Toxin profile of herbivorous zooplankton during a *Gonyaulax* bloom in the Bay of Fundy. *Bull. Jap. Soc. Sci. Fish.* **48**, 1673.

Hsu, C. P., Marchand, A., Shimizu, Y., and Sims. G. G. (1979). Paralytic shellfish toxins in sea scallops, *Placopecten magellanicus*, in the Bay of Fund. *J. fish. Res. Board Can.* **36**, 32–6.

Kotaki, Y., Oshima, Y., and Yasumoto, T. (1981). Analysis of paralytic shellfish toxins of marine snails. *Bull. Jap. Soc. Sci. Fish* **47**, 943–6.

——, ——, and —— (1985). Bacterial transformation of paralytic shellfish toxins in coral reef crabs and marine snails. *Bull. Jap. Soc. Sci. Fish.* **51**, 1009–13.

——, Tajiri, M., Oshima, Y. and Yasumoto, T. (1983). Identification of a calcerous red alga as the primary source of paralytic shellfish toxins in coral reef crabs and gastropods. *Bull. Jap. Soc. Sci. Fish.* **49**, 283–6.

Koyama, K., Noguchi, T., and Ueda, Y. (1981). Occurrence of neosaxitoxin and other paralytic shellfish poisons in toxic crabs belonging to the family xanthidal. *Bull. Jap. Soc. Sci. Fish.* **47**, 965.

Lin. Y., Risk, M., Ray, S. M., Van Egen, D., Clardy, J., Golik, J., James, J. C., and Nakanishi, K. (1981). Isolation and structure of brevetoxin B from the 'red tide' dinoflagellate *Ptychodiscus brevis* (*Gymnodinium breve*). *J. Am. chem. Soc.* **103**, 6773–5.

Mosher, H. S. and Fuhrman, F. A. (1984). Occurrence and origin of tetrodotoxin. In *Seafood toxins* (ed. E. P. Ragelis), pp. 333–44. American Chemical Society, Washington DC.

Mynderse, J. S., Moore, R. E., Kashiwagi, M., and Norton, T. R. (1977). Anti-leukemia activity in the Oscillatoriceae: isolation of debromoaplysiatoxin from *Lyngbya*. *Science* **196**, 538–40.

Oshima, Y., Buckley, L. J., Alam, M., and Shimizu, Y. (1977). Heterogeneity of paralytic shellfish poisons. Three new toxins from cultured *Gonyaulax tamarensis* cells, *Mya arenaria*, and *Saxidomus giganteus*. *Comp. Biochem. Physiol.* **57c**, 31–4.

Schantz, E. J. and Magnusson, H. W. (1964). Observations on the origin of the paralytic poison in the Alaska butter clam. *J. Protozool.* **11**, 239–42.

——, Mold, J. D., Stanger, D. W., Shavel, J., Reil, F. J., Bowden, J. P., Lynch, J. M., Wyler, R. S., Reigel, B. R., and Sommer, H. (1957). Paralytic shellfish poison. VI. A procedure for the isolation and purification of the poison from toxic clams and mussel tissues. *J. Am. chem. Soc.* **79**, 5230–5.

Schmitz, F. J., Prasad, R. S., Gopichand, Y., Hossain, M. B., Van der Heim, D. Z., and Schmit, P. (1981). Acanthifolicin, a new episulfide containing polyether carboxylic acid from extract of the marine sponge, *Pandaros acanthifolium*. *J. Am. chem. Soc.* **103**, 2467–9.

Shimizu, Y. (1982). Recent progress in marine toxin research. *Pure appl. Chem.* **54**, 1973–80.

—— (1984). Paralytic shellfish poisons. In *Progress in the chemistry of organic natural products* (ed. W. Herz, H. Griesback, and G. W. Kirby), Vol. 45, pp. 235–64. Springer, Vienna.

—— and Yoshioka, M. (1980). Transformation of paralytic shellfish toxins as demonstrated in scallop homogenates. *Science* **212**, 547–9.

——, Alam, M., Oshima, Y., and Fallon, W. E. (1975). Presence of four toxins in red tide infested clams and cultured *Gonyaulax tamarensis* cells. *Biochem. Biophys. Res. Commun.* **66**, 731–7.

——, Kobayashi, M., Genenah, A., and Ichihara, N. (1984a). Biosynthesis of paralytic shellfish toxins. In *Seafood toxins* (ed. E. P. Ragelis), pp. 151–60. American Chemical Society, Washington, DC.

——, Norte, M., Hori, A., Genenah, A., and Kabayashi, M. (1984b). Biosynthesis of saxitoxin analogues: the unexpected pathway. *J. Am. chem. Soc.* **106**, 6433–4.

Sommer, H. and Meyer, K. F. (1937). Paralytic shellfish poisoning. *Arch. Path.* **24**, 560–98.

Sullivan, J. J., Iwaoka, W. T., and Liston, J. (1983). Enzymatic transformation of PSP toxins in the littleneck (*Protothaca staminea*). *Biochem. Biophys. Res. Commun.* **114**, 465–72.

Tachibana, K., Scheuer, P. J., Tsukitani, Y., Kikuchi, H., Van Eugen, D., Clardy, J., Copichand, Y., and Schmitz, F. J. (1981). Okadaic acid, a cytotoxic polyether from two marine sponges of the genus *Halichondria*. *J. Am. chem. Soc.* **103**, 2469–71.

Yasumoto, T., Oshima, Y., and Yamauchi, M. (1978). Occurrence of a new type of shellfish poisoning in the Tohoku district. *Bull. Jap. Soc. Sci. Fish.* **44**, 1249–55.

——, ——, and Konta, T. (1981). Analysis of paralytic shellfish toxins of xanthid crabs in Okinawa. *Bull. Jap. Soc. Sci. Fish.* **47**, 943–59.

——, Murata, M., Oshima, Y., Matsumoto, G. K., and Clardy, J. (1984). Diarrhetic shellfish poisoning. In *Seafood toxins* (ed. E. P. Ragelis) pp. 207–14. American Chemical Society, Washington DC.

——, Oshima, Y., Sugawara, W., Fukuyo, Y., Oguri, H., Igarashi, Y., and Fujita, N. (1980). Identification of *Dinophysis fortii* as the causative organism of diarrhetic shellfish poisoning. *Bull. Jap. Soc. Sci. Fish.* **46**, 1405–11.

White, A. W. (1977). Dinoflagellate toxins as probable cause of an Atlantic herring kill and pteropods as apparent vector. *J. Fish. Res. Board Canada*, 2421–4.

Part IV

Effects of natural toxins on cells and tissues

9

The relationship between enzymatic activity and pharmacological properties of phospholipases in natural poisons

Philip Rosenberg

Introduction

While the enzymatic and pharmacological properties of phospholipase (PL) enzymes have been studied, a cause and effect relationship between the two has often been assumed to exist *a priori*, rather than being experimentally tested. In many cases where experimental evaluation of the relationship was studied, the conclusions went beyond those warranted by the data. In this review I shall evaluate those studies that have attempted to relate the enzymatic activity of a particular PL enzyme to a particular pharmacological property. My major purpose is to indicate the types of experiments that should be performed and to indicate why most of the experiments in the literature do not adequately test whether a cause and effect relationship exists between enzymatic activity and pharmacological actions. This review will be mainly concerned with PLA_2 (EC 3.1.1.4) enzymes, partly because many more studies attempting to define this relationship have been made with this enzyme than with other PL enzymes and partly because in my own research I have used snake venom PLA_2 enzymes.

In my earlier review (Rosenberg 1979) I discussed in detail the pharmacology of snake venom PLA_2 and attempted to relate pharmacological actions and enzymatic activity. Some of these earlier studies are also noted in this review if the authors used purified PLA_2 and studied both enzymatic and pharmacological activity. The theoretical relationships between amino acid sequence, conformation and pharmacological properties of PLA_2 enzymes has been discussed in two excellent articles (Dufton and Hider 1983; Dufton, Eaker, and Hider 1983).

Why are phospholipases currently of such interest?

Thudichum said, in 1884, that 'phosphatides are the centre, life and chemical soul of all bioplasm . . .'. What was said of phosphatides (phospholipids) then, is certainly true now for the catabolic enzymes that hydrolyse

129

phospholipids: phospholipases A_1, A_2, C, D, lysophospholipases, sphingo-myelinases, etc.

PLA_2 enzymes have been used for many years as enzymatic probes for studying the function of phospholipids in bioelectrically excitable and other tissues (Rosenberg 1966, 1971, 1972, 1976a; Narahashi 1974). More specifically, PL enzymes can help in evaluating the biological significance of the phospholipid methylation system, which may be of special significance in signal transduction and control of membrane fluidity (Hirata and Axelrod 1980, 1982; Mato and Alemany, 1983). Phospholipases, especially phosphatidylinositol specific PLC, have also been used in an effort to understand the wide-ranging effects attributed to phosphatidylinositol (PI) and poly-PI turnover (Shukla 1982; Fisher and Agranoff 1985; Berridge 1984; Nishizuka 1983; 1984; Hokin 1985; Van Rooijen, Fisher, and Agranoff 1985; Hirasawa and Nishizuka 1985; Farese 1983; Hawthorne 1983). Ca^{2+}-dependent PI breakdown is mediated through cytosolic and particulate PLC. PI-specific PLC also causes the release of certain membrane enzymes, indicating a specific interaction between PI and these enzymes. In these studies it was often assumed that effects of phospholipases were due to phosphlipid hydrolysis; the possible errors in such an assumption will be discussed later.

Phospholipases are valuable tools in studying the localization of phospholipids in biological membranes (Roelofsen 1982; Krebs 1982; Etemadi 1980; Van Deenen 1981). The asymmetric organization of red blood cell membranes has, for example, been demonstrated using phospholipases. Phospholipases have also been used as probes of the structural and functional organization of the red blood cell membrane and factors controlling haemolysis.

It has also been noted that activation of endogenous hydrolytic enzymes such as PLC and PLA_2 can lead to cellular membrane disruption and cell death (Shier 1982). Exogenous PL enzymes may, therefore, have usefulness as models for inducing pathological states that may mimic those induced *in vivo* upon activation of the endogenous enzyme. There is special concern about the activation of endogenous PLA_2 since this would lead to increased levels of arachidonic acid. This fatty acid is the substrate for the cyclooxygenase and the lipoxygenase enzyme systems that catalyze the synthesis of prostaglandins, thromboxanes, and leukotrienes (Samuelsson 1981; Vapaatalo and Parantainen 1978; Irvine 1982; Zahler, Kasermann, and Reist 1985). The biological control of the levels of these highly potent materials is of great current basic and clinical interest; a major controlling factor seems to be the level of free arachidonic acid. It has for example been suggested that a lipoxygenase product of arachidonic acid metabolism is responsible for mast cell degranulation induced by PLA_2 (Chi, Henderson, and Klebanoff 1982).

Another use of PLA$_2$ enzymes is to help us understand presynaptic control mechanisms associated with neurotransmitter release. The presynaptically acting snake venom toxins such as β-bungarotoxin, taipoxin, and notexin all have PLA$_2$ activity (for recent reviews see Fraenkel-Conrat 1982–83; Howard 1982; Karlsson 1979; Chang 1979). While the exact relationship between this enzymatic action and presynaptic neurotoxicity is uncertain and will be discussed later, these toxins may be useful as probes of transmitter release mechanisms. The actual and potential uses of PL enzymes are summarized in Table 9.1.

The use of exogenous PL is sometimes essential in our efforts to understand the functioning of intracellular endogenous PL. The amounts of mammalian intracellular enzyme (see Van den Bosch 1980) are so small that it is usually not possible to purify the enzyme and study its properties. By contrast, relatively large amounts of extracellular PLs are available from the pancreas, from snake and arthropod venoms and from bacteria, for studies of the types described in this review. PLA$_1$ activity has not been detected in snake venoms, although this enzyme is present in other tissues (Ansell, Hawthorne, and Dawson 1973).

PLA$_2$ (phosphatide acyl hydrolase) is found in almost all snake venoms (Rosenberg 1979; Fletcher, Elliott, Ishay, and Rosenberg 1979). PLB (lysophospholipase; lysolecithin acyl hydrolase, EC 3.1.1.5) has been reported in a number of snake, hymenoptera, and gila monster venoms

Table 9.1 Actual and potential usefulness of phospholipase enzymes from natural poisons.

---

1. To help evaluate the structural function of phospholipids and their role as mediators of biological processes, e.g.
  Phospholipid methylation system
  Phosphatidylinositol cycle
  Source of arachidonic acid (cyclooxygenase and lipoxygenase systems)
2. To determine asymmetric organization of phospholipids in biological membranes, e.g.
  Phospholipid asymmetry in red blood cells
3. As models of mammalian intracellular phospholipases which cannot be obtained in adequate amounts for certain enzymatic or pharmacological studies
4. As potential models of clinical disorders, e.g.
  Epilepsy (convulsant action)
  Haemolytic disorders (PLC, PLA$_2$)
  Coagulation disorders (anticoagulant action)
  Inflammation (increased levels of arachidonic acid)
5. To help understand presynaptic control mechanisms for neurotransmitter release, e.g.
  Use of β-bungarotoxin, notexin, taipoxin

(Fletcher *et al*. 1979; Rosenberg, Ishay, and Gitter 1977; Doery and Pearson 1964; Mohamed, Kamel, and Ayobe 1969). Phosphatidylcholine cholinephosphohydrolase (EC 3.1.4.3) and sphingomyelinase activity is present in mammalian tissue although the richest source of these enzymes is bacteria (Ikezawa, Taguchi, Asahi, and Tomita 1982–83). PLD activity has been found in high amounts in plants (Ansell *et al*. 1973), although the activity is also present in mammalian tissues and in bacteria. The distribution of PL enzymes is summarized in Table 9.2.

By 1981 the complete amino acid sequences of about 30 PLA_2 enzymes from pancreatic secretions and snake venoms were known (see Verheij, Slotboom, and De Haas 1981 for sequences and references). In this reference Verheij and co-workers also review the physicochemical, structural, and enzymatic properties of PLA_2. These phospholipases, although showing marked sequence homology, also have significant differences in amino

Table 9.2 Distribution of phospholipases.

PLA_1	<u>Mammalian tissues</u>
	Microsomes; plasma membranes,
	lysosomes
	Bacteria
PLA_2	Mammalian tissues
	Microsomes, plasma membranes,
	lysosomes, mitochondria
	<u>Pancreatic secretions</u>
	<u>Snake venoms</u>
	Bee and wasp venoms
	Bacteria
PLB —	Mammalian tissues
Lysophospholipase	Pancreatic secretions
	Snake venoms
	<u>Bee and Wasp venoms</u>
	Bacteria
PLC	Mammalian tissues
	<u>Bacteria</u>
	Plants
PLD	Mammalian tissue
	Bacteria
	<u>Plants</u>

Some of the richest sources are underlined. See following review articles for appropriate references: Shen and Lau 1979; Dennis 1983; Avigad 1976; Van den Bosch 1980.

acids, isoelectric points, and whether a monomer or a dimer is the active form. Even within a single venom many isoenzymes may be present; for example, up to 14 PLA_2 isoenzymes have been found in *N. naja* venom (Salach, Turini, Seng, Hanber, and Singer 1971; Shiloah, Klibansky, and DeVries 1973). PLA_2 enzymes also show marked differences in their stabilities, phospholipid substrate preferences, and enzymatic responses to various ions (Verheij *et al.* 1981; Rosenberg 1979). PLA_2 enzymes from snake venoms have six or seven disulphide bonds and 118 to 125 amino acids, of which 36 are invariant and another 29 to 45 have conservative substitutions. Homology is greatest between positions 25 to 52, which includes essential active-site amino acid residues including His-48, Tyr-52, and Asp-49. The homology is about the same between classical PLA_2 enzymes as it is between presynaptically acting neurotoxins from snake venoms that also have PLA_2 activity. A comparison of the amino acid sequence of *N. nigricollis* and *N. n. atra* PLA_2, which we have used extensively in our studies, with that of pancreatic PLA_2, and presynaptically acting toxins (notexin, caudoxin, and the A chain of B bungarotoxin) is shown in Table 9.3. The marked homology in their sequences is obvious.

Comparison of enzymatic and pharmacological potencies of phospholipases

While many reviews discuss the chemistry and the extremely varied and potent pharmacological actions of PL enzymes (Verheij *et al.* 1981; Rosenberg 1979; Shen and Lau 1979; Lee and Ho 1982; Randolph, Sakmar, and Heinrikson 1980; Dijkstra, Drenth, and Kalk 1981; Heinrikson 1982; Shukla 1982; Avigad 1976; Tu 1977) relatively few published articles have attempted to correlate enzymatic and pharmacological properties.

Possible mechanisms of pharmacological actions and critical factors to be considered when attempting to relate enzymatic and pharmacological potencies

Phospholipase enzymes can, theoretically, interfere with cellular functioning by:

(a) direct effects due to disruption of essential membrane phospholipids;

(b) indirect effects due to products released as a result of phospholipid hydrolysis;

(c) actions independent of phospholipid hydrolysis such as direct membrane disruption.

A more detailed description of possible mechanisms for PLA_2-induced actions is shown in Table 9.4.

The ideal experiments for evaluating critically whether PL enzymatic

Table 9.3 Amino acid sequence of PLA₂ and presynaptic PLA₂ neurotoxins.

```
                1           5          10          15          20          25          30          35          40          45
PLA₂
PAN        A L W G F R S M I K C A I P G S H P L M D F N N Y G C Y C G L G G S G T P V D E L D R C C
NOTEXIN    N * V * S Y L * Q * N H * K R * T W H Y M D * * * * * * * A * * * * * * * * * * * * * *
N. nig     N * Y * * K N * * H * T V * S — R * W W H * A D * * * * R * K * * * D * * * * * * * * *
N.n.a.     N * Y * * K N * * Q * T V * S — R S W W * * A D * * * * R * * * * * D * * * * * * * * *
β BT       N * I N * M E * * R Y T * * C E K T W G E Y A D * * * * A * * * * * R * I * A * * * * *
CAUDOXIN   N * I * * G N * S A M T G K * S — * — A Y A S * * * * W * K * Q * K * D T * * * *
                                            55|—       60          65          70          75          80         85        —90
PAN        E T H D N C Y R D A — K N L D S C K F L V D N P Y T E S Y S — C S N T E I T — C N S K N N — A
NOTEXIN    K I * * D * * G * — K — G * — — — * — * KMSA * D * Y — GENGPY — RNIKK — K
N. nig     Q V * * * E K * G * — M — G * — W — — — * — — * LTL * K — * QGKL * — SGG * S — K
N.n.a.     Q V * * * N E * E * — I S G * — W — — — * — — * FKT * E C S * QGTL * — * KGG * — *
β BT       Y V * * * * * G * E * — K H K * — — — — * — — * K * SQ * — K — LTKRT — I — * YGAAGGT
CAUDOXIN   F V * * C * * G K * D * — — — * — — — — S * KMIL * — K — FH * GN — V — * GD * — * — —
                  95         100         105         110         115         120         125
PAN        C E A F I C N C D R N A A I C F S K A — — P Y N K E H K N L D T K — K Y C
NOTEXIN    * L R * V * D * * V E * * F * A * * — * * N A N W I * * R * Q
N. nig     * G * A V * * L V * * N * * A G * — R * I D A N Y I N F * — R * Q
N.n.a.     * A * A V * D * L * * * * G C * * * D N N N Y I * L — A R * Q
β BT       — * R I V * D * * T * L * * G Q S — D I E * * I * A — R F * Q
CAUDOXIN   * K K K V * E * * V * * N K W R Y P S S — K — T G T A E K C
```

Gaps (—) have been introduced to get maximal alignment of half-cysteine and to get maximum homology. Note that gaps introduced in the pancreatic PLA₂ do not affect the numbering. Residues identical to corresponding residue in porcine pancreatic PLA₂ are indicated with an asterisk (*).

Abbreviations: PAN = Porcine pancreatic PLA₂; N. nig = N. nigricollis PLA₂; N.n.a. = Naja naja atra PLA₂; β BT = β-bungarotoxin (A chain).

A = Ala, C = Cys, D = Asp, E = Glu, F= Phe, G = Gly, H = His, I = Ile, K = Lys, L = Leu, M = Met, N = Asn, P = Pro, Q = Gln, R = Arg, S = Ser, T = Thr, V = Val, W = Trp, Y = Tyr.

References: PAN = Puijk et al. 1977; Notexin = Halpert and Eaker 1975; N. nigricollis = Obidairo et al. 1976; N. n. atra = Tsai et al. 1981; β Bt = Kondo et al. 1978, 1982; caudoxin = Viljoen et al. 1982.

Table 9.4 Possible mechanisms of PLA$_2$-induced pharmacological effects.

1. Hydrolysis of membrane phospholipids directly causing disruption of functions such as:
   (a) Selective permeability of membranes to ions, drugs, etc.
   (b) Enzymatic activities which are dependent upon phospholipids, e.g. Na, K-ATPase.
   (c) Receptor–ligand systems which may be dependent upon phospholipid coupling in their functioning, e.g. phosphatidylethanolamine methyl transferase system; Ca^{2+}-polyphosphoinositide turnover.
   (d) Intracellular sequestering of calcium within SR and mitochondria.
2. Hydrolysis of membrane phospholipids giving rise to pharmacologically active products that mediate PLA$_2$ action. Products would include:
   (a) Lysophospholipids and free fatty acids having detergent and other actions.
   (b) Arachidonic acid release causing formation of increased levels of thromboxanes, prostaglandins and leukotrienes.
3. Effects independent of phospholipid hydrolysis including for example direct membrane disruption, which could lead to:
   (a) Haemolytic action.
   (b) Cardiotoxicity.
   (c) Anticoagulant action.
   (d) Centrally induced convulsions.

activity and pharmacological potency are related would have to meet the criteria noted in Table 9.5.

An example of the importance of determining *in vitro* enzymatic activity in several different systems is shown in Table 9.6. (Barrington, Condrea, Soons, Yang, and Rosenberg 1984b). The marked difference of modified derivatives of *N. nigricollis* PLA$_2$, dependent upon the substrate utilized, is obvious, whereas there is no difference in *N. n. atra* PLA$_2$ activity.

In most studies, the pharmacologic effects of the hydrolytic products (lysophosphatides, free fatty acids) produced as a result of the action of PLA$_1$ or PLA$_2$ on phospholipids have not been evaluated. Incorrect conclusions may, therefore, be drawn about phospholipid function since it may be supposed that pharmacological effects are directly due to hydrolysis of phospholipids, whereas they are actually due to the toxic actions of the hydrolytic products. For example, lysophosphatides have detergent properties and affect many tissues including nerve (Zeller 1951; Tobias 1955; Morrison and Zamecnik 1950; McArdle, Thompson, and Webster 1960; Rosenberg and Condrea 1968). One should also test whether PLA$_2$ effects are due to alterations in levels of products derived from arachidonic acid (prostaglandins, etc.). Although products produced by the actions of other PL enzymes (e.g. diglycerides, phosphatidic acid, phosphorylated bases)

Table 9.5 Critical factors in attempting to correlate pharmacological and enzymatic activities of phospholipase (PL) enzymes.

---

1. Use pure PL enzymes, preferably of known amino acid sequence.

2. Determine enzymatic activity *in vitro* in several systems (lecithin–triton mixed micelles, egg yolk, homogenates of tissue of interest, etc.).

3. Quantitate the extent of phospholipid hydrolysis in the tissue upon which pharmacological measurements are made.

4. Measure pharmacological potency *in vivo* under conditions where enzymatic activity would and would not be expected to be present (e.g. presence or absence of Ca^{2+}, use of enzymes chemically modified at His-48). Confirm expected effects on enzymatic activity (points 2 and 3 above).

5. Test whether pharmacological effects are actually due to hydrolytic products of PL action.

6. Check how known chemical modification of the enzyme affects enzymatic and pharmacological properties.

7. Observations with one particular PL enzyme cannot necessarily be generalized.

---

are not generally thought to be potent in their effects, they should be tested in the particular system under investigation.

To quantitate and compare the pharmacological potencies for PL enzymes and relate them to enzymic activities, it is best to quantitate the actual extent of phospholipid hydrolysis in the biologic preparation to which PLA_2 is added. It is then possible to express enzymic potency in terms of weights of the enzyme preparations which give comparable extents of phospholipid hydrolysis. If pharmacologic potency is due to phospholipid hydrolysis, one might expect to find similar pharmacological and enzymic ratios of potency for the different preparations of enzyme. It is impossible to evaluate the essential involvement of phospholipids for a particular pharmacologic action without determining the extent of phospholipid splitting. Nevertheless, many investigators reach conclusions concerning phospholipid function or PL action without ever measuring the extent of phospholipid hydrolysis in the tissue of interest.

In our studies we have attempted to adhere to all seven criteria noted in Table 9.5, and examples of our data are given elsewhere in this chapter. It will become obvious that there is no direct relationship between enzymatic activity and pharmacologic potency of several different PLA_2 enzymes. A few examples of dissociation between pharmacological and enzymatic activity which we have observed in our studies are shown in Table 9.7.

Lethal potency

We have extensively studied the pharmacological and enzymatic properties of the basic PLA_2 from *N. nigricollis*, the acidic PLA_2 from *N. n. atra* and

Table 9.6 Effects of carboxyl group modification on *N. n. atra* and *N. nigricollis* phospholipase A_2 on lethal potencies and enzymatic activities.

		Enzymatic activity (per cent of native activity) on:				Lethal potency	
				Homogenates of:			
		PC +	Egg			i.v.	i.v.r.
Modification	pI	Triton	yolk	Heart	Diaphragm	(% of native)	
N. n. atra							
Native	5.2						
pH 3.5	9.4	2	2	3	3	—	29
pH 5.5	8.0	2	5	4	4	—	29
pH 5.5 +							
Ca^{2+}	8.0	12	17	17	17	100	500
N. nigricollis							
Native	10.6						
pH 3.5	>11	<1	9	8	8	<12	5
pH 5.5	>11	<1	11	10	10	<12	5
ph 5.5 +							
Ca^{2+}	>11	22	61	100	100	17	33

The per cent of native (unmodified) enzymatic activity values shown in the table are means of two to three determinations that varied less than 20 per cent. The activities of the native enzymes on the various substrates, expressed as means of two to four determinations which varied less than 20 per cent were as follows (μEq free fatty acids liberated per min per mg): *N. n. atra*: PC + Triton, 500; egg yolk, 2000; rat heart, 1585; rat diaphragm, 1263. *N. nigricollis*: PC + Triton, 190; egg yolk, 378; rat heart, 488; rat diaphragm, 330.

The i.v. LD_{50} values in mice for native *N. n. atra* and *N. nigricollis* PLA_2 are 8.6 and 0.6 mg/kg^{-1}, respectively. The i.v.r. LD_{50} values for native *N. n. atra* and *N. nigricollis* PLA_2 are 7.5 and 0.5 μg rat^{-1} rat, respectively.

Of the nine free carboxyls in *N. nigricollis* PLA_2 (7 Asp, 1 Glu, 1 COOH terminal) and the fifteen in *N. n. atra* PLA_2 (10 Asp, 4 Glu, 1 COOH terminal) we would expect all to be modified except Asp 99 at pH 3.5, Asp 99 + 39 at pH 5.5, and Asp 99 + 39 + 49 at pH 5.5 in the presence of Ca^{2+} (Barrington *et al.* 1984b).

Abbreviations: PC = phosphatidylcholine; i.v. = intravenous, i.v.r. = intraventricular.

the neutral PLA_2 from *H. haemachatus* venoms. As shown in Table 9.8, their lethal potency is apparently inversely related to their *in vitro* enzymatic activity. For example, *N. nigricollis* PLA_2 has the greatest lethal potency but the least enzymatic activity (Rosenberg, Condrea, Fletcher, Rapuano, and Yang 1983b; Fletcher, Rapuano, Condrea, Yang, Ryan, and Rosenberg 1980: Condrea, Yang, and Rosenberg 1980; Condrea, Fletcher, Rapuano, Yang, and Rosenberg 1981a). This lack of relationship is even more dramatic when one considers the extensive amino acid sequence homology in these three enzymes; about 80 of the approximately 120 amino acid residues are identical in sequence for all three PLA_2 enzymes (Joubert

Table 9.7 Lack of association between pharmacological potency and *in vivo* phospholipid hydrolysis.

Condition — PLA$_2$	Ph'col. action	% hydrolysis		
		PC	PE	PS
Langendorff heart				
N. nigricollis, 120 μg	+ +	3	2	5
N. n. atra, 1620 μg	—	6	38	5
Phrenic — diaphragm				
N. nigricollis 12 μg ml^{-1}	+ +	30	38	45
O Ca^{2+} + Sr^{2+}				
N. n. atra 12 μg ml^{-1}	—	43	64	34
O Ca^{2+} + Sr^{2+}				
A. p. piscivorus[a] — Asp 49	+	43	50	30
A. p. piscivorus[a] — Lys 49	+ +	4	0	10
Brain — SPM				
N. n. atra 12 μg rat^{-1}	+ +	0	10	8
N. n. atra 225 μg rat^{-1}	—	2	10	8
Lysine fr. 5				
Plasma — coagulation				
N. nigricollis 0.25 μg ml^{-1}	+ +	14	35	—
N. n. atra 2.5 μg ml^{-1}	±	93	100	—

    Pharmacological actions include ventricular fibrillation (Langendorff), block of direct and indirect contraction (phrenic diaphragm), lethal potency (brain-SPM) and anticoagulant action (plasma coagulation).
    [a] Concentration = 35 μg ml^{-1}.
    Abbreviations: SPM = synaptic plasma membranes; PC = phosphatidylcholine; PE = phosphatidylethanolamine; PS = phosphatidylserine.
    Based upon data contained in joint publications by Rosenberg, Condrea, Yang, Fletcher, Rapuano, and Soons (see references).

1975; Obidairo, Tampitag, and Eaker 1976; Tsai, Wu, and Lo 1981). To study this apparent lack of relationship between enzymatic activity and lethal potency, we investigated some other enzymatic properties of these PLA$_2$ enzymes. The pH dependencies of the *N. nigricollis* and *H. haemachatus* enzymes were similar showing a broad bimodal pH optimum at pH 6 and 9 (Condrea *et al.* 1980). These same PLA$_2$ enzymes showed increased hydrolytic activity as the temperature was increased between 10 and 70°C and both favoured substrates in the liquid crystalline state (Condrea *et al.* 1980). Differences in substrate specificities were as follows: *N. nigricollis*, phosphatidylethanolamine (PE) ≥ phosphatidylserine (PS) >> phosphatidylcholine (PC); *H. haemachatus*, PE > PC > PS; *N. naja atra*, PE > PS > PC (Condrea *et al.* 1980, 1981a). These differences in substrate specificity cannot, however, explain the differences

Table 9.8 Kinetic parameters and lethalities of phospholipases A_2 (PLA$_2$).

PLA$_2$	pI	V_{max}[a]	K_m (mM)	LD$_{50}$ i.v.r. (μg rat^{-1})	LD$_{50}$ i.v. (mg kg mouse^{-1})
N. n.	10.6	256	4.2	0.5	0.6
N. n. a.	5.2	500	5.3	7.5	8.6
H. h.	7.4	1000	2.2	15.0	8.6

[a] Activity on lecithin–triton mixed micelles (μeq min^{-1} mg^{-1}.

Abbreviations: *N. n.*, *Naja nigricollis*; *N. n. a.*, *Naja naja atra*: *H. h.*, *Hemachatus haemachatus*; i.v.r. = intraventricular into right lateral ventricle; i.v. = intravenous into tail vein.

in lethal potency, since measurements of actual phospholipid hydrolysis in various organs *in vivo* do not correlate with the lethal potency or other pharmacological actions (see following sections of review). Death appeared due to congestion, haemorrhage, and oedema in the lungs. Consideration of dosages required and times until onset of action suggests that, dependent upon the route of administration, the effect is either mediated via a central action or is due to a direct effect on the cardiac and/or respiratory system in the periphery. The pattern and extent of phospholipid hydrolysis in various brain regions was similar following intraventricular injection of the two phospholipases, so that no relationship between phospholipid hydrolysis and lethal potency could be established (Fletcher *et al.* 1980). The PLA$_2$ enzymes cannot cross the blood–brain barrier to a significant extent in either direction, so lethal effects following intravenous and intraventricular injection are due, respectively, to peripheral and central effects (Fletcher, Rapuano, Condrea, Yang, and Rosenberg 1981). Thus, while it is often assumed that enzyme activity is essential for the lethal potency of PLA$_2$ enzymes, a comparison of LD$_{50}$ values with enzyme activity (Lee and Ho 1982) shows no relationship between these two parameters (taipoxin LD$_{50}$ = 2 μg kg^{-1} mouse with enzyme activity of 406 μmol min^{-1} mg^{-1} while the neutral PLA$_2$ from *N. nigricollis* venom has an LD$_{50}$ of 10 200 μg kg^{-1} mouse and an enzymatic activity of 733 μmol min^{-1} mg^{-1}.

Effects on bioelectrically excitable tissues

Axonal actions

The purified PLA$_2$ fractions from *H. haemachatus* and *A. p. piscivorus* venoms have been found to increase permeability of squid and lobster axons to poorly penetrating compounds such as curare and acetylcholine and render the axons sensitive to the effects of these synaptically active drugs, which normally do not act upon axons (Rosenberg and Ehrenpreis 1961; Rosenberg and Podleski 1962, 1963; Rosenberg and Hoskin 1963; Rosenberg and Ng 1963; Rosenberg 1965; 1971, 1976a, Hoskin and Rosenberg 1965; Rosenberg and Mautner 1967, Condrea, Rosenberg, and Dettbarn 1967; Rosenberg and Condrea 1968; Martin and Rosenberg 1968). These effects were not directly due to splitting of phospholipids since the percentage of the squid giant axon phospholipid hrdrolysed was identical in finely dissected squid giant axons, where the venoms and the purified PLA_2 were inactive, and in the crudely dissected axons, where PLA_2 and the venoms induced all of the effects described above. In the finely dissected axons, however, there is much less phospholipid substrate and, therefore, less lysophosphatide produced. Indeed, a mixture of natural or synthetic lysophosphatides mimicked the action of PLA_2 (Rosenberg and Condrea 1968). Therefore, the results indicate that in the nonmyelinated lobster axon and squid giant axon, the effects of venoms are due to their PLA_2 component hydrolysing the axonal phospholipids and liberating lysophosphatides, which exert marked effects on axonal functioning. That the effects are not due to phospholipid splitting *per se* has been supported by later studies showing that a much greater percentage of phospholipid hydrolysis by PLC than by PLA_2 did not give rise to blocking of conduction or the other effects produced by PLA_2 (Rosenberg and Condrea 1968; Rosenberg 1970). In our studies on the squid giant axon, PLA has been an extremely useful tool for studying whether phospholipids are essential in axonal conduction (Rosenberg 1966, 1971, 1976). It has been possible to conclude that most membrane phospholipids are not essential for axonal conduction. Normal function can apparently be maintained even when most of the phospholipids have been hydrolysed.

Synaptic actions

The actions of both classical PLA_2 enzymes, such as *N. nigricollis* and *N. n. atra* PLA_2, and presynaptically acting toxins from snake venoms that have PLA_2 activity will be considered in this section. The percentage of sequence homology between a classical PLA_2 enzyme and a toxin is about the same as between two enzymes or two toxins, e.g.:

  N. nigricollis — *n. n. atra* PLA_2 = 75 per cent homology;
  Notexin — A chain of β bungarotoxin (BT) = 52 per cent;
  N. nigricollis — Notexin = 61 per cent;
  N. nigricollis — A chain of β BT = 52 per cent.

On the isolated single electroplax of the electric eel (*Electrophorus electricus*), a purified preparation of PLA_2 from *A. p. piscivorus* venom and lysophosphatidylcholine caused depolarization and block of both direct and indirect stimulation at concentrations of 0.1–0.5 mg ml^{-1} (Bartels and

Rosenberg 1972). The endplate potential was depressed prior to failure of junctional transmission. Block of electrical activity by PLA_2 was associated with 80–100 per cent hydrolysis of phosphatidylcholine (PC), phosphatidylethanolamine (PE), and phosphatidylserine (PS) the three major phospholipids of the cell. This may have either been directly responsible for the pharmacological effects, or the lysophosphatides produced as a result of PLA_2 action may have mediated the pharmacological effects. Lower concentrations of PLA_2 that did not block electrical activity hydrolysed approximately the same percentage of PE and PS, but only about one-third of the PC. Block of excitability and extensive phospholipid hydrolysis was also associated with a two to threefold increase in permeability to ^{14}C choline (Rosenberg 1973a). Purified PLA_2 (0.2 and 2.0 mg ml^{-1}) caused mitochondrial swelling and a pinching off of the membrane in pocketings of the electroplax to form clusters of small, rounded vesicles external to the membrane. Lysophosphatidylcholine had much less of an effect on the membrane ultrastructure (Rosenberg 1976b). These results provide evidence that phosphlipids may be essential for the functioning of this synapse-containing preparation, a conclusion also reinforced by the findings that both the application of acetylcholine and electrical stimulation increase the incorporation of ^{14}C glucose and ^{32}P inorganic phosphate into the phospholipids of the electroplax (Rosenberg 1973b). The observations on the membrane ultrastructure suggest that the binding between phospholipids and proteins is primarily hydrophobic in nature and is disrupted by PLA_2-induced hydrolysis of the β fatty acid ester of the phospholipid.

N. nigricollis PLA_2, while having much greater lethal potency and haemolytic, anticoagulant, and cardiotoxic activity than *H. haemachatus* and *N. n. atra* PLA_2 enzymes (see other sections of this review), was about equipotent with the latter two enzymes in terms of their potency on the electroplax and phrenic nerve–diaphragm neuromuscular junction (Fletcher *et al.* 1980, 1981). For example, concentrations of 5 and 10 μg ml^{-1} of the *N. nigricollis* and *H. haemachatus* phospholipases, respectively, were required to block electrical activity of the isolated single electroplax. The ultrastructural changes produced by both phospholipases were also similar. *N. nigricollis* phospholipase produced only slightly greater overall hydrolysis in the innervated and non-innervated membranes of the electroplax than did *H. haemachatus* phospholipase. The results suggest that these two phospholipases do not have a specific junctional effect and that the small difference in potency on the junction cannot be responsible for the large difference in lethal effect observed in mammalian species (Fletcher *et al.* 1980).

All three PLA_2 enzymes (12 μg ml^{-1}) abolish the directly and indirectly elicited muscle twitches of the rat phrenic nerve–diaphragm preparation. This block, in normal or altered bathing media, appeared to correlate with the level of phospholipid hydrolysis for the *N. naja atra* enzyme, but not for the *N. nigricollis* enzyme. These results suggest that *N. nigricollis* PLA_2 acts by another mechanism in addition to phospholipid hydrolysis (Fletcher *et al.* 1981). No evidence for a specific presynaptic effect was obtained, since the directly and indirectly evoked contractions of the diaphragm were equally affected, suggesting a primary action on the muscle membrane (Fletcher *et al.* 1981). Replacement of Ca^{2+} by Sr^{2+} in this preparation blocked the effects on contraction of *N. n. atra* but not *N. nigricollis* PLA_2. Since Ca^{2+} is essential for venom PLA_2 enzymatic activity (Verheij *et al.* 1981), these results initially suggested that *N. nigricollis* PLA_2, but not *N. n. atra* PLA_2 has no action independent of phospholipid hydrolysis. However, phospholipid hydrolysis was shown to occur in the diaphragm even in the presence of Sr^{2+} (and absence of Ca^{2+}), no doubt due to membrane-bound Ca^{2+} in the tissue (Fletcher *et al.* 1981). No relationship between pharmacological potency and extent of phospholipid hydrolysis could be demonstrated. Lee, Ho, and Eaker (1977) reported that *N. nigricollis* phospholipase A_2 exhibits the characteristics of a cardiotoxin on the resting membrane potential of the isolated rat diaphragm and that these characteristics are inhibited by high (10 mM) Ca^{2+} concentrations. However, our results show an enhanced effect of the *N. nigricollis* phospholipase on the diaphragm muscle twitch in high Ca^{2+} medium, in contrast to the inhibition of cardiotoxin-induced contractures in the presence of 10 mM Ca^{2+}.

The relationship between the chemistry of the presynaptically active toxins and their neurophysiological effects may be found in several review articles (Lee and Ho 1982; Karlsson 1979; Chang 1979: Fraenkel-Conrat 1982–83; Howard and Gundersen 1980; Howard 1982). β-bungatotoxin liberated fatty acids from synaptosomal preparations of the rat cerebral cortex, thereby inhibiting oxidative phosphorylation in the mitochondria of the nerve terminals and causing an efflux from the synaptosomes of previously accumulated γ-aminobutyric acid and 2-deoxy-D-glucose (Wernicke, Vanker, and Howard 1975). The effect on efflux required the presence of Ca^{2+} and was inhibited by Mg^{2+} and Mn^{2+}, while the uncoupling of oxidative phosphorylation by the toxin was prevented by bovine serum albumin, which binds free fatty acids. These observations support the suggestion that the pharmacological effects of the toxin may be due either to the direct hydrolysis of phospholipids or to the fatty acids and lysophosphatides liberated as a result of PLA_2 activity. A Ca^{2+} requirement is a common characteristic of PLA_2 enzymes from various sources, and it is, therefore, of interest that low Ca^{2+} in the medium markedly increases the time required for neuromuscular block with β-bungarotoxin (Lee and Chang 1966). It was suggested by Wernicke and co-workers that the initial phase of increased rate of spontaneous acetylcholine release followed by neuromuscular block after exposure to β-bungarotoxin could be due to a PLA_2-induced inhibition of oxidative phosphorylation. β-bungarotoxin inhibited calcium accumulation into subcellular fractions of rat brain, an effect apparently due to an action on the mitochondria (Wagner, Mart, and Kelly 1974). The possible importance of inhibition of choline transport by these toxins has also been discussed (Dowdall, Fohlman, and Watts 1979).

The relationship of PLA_2 activity to toxicity of β-bungarotoxin has been noted by Tobias, Donlon, Shain, and Catravas (1976). Both the major bungarotoxin peak and another minor peak showed Ca^{2+}-dependent PLA_2 activity, which was destroyed by boiling at pH 8.6. Material from both peaks inhibited ADP-dependent oxygen consumption in mitochondria but the minor peak did not require Ca^{2+} for this effect. The data on binding to mitochondrial and synaptosomal fractions suggest that toxicity is related to PLA_2 activity. Strong, Goerke, Oberg, and Kelly (1976) also demonstrated that strontium inhibited both the PLA_2 activity and the effects of β-bungarotoxin on neuromuscular transmission. In comparing the PLA_2 activity and the minimum lethal dose of β-bungarotoxin with those of *N. naja* and *V. russelli* the following PLA_2 results were obtained: μEq free fatty acids liberated per min per mg protein were 133, 76, and 424 for β-bungarotoxin, and *N. naja* and *V. russelli* PLA_2 respectively. The minimal lethal doses in mice were 0.01, 4, and 0.48 mg kg^{-1}, respectively, showing the much greater lethal potency of β bungarotoxin than the usual acidic PLA_2 preparations. Certainly, ability to liberate free fatty acids in artificial *in vitro* assay systems cannot be correlated with *in vivo* biologic potency.

The findings with β-bungarotoxin were not the first indication that some snake venom PLA_2 preparations may be associated with a presynaptic site of action. The basic *Crotalus* PLA_2 was reported to have a presynaptic action on the frog sartorius nerve–muscle preparation, causing an increase in the frequency of miniature end-plate potentials (Brazil, Excell, and De Sa 1973). A neuromuscular blockade and a myotoxic effect has also been noted in mammalian systems (Breithaupt and Habermann 1973). PLA_2–crotapotin complexes decreased the contractions of isolated phrenic hemidiaphragms of rats to direct and indirect stimulation. A similar block of neuromuscular transmission was also observed *in vivo* (Breithaupt 1976). Crotoxin is a very potent neurotoxin, probably most active in the dimeric form. It has PLA_2 activity and differs from the other presynaptic neurotoxins in that it has both pre- and postsynaptic actions; postsynaptically it stabilizes the acetylcholine receptor–ionophore complex in the desensitized state (Slotta and Fraenkel-Conrat 1938; Bon, Changeux, Jeng, and Fraenkel-Conrat 1979; Radvanyi and Bon 1984). Irreversible inactivation of its PLA_2 activity by chemical modification, or reversible inactivation replacement of Ca^{2+} with Sr^{2+} in the medium, prevents the physiological action of crotoxin (Marlas and Bon 1982). On the eel electroplax it was suggested that the postsynaptic action is due to phospholipid hydrolysis at critical sites, perhaps closely related to the acetylcholine receptor (Marlas and Bon 1982). Several different methods were used to assess the importance of PLA_2 activity to the postsynaptic blocking action. Unfortunately, actual phospholipid hydrolysis in the electroplax was not measured; correlations were drawn between postsynaptic potency and *in vitro* PLA_2 activity on egg PC or on Torpedo receptor rich membrane fragments.

Eaker and his collaborators have carried out studies clarifying the relationship between the presynaptic neurotoxic activity of notexin, the neurotoxin from the venom of the Australian tiger snake *Notechis scutatus scutatus*, and its PLA_2 activity. The complete amino acid sequency of notexin, which exhibits weak PLA_2 activity, is homologous to porcine pancreatic PLA_2, a PLA_2 from *N. melanoleuca venom*, one of the subunits of β-bungarotoxin and one of the subunits of crotoxin (Halpert and Eaker 1975). Some evidence has been obtained that the neurotoxic activity of notexin may be associated with its PLA_2 activity. The modification of one histidine residue in notexin by the use of *P*-bromophenacyl bromide caused a 99.8 per cent loss of both PLA_2 activity and lethal neurotoxicity (Halpert, Eaker, and Karlsson 1976).

The above results suggested to the authors of these various publications that PLA_2 activity is implicated in the neurotoxicity caused by these toxins. More specifically it has been suggested that the initial binding to the presynaptic nerve terminal is not dependent on PLA_2 activity, whereas the subsequent alterations in transmitter release are PLA_2-dependent reactions (Kelly, Von Wedel, and Strong 1979; Su and Chang 1984). Selectivity and potency of the toxins may be related to the initial binding step. These binding sites appear to differ from one toxin to another (Chang and Su 1980). It is thus suggested that there is a disruption in the presynaptic membrane due to the PLA_2 activity of the toxin, which results in increase then failure of transmitter release. Howard (1982) and Howard and Gundersen (1980) point out that there is no evidence that these neurotoxins enter the cell and suggest as a likely mechanism of action the alteration of calcium transport across the plasma membrane. It was suggested that specificity of binding sites confers specificity of action upon these toxins. The nature of these binding sites, however, remains unclear. For convenience, synaptosomes have often been used as model systems upon which to study the action of presynaptic toxins. Disruption of the synaptosomal membrane associated with depolarization and inhibition of choline uptake were noted and suggested to be responsible for increased release of acetylcholine (Sen, Baba, Sehulz, and Cooper 1978). In a recent review (Lee and Ho 1982) it was claimed that PLA_2 activity of these presynaptically acting toxins is responsible for their neurotoxicity, because:

(a) these toxins are basic PLA_2 enzymes;

(b) inhibition of catalytic activity either by replacement of Ca^{2+} with Sr^{2+} or by acylation of His 48 (enzymatic inactivation) results in a corresponding loss of neurotoxicity;

(c) ultrastructural changes occur in subcellular membranes.

While suggestive, these criteria are not sufficient for reaching a firm conclusion. Indeed it was concluded (Chang and Su 1982) that histidine-modified, PLA_2 inactive β-bungarotoxin, crotoxin, and notexin have their own presynaptic effects, unrelated to enzymatic activity, although the physiological actions were greatly enhanced by the presence of PLA_2 activity; once again phospholipid hydrolysis in the tissue was not measured. Moreover, there is no quantitative relationship between PLA_2 activity and presynaptic potency.

Other criticisms can be made of the presently available evidence. Our own studies, as outlined elsewhere in this review, show that:

1. Bound Ca^{2+} in the tissue may allow PLA_2 activity to occur even in a supposed zero $Ca^{2+} + Sr^{2+}$ medium;

2. The loss of toxic potency upon substituting Ca^{2+} with Sr^{2+} may have nothing to do with inhibition of PLA_2 activity, but may imply that the biological effect is mediated via Ca^{2+};

3. While modification of His 48 does abolish both enzymatic and pharmacological activity, other chemical modifications may selectively affect one activity or the other. Manoalide, which is isolated from a sponge, is a potent PLA_2 inhibitor that can decrease the presynaptic action of β-bungarotoxin (De Freitas, Blankemeir, and Jacobs 1984). No relationship was found between the concentrations required to inhibit PLA_2 enzymatic activity *in vitro* and to block neurotoxicity of β-bungarotoxin.

4. Ultrastructural changes need not be due to PLA_2 action but could be associated with a direct membrane disruptive action as we suggest occurs with *N. nigricollis* PLA_2.

In conclusion while I would agree with those investigators who say that potency and specificity of action may be due to specific binding sites in the presynaptic terminal while the PLA_2 activity of the toxins may be essential for the alterations in neurotransmitter release, I would qualify this by saying that this conclusion has not been unequivocally demonstrated. Some uncertainty will remain until a suitable preparation has been found where the degree of phospholipid hydrolysis at the site of action can be correlated with relative neurotoxic potency. Even if PLA_2 activity is essential, the role of secondary products of its action (thromboxanes, fatty acids, etc.) must be more thoroughly evaluated.

Central nervous system effects

A purified preparation of PLA_2 from *N. nigricollis* venom reduced the uptake of acetylcholine and increased the release of radioactive acetylcholine from preloaded slices of mouse cerebral cortex (Heilbronn 1969). The PLA_2 also caused vacuolization and the formation of electron-dense particles in the cortex slices. Histidine uptake into mouse brain slices was also reduced by a purified PLA_2 isolated from *Hemachatus haemachatus* venom (Kirschmann, Ten-Ami, Smorodinski, and De Vries 1971), an effect which was associated with a 10–30 per cent hydrolysis of the brain phospholipids. A partially purified PLA_2 from *V. russelli* venom markedly inhibited the uptake of norepinephrine into synaptosomes from the guinea-pig cerebral cortex and inhibited (Na + K)-ATPase activity (Sun 1974). Lysophosphatidylcholine had similar effects but the synaptosomal particles were not disrupted after PLA_2 treatment. It is unclear whether these are direct effects or are caused by a detergent action of liberated lysophosphatides.

There have been a few studies concerned with the ability of PLA_2 to alter ligand/receptor binding in the central nervous system. Pasternak and Snyder (1974) studied the effects of various enzymes, including PLA_2, on the stereospecific binding of (^{3}H)-naloxone to rat brain homogenates. Relatively low concentrations of PLA_2 inhibited binding, but high concentrations of lysophosphatidylcholine were required for the same effect. Purified PLA_2 isolated from bee venom markedly decreased the binding of γ-aminobutyric acid (GABA) to junctional complexes isolated from the rat cerebellum (Giambalvo and Rosenberg 1976). Inhibition of binding was correlated with the extent of splitting of phospholipids, and lysophosphatidylcholine had effects identical to those of PLA_2. In this same study it was found that hydrolysis of the polar head groups of the phospholipids with PLC markedly increased GABA binding to synaptosomes. Venom PLA_2 inhibited spiperone binding to dopamine receptors in microsomal membranes from sheep caudate nucleus (Oliveira, Duarte, and Carvalto 1984), but the actions of PLA_2 seemed to be due to an alteration of the membrane by lysophospholipids.

Following intraventricular injection into the brain, presynaptic toxins cause neuronal degeneration, an increased efflux, and inhibit influx of choline, acetylcholine, noradrenalin, GABA, and serotonin in brain minces or synaptosomes (Sen, Grantham, and Cooper 1976: Sen and Cooper 1975; Wernicke, Oberjat, and Howard 1974; Hawley and Emson 1979).

N. nigricollis, *N. n. atra*, and *H. haemachatus* PLA_2 induce, after a 2–4 hour latency, recurrent convulsant episodes lasting several hours. *N. nigricollis* PLA_2 is, however, effective in about one-tenth the dose of the other two enzymes (Fletcher *et al.* 1980). There was no significant difference in phospholipid hydrolysis in the various brain regions to explain the difference in potency (Fletcher *et al.* 1980). Even in isolated synaptic plasma membrane fractions obtained from brain following intraventricular PLA_2 injection, there is no relationship between lethal potency and phospholipid hydrolysis (Condrea *et al.* 1981a). What appears, however, to be directly related to the lethal potency of the phospholipases, is their ability to bind to synaptic plasma membranes *in vivo* or *in vitro* (Rapuano, Yang, and Rosenberg, unpublished observations). Multiple specific and non-specific binding components were demonstrated for both iodinated *N. nigricollis* and *N. n. atra* PLA$_2$ enzymes, but the binding of the *N. nigricollis* enzyme was about tenfold greater than that of the *N. n. atra* enzyme, measured either in the presence or absence of Ca^{2+} (Fig. 9.1). The binding in the presence and absence of Ca^{2+} was very similar, suggesting that binding is independent of phospholipid hydrolysis (especially since EDTA was present in the Ca^{2+}-free medium, assuring that no phospholipid hydrolysis occurred). The effects of heat and enzyme (trypsin, chymotrypsin, etc.) treatment suggest that the phospholipases bind to phospholipids rather than proteins. Carbamylation of lysine residues in the two PLA$_2$ enzymes reduced binding (Fig. 9.1) and lethal potency (Table 9.9) equally, while having little effect

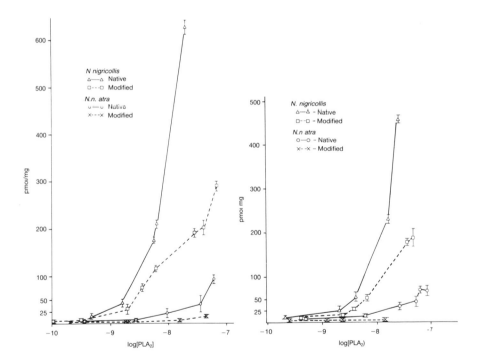

Fig. 9.1 Total binding to brain synaptic plasma membranes of radioiodinated native and carbamylated (modified *N. nigricollis* (8.2 of 10 lysines modified) and *N. n. atra* (3.2 of 5 lysines modified) PLA$_2$ *in vitro* in a normal calcium medium (left) or a calcium-free medium containing EDTA (right). Values are presented as means ± SE ($n = 3$). (Rapuano, Yang, and Rosenberg, unpublished observations.)

Table 9.9 The effects of modification of *N. nigricollis* and *N. n. atra* PLA$_2$ on V_{max} and lethal potency.

Modification		V_{max}		IVR lethality (per cent of native)	
		N.nig	*N.n.atra*	*N.nig.*	*N.n.atra*
His–48					
Alkylation		0.8	0.2	2	<2
Methylation		1.0	0.2	<3	<2
Arginines					
pH 7.5		—	62	—	63
pH 8.5		—	42	—	<13
Lysines					
Carbamylation	(a)	89	90	57	7
	(b)	49	87	13	<3
Acylation	(c)	28	43	13	12
	(d)	40	69	13	25
Guanidination	(e)	108	113	13	67
Aspartic acids					
pH 3.5	(f)	<1	1	5	29
pH 5.5		<1	2	5	29
pH 5.5 + Ca^{2+}		16	13	33	550
Tryptophan	(g)	64	51	67	54
Tyrosine					
3	(h)	49	47	50	625
62(63)		22	11	2	<12
3 + 62(63)		9	6	5	<12

(a) = 7.4 of 10 (*N.n.*) and 1.2 of 5 (*N.n.a.*) modified.
(b) = 9.0 of 10 (*N.n.*) and 4.2 of 5 (*N.n.a.*) modified.
(c) = EOFA (ethoxyformic anhydride) 20 mM (*N.n.*) and 10 mM, fr. b (*N.n.a.*).
(d) = EOFA 20 mM + dihexanoyl lecithin (DiC$_6$) (*N.n.*) and EOFA 10 mM + DiC$_6$, Fr. 2 (*N.n.a.*).
(e) = 9.4 of 10 (*N.n.*) and 4.5 of 5 (*N.n.a.*) modified.
(f) = All carboxyl groups of glutamic and aspartic acid modified except Asp 99 (pH 3.5), Asp 99 + 39 (Asp 5.5), Asp 99 + 39 + 49 (pH 5.5 + Ca^{2+}).
(g) = 2.4 of 3 (*N.n.*) and 3.0 of 3 (*N.n.a.*) modified.
(h) = Tyr. 3, 62(3), or 3 + 62(63) modified.

on enzymatic activity (Table 9.10; Condrea *et al.* 1981a; Rapuano, Yang, and Rosenberg, unpublished observations).

Actions on muscle

Pure PLA$_2$ from bee venom depolarized and decreased the resistance of the extensor digitorum longus and soleus muscles of the rat, effects that were mimicked by lysophosphatidylcholine (Albuquerque and Thesleff 1968). There was, however, little effect on membrane excitability or on sensitivity

Table 9.10 Effects of modification of *N. nigricollis* and *N. n. atra* PLA$_2$ on haemolytic and anticoagulant activity.

	V_{max}		Haemolytic (per cent of native)		Anticoagulant (per cent of native)	
	N.nig.	*N.n.atra*	*N.nig.*	*N.n.atra*	*N.nig.*	*N.n.atra*
His–48						
Alkylation	0.8	0.2	10	—	—	—
Methylation	1.0	0.2	10	0	2	<4
Arginines						
pH 7.5	—	62	—	—	8	63
pH 8.5	—	42	—	—	—	21
Lysines						
Carbamylation (a)	89	90	100	—	—	—
(b)	49	87	<50	—	3	<5
Acylation						
—EOFA 10 mM	43	43	—	—	—	50
—EOFA 20 mM	33	69	—	—	—	10
Guanidination (c)	108	113	100	—	50	—
Aspartic acids						
pH 3.5 (d)	<1	1	20	35	5	<5
pH 5.5	<1	2	20	25	1	<3
pH 5.5 + Ca^{2+}	16	13	65	<100	50	50
Tryptophan (e)	64	51	29	—	50	—
Tyrosine						
3 (f)	49	47	77	+	50	100
62(63)	22	11	40	0	50	25
3 + 62(63)	9	6	—	0	12	25

Haemolytic activity only observed with high concentrations of *N.n.atra* PLA$_2$, long periods of incubation, and dilute solutions of red blood cells.
  (a) = 7.4 of 10 (*N.n.*) and 1.2 of 5 (*N.n.a.*) modified.
  (b) = 9.0 of 10 (*N.n.*) and 4.2 of 5 (*N.n.a.*) modified.
  (c) = 9.4 of 10 (*N.n.*) and 4.5 of 5 (*N.n.a.*) modified.
  (d) = All carboxyl groups of glutamic and aspartic acid modified except Asp 99 (pH 3.5), Asp 99 + 39 (pH 5.5), Asp 99 + 39 + 49 (pH 5.5 + Ca^{2+}).
  (e) = 2.4 of 3 (*N.n.*) and 3.0 of 3 (*N.n.a.*) modified.
  (f) = Tyr 3, 62(63), or 3 + 62(63) modified.

of denervated fibres to acetylcholine. *Crotalus* PLA$_2$ alone in combination with crotapotin decreased contractions of the isolated chick biventer cervicis muscle, but did not cause a contracture (Breithaupt 1976), indicating that they are not depolarizing blockers. Sket and Gubensek (1976), found that two PLA$_2$ fractions, isolated from *V. ammodytes* venom, caused a contracture of the guinea pig ileum in very low concentrations (6.6×10^{-9} M). A possible mechanism of action involving the formation of prostraglandins was suggested in this smooth muscle preparation, but not proven.

PLC will block conduction in muscles with sodium-generated action potentials, but has no effect on muscles with calcium-generated action potentials (Johansson and Thesleff 1968). These findings were related to the extent of phospholipid hydrolysis in sarcolemmal preparations purified from various muscles (Knickelbein and Rosenberg 1980). Whereas sphingomyelin (SM), phosphatidylcholine (PC), and phosphatidylethanolamine (PE) were extensively hydrolysed in all of the sarcolemmal preparations, PI and PS were only hydrolysed in muscles with sodium generated action potentials and hydrolysis was less in the presence of tetrodotoxin. These results suggest that phosphatidylinositol (PI) and phosphatidylserine (PS) may be associated with the sodium and calcium channels but that only in the sodium channels are the phospholipids accessible to PLC.

PLC (*C. perfringens*) stimulates NA^+-dependent Ca^{2+} uptake in purified cardiac sarcolemmal vesicles, when 10 to 70 per cent of the membrane phospholipid (PC, PE, SM) is hydrolysed (Philipson *et al*. 1983). The acidic phospholipids PS and PI were not hydrolysed and seem to be sufficient to ensure adequate Na^+-Ca^{2+} exchange activity, even in the presence of gross morphological changes induced by PLC.

The approximately fifteenfold greater intravenous lethal potency of *N. nigricollis* PLA_2 relative to *N. n. atra* or *H. haemachatus* PLA_2 (Table 9.8) appears to be due to a specific, more potent cardiotoxic action possessed by the *N. nigricollis* enzyme (Fletcher *et al*. 1981; Fletcher, Yang, and Rosenberg 1982).

In the above and in many other studies it has been consistently demonstrated that the cardiotoxic action of *N. nigricollis* PLA_2 in rat heart is due to a direct non-enzymatic action (Fletcher *et al*. 1980, 1981, 1982; Soons, Yang, and Rosenberg, 1984; Barrington, Yang and Rosenberg, 1984a; Barrington *et al*. 1984b; Condrea, Soons, Barrington, Yang, and Rosenberg 1985). This has been determined by direct comparisons of cardiotoxicity and phospholipid hydrolysis.

To see if differing cardiotoxic potency was related to differences in the extent of binding, iodinated *N. nigricollis* and *N. n. atra* PLA_2 enzymes were incubated with isolated rat ventricle preparations (Soons *et al*. 1984). Both enzymes bound to a similar number of partially overlapping binding sites. A 100-fold excess of non-radioactive *N. n. atra* PLA_2 decreased the binding of radioactive *N. n. atra* enzyme, as expected, due to displacement of specific binding. In a marked and unexpected contrast to this, a 100-fold excess of cold *N. nigricollis* PLA_2 more than doubled the binding of the radioactive *N. nigricollis* enzyme. This effect was not dependent upon enzymatic activity since the same effect was observed in the presence or absence of Ca^{2+}; under these conditions very low ($+ Ca^{2+}$) or no ($- Ca^{2+}$) *in vivo* phospholipid hydrolysis was observed. Also, this effect of the non-radioactive *N. nigricollis* PLA$_2$ could be mimicked by the cationic detergent cetyltrimethyl ammonium bromide. The ability of the non-radioactive *N. nigricollis* PLA$_2$ to expose additional binding sites to the radioactive enzyme appears to be due to a disruptive action, which may also be responsible for the direct haemolytic action of the enzyme (Condrea *et al.* 1980).

Since cardiac tissue has a high content of arachidonic acid at the Sn-2 position of the major membrane phospholipids, it was of interest to test whether increased prostaglandin synthesis could contribute to the cardiotoxic effects of *N. nigricollis* PLA$_2$ (Barrington, Soons, and Rosenberg, unpublished observations). Intracellular action potentials and cardiac contractility were monitored in the isolated right ventricular wall of a rat heart exposed for 1 h to *N. nigricollis* PLA$_2$, with or without indomethacin, or to arachidonic acid. The tissues were homogenized, prostaglandins were extracted, and the 6-keto PGF$_1$ and PGE$_2$ contents of the hearts were determined. The physiological effects and prostaglandin content of hearts treated with *N. nigricollis* PLA$_2$ were not altered by indomethacin nor mimicked by concentrations of arachidonic acid comparable to that present in *N. nigricollis* PLA$_2$-treated tissue. The effects of *N. nigricollis* PLA$_2$, indomethacin, and arachidonic acid on peak amplitude of cardiac contraction and resting tension are shown in Fig. 9.2. These results support our previous suggestion that exogenously applied *N. nigricollis* PLA$_2$ causes cardiotoxic effects by a mechanism that is independent of phospholipid hydrolysis.

The direct effects on muscle of these PLA$_2$ enzymes somewhat resemble the actions of cardiotoxins from venoms on excitable cells (Condrea 1974, 1979; Chang 1979); that is, the PLA$_2$ molecule may possess independent sites responsible for cardiotoxicity and enzymatic activity. Under conditions where a PLA$_2$ enhanced the haemolytic action of cardiotoxins, it had no effect on the contactures induced by cardiotoxin in chick muscle (Harvey, Hider, and Khader 1983).

Some presynaptic toxins with PLA$_2$ activity, such as notexin and taipoxin, are myotoxic causing necrosis of skeletal muscle, independent of their effects on nerve (Harris, Johnson, and Karlsson 1975; Lee, Chen, and Karlsson 1976; Harris and Johnson 1978; Harris and Maltin 1982). Covalent modification of histidine at the enzymatic active site causes a decrease of both PLA$_2$ activity and myotoxicity (Harris and Johnson 1978). However, in this study the loss in myotoxicity was only about one-tenth the loss in enzymatic activity. As discussed elsewhere, observations with covalent modification of His 48 alone are insufficient to reach a conclusion as to whether phospholipid hydrolysis is essential to the toxin's action. Crotoxin, from the South American rattlesnake, has both pre- and postsynaptic physiological effects (including myotoxicity, which was suggested as being due to disruption of the sarcolemmal membrane), mitochondrial changes,

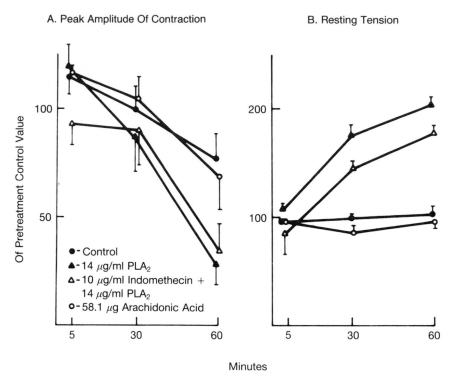

Fig. 9.2 The sequence of contractile changes in right ventricular wall of the rat heart following PLA$_2$ and arachidonic acid. the time courses are presented for: 14 μg *N. nigricollis* PLA$_2$ per ml (▲, $n = 8$); 58.1 lμg ml^{-1} arachidonic acid (0, $n = 5$); 10 μg indomethacin plus 14 μg PLA$_2$ per ml (△, $n = 5$); and control (●, $n = 6$). All points are means ± SE (Barrington, Soons, Yang, and Rosenberg, unpublished observations).

and internal calcium ion accumulation (Gopalakrishnakone, Dempster, Hawgood, and Elder 1984). The involvement of phospholipid hydrolysis in these effects was presumed but not proven.

Effects on blood

The haemolytic action of PLC enzymes from various bacterial organisms has been extensively studied (for review see Ikezawa *et al.* 1982–83). Their haemolytic potency is dependent upon the substrate specificity of the enzyme, the phospholipid composition and the distribution of phospholipids within the red cell membrane. The erythrocytes from various species differ in their sphingomyelin content; those with the highest content are most liable to lysis. Some PLC enzymes cannot hydrolyse phospholipids in the intact erythrocyte. There is thus a clear relationship between the extent of phospholipid hydrolysis in the erythrocyte membrane and the haemolytic potency of PLC enzymes.

Various physiological agonists such as thrombin and platelet activating factor induce platelet activation by stimulation of endogenous PLC, an effect that is independent of liberation or metabolism of arachidonic acid (Lapetina and Siess 1983; Siess, Weber, and Lapetina 1984). The PLC-induced activation of platelets is dependent on PI hydrolysis and associated Ca^{2+} mobilization, but not dependent on phosphatidic acid production, thromboxane, or ADP secretion (Billah and Lapetina 1983; Navran, Romstedt, Chang, Miller, Feller, and Akbar 1984). Platelet activating factor (1-*O*-alkyl-2-acetyl-*sn*-glycero-3-phosphocholine) is a bioactive phospholipid released from leukocytes which in addition to a hypotensive action, activates and degranulates platelets and stimulates PLA_2 and PLC activities in platelets and fibroblasts (Kawaguchi and Yasuda 1984).

The ability of *N. nigricollis* PLA_2 to haemolyse red blood cells directly (Condrea *et al.* 1980) and exert a potent anticoagulant action (Condrea, Yang, and Rosenberg 1981d, 1982, 1983c) contrasts markedly with the relatively weak haemolytic and anticoagulant activity of *N. n. atra* and *H. haemachatus* PLA_2. *N. nigricollis* enzyme haemolyses and hydrolyses phospholipids of fresh guinea pig cells and of human red cells separated from stored outdated blood. Previous reports on a direct lytic effect of the *N. nigricollis* PLA_2 have appeared in the literature (Dumarey, Sket, Joseph, and Boquet 1975; Lee, Ho, and Eaker 1977). Another basic PLA_2 from *Agkistrodon halys blomhofii* venom directly haemolysed and induced phospholipid hydrolysis in human red cells when the reaction was carried out at elevated pH or at increased Ca^{2+} (Martin, Luthra, Wells, Watts, and Hanahan 1975). The direct lytic and phospholipid splitting ability of the *N. nigricollis* enzyme resembles the synergistic effects induced by a combination of direct lytic factor and PLA_2 (Condrea 1979). It seemed an attractive speculation that the *N. nigricollis* PLA_2, a protein with both positive charge and enzymatic activity, combines the properties of the direct lytic factor and PL activity in the same molecule. The question of whether the direct lytic and phospholipid splitting ability of the *N. nigricollis* enzyme resembles the synergistic effects induced by a combination of direct lytic factor and PLA_2 (Condrea, 1979). It seemed an attractive speculation that the *N. nigricollis* PLA_2, a protein with both positive charge and enzymatic activity, combines the properties of the direct lytic factor and PL activity in the same molecule. The question of whether the direct lytic property is unique to basic phospholipases has been asked before. Reports by Martin *et al.* (1975) and by Haest and Deuticke (1976) document the fact that an acidic phospholipase isolated from *N. naja* is also capable of inducing direct haemolysis and phospholipid hydrolysis of human erythrocytes at elevated pH and 40 nM Ca^{2+} or at neutral pH and 10 mM Ca^{2+} following preincubation of the cells for 24 h in glucose-free medium. Both the *Crotalus adamanteus* enzyme and the acidic phospholipase from *A. h. blomhofii* were inactive in the above conditions (Martin *et al.* 1975).

The relationship between haemolytic activity and phospholipid hydrolysis in erythrocytes has been reviewed by Condrea (1979), Avigad (1976) and Alouf (1977). Hydrolysis of the phospholipids on the inner leaflet of the red cell membrane bilayer is associated with haemolysis whereas non-haemolytic PL enzymes attack only the external phospholipids. It must be born in mind, however, that the ability of a PL enzyme to reach the inner phospholipids in the intact erythrocyte may be determined by properties other than enzymatic activity, for example, direct lytic, detergent, or other membrane perturbing effects may be involved. Thus, *N. nigricollis* PLA$_2$ can hydrolyse the inner phospholipids of the red cell membrane, whereas *N. n. atra* PLA$_2$ cannot, even though *N. nigricollis* PLA$_2$ has lower enzymatic activity and no unique phospholipid specificity as compared to *N. n. atra* PLA$_2$.

The differences in anticoagulant potency between *N. nigricollis* and several other PLA$_2$ enzymes could not be related to differences in phospholipid hydrolysis; for example, *N. nigricollis* is a potent anticoagulant at doses which cause less phospholipid hydrolysis than is caused by non-anticoagulant doses of *N. n. atra* or *H. haemachatus* PLA$_2$ (Table 9.11).

It appeared that the differences between the phospholipases had to be in their differing abilities to disrupt organized membrane (surface) structures, rather than in differences in enzymatic activity. Evidence for such an explanation was found in studies on plasma lipoproteins (Zan, Condrea, Yang, and Rosenberg 1983). *N. nigricollis* PLA$_2$ showed almost equal ability to hydrolyse phospholipids (PC and PE) in the more organized structure of high density lipoprotein (HDL) and the less constrained phospholipids in very low density lipoprotein (VLDL), whereas *N. n. atra* PLA$_2$ hydrolysed the phospholipids much more effectively in VLDL than in HDL. Detergent treatment of HDL and VLDL eliminated this difference between the *N. nigricollis* and *N. n. atra* enzymes. The direct membrane-penetrating ability of these phospholipases is important in determining the overall hydrolytic rate on organized structures. The *N. nigricollis* PLA$_2$ probably exerts its anticoagulant action by formation of a complex between the enzyme and plasma phospholipids, rendering the latter unavailable as catalytic surfaces for the coagulation proteins (Boffa and Boffa 1976; Boffa, Delori, and Soulier 1972; Boffa, Verheij, and De Haas 1982; Prigent-Dachary, Boffa, Boisseau, and Dufourcq 1980). Strong inhibitors of coagulation bind to phospholipids, especially PS, and do not require Ca^{2+} for this interaction (Prigent-Dachary *et al.* 1980). Whether phospholipid hydrolysis is essential to the coagulant action was not considered in this study.

Our conclusion that anticoagulant potency is not related to phospholipid

Table 9.11 Phospholipid hydrolysis and anticoagulant activity of PLA$_2$ on rabbit platelet-poor plasma.

Phospholipases		Lipids	Per cent hydrolysis at:				
			45 s	1 min 45 s	4 min 30 s	9 min	30 min
N.n.	0.062 μg	PC	1	3	2̲	9	30
		PE	0	7	1̲3̲	14	50
		TPL	0.7	2	2̲	7	23
	0.250 μg	PC	10	14		53	86
		PE	34	35		69	100
		TPL	9	11		40	64
N.n.a.	0.5 μg	PC	61	75	8̲9̲	95	100
		PE	75	83	1̲0̲0̲	100	100
		TPL	46	56	6̲6̲	71	74
	5.0 μg	PC	92	97		99	100
		PE	100	100		100	100
		TPL	68	72		73	74
H.h.	1.0 μg	PC	27	46	7̲0̲	78	90
		PE	45	59	7̲9̲	100	100
		TPl	?1	35	5̲3̲	59	67
	5.0 μg	PC	84	90		100	100
		PE	90	96		100	100
		TPL	62	67		74	74

One-millilitre plasma samples were supplemented with enzyme, recalcified, and extracted for lipids at the times indicated. Recalcification time of control plasma was 1 min 45 s. The values underlined show the extent of phospholipid hydrolysis at the time of clotting. Note that the highest concentration of each phospholipase shown was the minimal concentration required to prevent clotting (730 min). The sum of hydrolysable substrates in plasma is 74 per cent of TPL. Values are means of duplicate samples, the individual values being within ± 1 per cent of the means shown.

Abbreviations: *N.n.*, *Naja nigricollis*; *H.h.*, *Hemachatus haemachatus*; *N.n.a.*, *Naja naja atra*; PC, phosphatidylcholine; PE, phosphatidylethanolamine; TPL, total phospholipid.

(Table modified from Condrea, Fletcher, Rapuano, Yang, and Rosenberg (1981c).

hydrolysis was questioned (Verheij, Boffa, Rotnen, Bryckaert, Verger, and De Haas 1980; Boffa *et al.* 1982) on the basis of experiments using added rather than endogenous phospholipids and because in our first studies we had not monitored hydrolysis of PS, the major procoagulant phospholipid. However, results with *N. nigricollis* PLA$_2$ in which lysines were carbamylated (Condrea *et al.* 1982), showed that anticoagulant activity was lost while enzymatic activity was unaffected, and studies in which we monitored PS hydrolysis (Condrea *et al.* 1983c) strengthened our conclusion that the extent of phospholipid hydrolysis is not directly related to anticoagulant potency. Our conclusion was strengthened by the finding of Boffa, Barbier, and de Angulo (1983) that cardiotoxins have anticoagulant activity even though they do not have any PLA_2 activity. The cardiotoxins do, however, have all the other features that distinguish non-anticoagulant PLA_2 enzymes from anticoagulant (e.g. *N. nigricollis* PLA_2) enzymes, i.e. basicity, high penetrability, and preference for interacting with negatively charged phospholipids.

Effects of chemical modification on enzymatic and pharmacological properties of phospholipases

An excellent review of the effects of chemical modification on the enzymatic properties of PLA_2 appeared in 1981 (Verheij *et al.* 1981). The effects of chemical modification on pharmacological properties were, however, not discussed, since there have been few systematic studies on the relationship between PLA_2 enzymatic activity and pharmacological properties subsequent to chemical modification.

Our approach in studying the relationship between enzymatic and pharmacological properties was to see if by chemical modifications of various amino acid residues in the PLA_2 we could selectively decrease enzymatic activity or pharmacological and lethal properties. A summary of the chemical modifications which we have made in the amino acid side chains of *N. nigricollis* and *N. n. atra* PLA_2 enzymes is shown in Table 9.10. A summary of how chemical modification affects and enzymatic activity (lecithin–triton, 1:2, mixed micelles) and intraventricular lethal potency in rats is shown in Table 9.9. The effects of chemical modification on hemolytic and anticoagulant activity and the relationship to PLA_2 activity are shown in Table 9.10.

In agreement with results of others (see Verheij *et al.* 1981 for references) we found that bromphenacylation of histidine 48 at the active site in the PLA_2 enzymes from *N. nigricollis*, *H. haemachatus*, and *N. naja atra* snake venoms reduced the enzymatic activity to 0.2–0.8 per cent that of the native species, while the K_m values remained practically unchanged (Condrea *et al.* 1981c). Also unchanged following modification were the characteristic substrate specificities of the three enzymes. It appears most likely that the residual activity of the modified enzymes originates from contamination by non-modified species. The decrease in enzymatic activity was accompanied by a decrease in all other biochemical and physiological parameters studied such as direct haemolysis (for *N. nigricollis* PLA_2), ability to hydrolyse red cell phospholipids, intravenous LD_{50} in mice, intraventricular LD_{50} in rats, brain phospholipid hydrolysis, and ability to block action potentials in eel electroplax. The effect of methylation of the histidine 48 position of *N. nigricollis* and *N. n. atra* PLA_2 was also determined (Condrea,

Rapuano, Soons, Yang, and Rosenberg 1983b). Following methylation a very low residual enzymatic activity (0.4–1 per cent of control) was accompanied by a parallel loss in intraventricular lethality, anticoagulant potency, direct haemolytic action, and ability to block directly and indirectly evoked contractions of the mouse phrenic nerve diaphragm preparation. Since methylation does not impair the enzyme's ability to bind monomeric or micellar substrates or Ca^{2+}, the results suggest that the pharmacologically active region of the molecule is different from the micellar substrate binding site but strongly influenced by the invariant histidine-48 located at the enzymatic active site. These results if considered alone would suggest that catalytic activity is essential for the lethal and pharmacological actions of these PLA_2 enzymes. However, our results, described previously with the native enzymes, suggested that some pharmacological actions of these PLA_2 enzymes (e.g. cardiotoxicity, anticoagulant activity) are not due to phospholipid hydrolysis. The possibility existed, therefore, that the enzymatic and pharmacological properties of the enzymes were determined by two separate active sites of the protein, but these sites overlapped in the region of histidine-48. Alternatively, modification at the known enzymatic active site at histidine-48 could cause changes in the configuration of the molecule at separate pharmacologically active sites, some distance from the enzymatic active site. It was, therefore, thought essential to carry out other amino acid side chain modifications to see if any change gave rise to a dissociation between pharmacological and enzymatic activity.

We found that modification of basic amino acid residues (arginine, lysine) using several different types of reagents (Table 9.12) decreases pharmacological activity more than enzymatic activity (Tables 9.9 and 9.10). The extent of arginine modification is greater at pH 8.5 than at pH 7.5 and at this more alkaline pH lethal and anticoagulant potency were decreased to a greater extent than enzymatic activity (Condrea, Rapuano, Fletcher, Yang, and Rosenberg 1981b). These results suggested that extensive modification of catalytically non-essential residues may influence the pharmacological functions of the molecule. A more marked dissociation between pharmacological and enzymatic activity was noted when the basic side chain residues of lysine were carbamylated (Condrea *et al.* 1981a), ethoxyformylated or guanidinated (Condrea, Rapuano, Fletcher, Yang, and Rosenberg 1983a; Tables 9.11 and 9.12). Carbamylation of nine out of ten lysine residues in the toxic PLA_2 from *N. nigricollis* venom decreased its lethality at least eightfold and abolished its direct haemolytic and anticoagulant activities, while the enzymatic activity, as measured on purified substrates, fell by 50 per cent. Likewise, carbamylation of three out of five lysines in the relatively less toxic *N. naja atra* PLA_2, induced detoxification and caused a loss of its blocking activity on the phrenic nerve diaphragm preparation, while its enzymatic activity on purified substrates was

Table 9.12 Amino acid residue modification of phospholipases.

Group modified	Treatment	Result
Histidine-48	p-bromophenacyl bromide	Alkylation
Histidine-48	Methyl-p-nitrobenzene-sulfonate	Methylation
Lysines	Potassium cyanate	Carbamylation
Lysines (+ histidine?)	Ethoxyformic anhydride	Acylation
Lysines	O-methylisourea	Guanidination lysines-homoarginine
Arginines	Phenylglyoxal	Diphenylglyoxalation
Aspartic and glutamic acids (free carboxyls)	1-ethyl-3(3-dimethylaminopropyl) carbodiimide + semicarbazide	Semicarbazide addition
Tryptophan	2-hydroxy-5-nitrobenzylbromide	Alkylation
Tyrosine	p-nitrobenzene-sulphonyl fluoride	Nitrobenzene sulphonylation

unaltered. Results obtained when seven out of ten lysines in *N. nigricollis* PLA$_2$ were carbamylated indicate that basicity is not an absolute requirement for high lethal potency, haemolytic activity, or cardiotoxicity. The enzymatic and pharmacological potencies of this derivative were hardly affected, even though the isoelectric point of the *N. nigricollis* PLA$_2$ decreased from pH 10.6 to pH 5.4. The extent of phospholipid hydrolysis induced in erythrocytes, rabbit plasma, phrenic nerve diaphragm preparation, brain minces, and brain synaptic plasma membranes by incubation with the carbamylated enzymes was in agreement with their enzymatic activities as measured on purified substrates. Levels of phospholipid hydrolysis in heart, lung, and kidney of mice given phospholipase intraventricularly, showed that carbamylated derivatives of *N. nigricollis* PLA$_2$ lost their ability to reach and/or hydrolyse substrates *in vivo*. However, the decrease in phospholipid hydrolysis *in vivo* did not correlate with the decrease in toxicity, since at comparably low levels of phospholipid hydrolysis some phospholipases were lethal and others were not. Moreover, when intraventricular administration was used, both lethal amounts of the native *N. naja atra* enzyme and its non-lethal carbamylated derivatives produced equally low levels of hydrolysis of synaptic membrane phospholipids. Lysine residues were also modified by acylation with ethoxyformic anhydride (in the presence or absence of the substrate dihexanoyl lecithin) or guanidination with O-methylisourea. Ethoxyformylation gave rise to some protein fractions in which enzymatic activity was preserved to a greater degree than intraventricular lethality. Guanidination had little effect on the isoelectric point of catalytic activity of either enzyme or on the lethal potency of the *N. n. atra* enzyme. However, the intraventricular lethality of the *N. nigricollis* enzyme was decreased much more than were its intravenous lethality, direct haemolytic potency, anticoagulant activity, or cardiotoxic action on rat atrium. When these results are compared to those previously obtained when the lysines in these two enzymes were carbamylated with potassium cyanate (a procedure that markedly decreased the isoelectric point of the enzymes) it can be concluded that charge alone does not account for differences in toxicity. The data also indicates that there are at least two distinct active sites in both enzymes, one being primarily responsible for enzymatic activity and the other(s) associated with lethal and pharmacological effects of the protein. Modification of lysines affects the latter site(s), while having little or no effect on enzymatic activity. Ethoxyformylation in the presence and absence of the phospholipid substrate DiC_6 (to protect the enzymatic active site against acylation) has been used in attempting to evaluate whether enzymatic activity is essential for the lethal and pharmacological properties of proteins having phospholipase activity. Ethoxyformylation would be primarily expected to acylate histidine and lysine residues (Spande, Witkop, Degani, and Patchornik 1970; Melchior and Fahrney 1970; Halpert 1979). It is not likely that histidine-48 at the enzymatic site of the enzyme is acylated, since our previous results showed that this would lead to complete loss of both enzymatic and pharmacological effects (Condrea *et al.* 1981c), whereas Condrea *et al.* (1983a) showed only partial loss of these activities. This finding is also in agreement with previous conclusions that any histidines modified are not at the active site (Halpert 1979). Treatment of Eastern diamondback rattlesnake (*Crotalus adamanteus*) PLA_2 with 30 nM ethoxyformic anhydride (EOFA) induced enzymatic inactivation upon acylation of one lysine residue per dimer, while histidine residues did not react (Wells 1973). Halpert (1979) found, following treatment of notechis II-5 and notexin (two presynaptically acting neurotoxins that have PLA_2 activity) with EOFA, that one histidine residue (not at the enzymatic active site) and one lysine residue were ethoxyformylated. Associated with the moficiations were loss of both enzymatic activity and lethality. Likewise, EOFA treatment inactivated both PLA_2 activity and neurotoxicity of β-bungarotoxin, a presynaptically acting toxin (Howard and Truog 1977; Ng and Howard 1978). EOFA treatment of a nonneurotoxic PLA_2 enzyme of relatively low lethality also caused the loss of enzymatic activity, as well as its ability to inhibit GABA uptake into synaptosomes and Ca^{2+} uptake into sarcoplasmic reticulum (Ng and Howard 1978, 1980). Of special interest is the observation that if ethoxyformylation was carried out in the presence of the phospholipid substrate DiC_6, the PLA_2 activity was conserved while the lethality and neurotoxicity of β-bungarotoxin (Howard and Truog 1977; Ng and Howard 1978, 1980) and notexin (Halpert 1979) was decreased or lost. Ethoxyformylation in the presence of substrate therefore converted neurotoxic into non-neurotoxic phospholipases. In contrast, treatment of a non-neurotoxic PLA_2 of relatively low lethal potency with DiC_6 completely protected enzyme activity as well as pharmacological actions against the inhibitory actions of EOFA (Ng and Howard 1978, 1980). The above results suggested to the authors that EOFA modifies two sites on the neurotoxic phospholipases, one of which is responsible for enzymatic activity, while the other is primarily responsible for neurotoxicity. In contrast, non-neurotoxic phospholipases were suggested to have only a single active site, the enzymatic site, with all pharmacological effects being directly related to enzymatic activity. We found a greater preservation of enzymatic activity than of intraventricular lethality following EOFA or EOFA plus DiC_6 treatment of *N. nigricollis* and of *N. n. atra* PLA_2. These results reinforce our previous conclusion (Condrea *et al.* 1981a) that it is possible to dissociate enzymatic activity from pharmacological effects in both the highly toxic *N. nigricollis* enzyme and in the less toxic *N. n. atra* enzyme, suggesting the presence of at least two distinct active sites in both enzymes.

The opposite type of association was observed when the free carboxyl groups of aspartic and glutamic acid were modified (Tables 9.11 and 9.12; Rosenberg, Condrea, Rapuano, 1983a; Barrington *et al.* 1984b). For the first time, derivatives of PLA_2 were obtained that retained greater pharmacological than enzymatic activity. By treating *N. nigricollis* PLA_2 with carbodiimide and semicarbazide, we obtained derivatives having varied numbers of modified carboxylate groups. When tested on artificial and natural substrates, derivatives of both enzymes with a modified carboxylate group at the active site (Asp-49) retained little enzymatic activity (<1–10 per cent) and also lost most of their lethal potency (5–29 per cent of native enzyme). Carboxyl modification with protection of Asp-49 in *N. n. atra* enzyme resulted in a derivative with lethal potency equal to or greater than the native enzyme and enzymatic activity that was low on all substrates (12–17 per cent of native enzyme). Similar protection of Asp-49 at the active site in *N. nigricollis* enzyme produced a derivative with decreased enzymatic activity on artificial substrate (22 per cent of native enzyme) and decreased lethality (17–33 per cent of native enzyme), but with full enzymatic activity on natural substrates. This difference in enzymatic activity, dependent on the substrate employed (Table 5.6), has already been commented upon. When tested on electrical and mechanical properties of the isolated perfused heart and the isolated ventricle muscle wall, the derivatives of both enzymes retained considerably more of the cardiotoxic activity than would have been expected on the basis of their residual enzymatic activity. The one exception occurred with the least-modified *N. nigricollis* derivative, which had an unaltered Asp-49; this enzyme retained both cardiotoxic activity and full enzymatic activity on natural substrates. The extent of phospholipid hydrolysis following treatment was measured in the isolated heart preparation and in hearts removed from mice following i.v. injection of the phospholipases. Very low levels of phospholipid hydrolysis were observed, and no correlation could be made between the extent of hydrolysis and the pharmacological potencies of these enzymes. Modification of the enzymatic active site, whether of Asp-49 in this study or of His-48 in prior studies, leads to a large decrease in both enzymatic activity and lethal potency. Asp and Glu residues outside the enzymatic site contribute significantly to the lethal potency of the *N. nigricollis* enzyme and to the enzymatic activity of the *N. n. atra* enzyme. Based on these data we once again conclude that changes in isoelectric points are not responsible for altered lethal potencies following chemical modification and that some pharmacological effects of snake venom PLA$_2$ are due to a non-enzymatic action, suggesting two distinct but perhaps overlapping active sites.

In contrast to the marked dissociations we have noted when the basic or acidic amino acid residues were modified, there was no dissociation when the tryptophan residues were modified (Tables 9.11 and 9.12; Condrea, Soons, Barrington, Yang, and Rosenberg 1985). Tryptophan residues may be involved in substrate binding, although some phospholipases have no tryptophan. We investigated the effect of alkylating the tryptophans in *N. nigricollis*, *N. n. atra*, and *H. haemachatus* PLA$_2$ with 2-hydroxy-5-nitrobenzyl bromide. Chemical modification caused decreases in enzymatic activity, although the extent of inactivation varied with the enzyme and with the substrate (lecithin micelles, egg yolk, heart homogenates). The specificity of the enzymes for individual phospholipid substrates was not affected. Alkylation of the tryptophans also caused decreases in lethal, haemolytic, anticoagulant, and cardiotoxic potencies, which were similar to the extents of decrease in enzymatic activity. Our results suggest that tryptophans are not specifically associated with either the enzymatic or the pharmacological active site nor are essential for either activity.

Using *p*-nitrobenzenesulphonyl fluoride (Table 9.12) we modified one or two tyrosine residues out of the nine present in *N. nigricollis* or *N. n. atra* PLA$_2$ (Tables 9.9 and 9.10; Rosenberg, Condrea, Soons, and Yang, unpublished observations). Tyrosines 3 and 62 (63) in cobra venom phospholipases are invariant and it has been suggested that they are associated with the Ca^{2+} and substrate binding site. It was, therefore, of interest to check the effects of chemical modification. Residual enzymatic activity was maintained upon chemical modification of the side chain, suggesting that these tyrosines are not essentially involved at the enzymatic active site; modification of tyrosine 62 causes a greater loss of activity than modification of tyrosine 3. A marked dissociation between enzymatic activity and lethal

potency was noted upon modification of tyrosine 62 in *N. nigricollis* PLA$_2$
and tyrosine 3 in *N. n. atra* PLA$_2$; in the former case a greater loss of lethal
potency than of enzymatic activity was observed, whereas in the latter case a
sixfold increase in lethal potency was associated with about a 50 per cent
decrease in enzymatic activity. The residual haemolytic and anticoagulant
potencies corresponded approximately to the residual enzymatic activity,
whereas the effects of the derivatives on contractile tension of heart muscle
were greater than would be expected given the level of residual enzymatic
activity and the very low levels of phospholipid hydrolysis in the heart.

We are now engaged in studying the relationship between enzymatic and
pharmacological activity in an unusual PLA$_2$ enzyme from *Agkistrodon
p. piscivorus* venom, which in contrast to other PLA$_2$ enzymes has a lysine-
replacing aspartic acid at position 49 (Maraganore, Merutka, Cho, Welches,
Kezdy, and Heinrikson 1984). The C-terminus of this lysin 49 enzyme is also
enriched in lysines (7 of the last 17 residues). As a result of this substitution
the usual order of addition, i.e. Ca^{2+} before phospholipid, is altered so that
the lysine 49 enzyme binds phospholipid before Ca^{2+}. The *in vitro* rate
constants of the two enzymes are, however, very similar (Maraganore *et al.*
1984). In contrast to an Asp-49 PLA$_2$ from the same venom, the Lys-49
PLA$_2$ had much less lethal potency (intravenous in mice or intraventricular
in rats) even though it is more basic (pI 11.0 vs 9.6). The cardiotoxic effects
and effects on contraction of the phrenic nerve diaphragm preparation by
the lysine 49 enzyme were similar to those of the Asp-49 enzyme (Dhillon,
Maraganore, Heinrikson, and Rosenberg, unpublished observations). Of
special interest was the finding that the lysine 49 enzyme caused no significant *in vivo* phospholipid hydrolysis in the heart or diaphragm even at a dose
(35–70 µg ml^{-1}) having marked pharmacological effects, while the aspartate
49 enzyme caused significant hydrolysis (Rosenberg, Maraganore, Dhillon,
and Benjamin, unpublished observations). Some of the phrenic nerve
diaphragm results are shown in Table 9.7. This once again shows that
pharmacological effects of PLA$_2$ enzymes may occur independent of phospholipid hydrolysis.

Conclusions

The emphasis in this review has been on the snake venom PLA$_2$ enzymes
because more information is available on the relationship between
enzymatic and pharmacological properties of this enzyme and because my
personal research in this area has mainly used snake venom PLA$_2$ enzymes.

Snake venom PLA$_2$ enzymes are extensively used as enzyme probes with
which to study phospholipid organization and asymmetry in biological

membranes. It has often been assumed in these studies that the pharmacological properties of PLA_2 enzymes can be explained by their enzymatic activity, that is phospholipid hydrolyses. This assumption must be re-evaluated for the following reasons:

1. Basic PLA_2 enzymes and so-called presynaptic acting toxins (which are also PLA_2 enzymes) tend to be more toxic than acidic PLA_2 enzymes even though their enzymatic activity may be less.

2. There is little correlation between pharmacological effects (e.g. cardiotoxicity, neurotoxicity, anticoagulant potency) and the extent of hydrolysis of phospholipids measured in heart, diaphragm, or plasma.

3. Chemical modification of lysines and arginines in a basic and an acidic PLA_2 cause under certain conditions a much greater loss of pharmacological activity than of enzymatic activity, whereas the reverse dissociation is observed upon modification of carboxyl groups in glutamic and aspartic acid residues. Dissociation is also observed between enzymatic and pharmacological properties in tyrosine-modified derivatives, although not consistently in one direction. Modification of histidine 48 or tryptophan causes decreases in pharmacological properties, which parallel the decreases in enzymatic activity.

The above considerations lead us to suggest that two separate but perhaps overlapping regions exist within the molecule. These regions are respectively responsible for the pharmacological and the enzymatic properties of the enzyme. The enzymatic active site(s) would be concerned with substrate and calcium binding as well as the hydrolytic reaction itself. The pharmacological active site might be concerned with binding of the enzyme to biological membranes and events subsequent to binding (e.g. direct membrane disruptive action could be responsible for haemolytic activity and the disruption of organized lipoprotein structures could be responsible for anticoagulant potency). It appears that basic groups, lysines and arginines, may be primarily located at the pharmacological active site whereas acidic amino acids, such as aspartic acid, are more associated with the enzymatic active site. Charge alone, however, is not the major determinant of pharmacological or lethal potency. For example the pH 5.5 and pH 5.5 + Ca^{2+} carboxylate modified derivatives of *N. nigricollis* have isoelectric points of > 11, while these derivatives of *N. n. atra* PLA_2 also have identical isoelectric points (pI = 8). Despite this the pH 5.5 derivatives shown must lower lethal potencies (Table 9.9; Rosenberg *et al.* 1983a; Barrington *et al.* 1984b). This agrees with our finding that both carbamylation and guanidination of lysines decrease lethal potency, although only the former modification decreases the isoelectric point.

In reviewing the sequences and the conformational properties of snake venom PLA_2 enzymes Dufton *et al.* (1983) and Dufton and Hider (1983) considered the properties that allowed a PLA_2 molecule to penetrate lipid monolayers. *N. nigricollis* PLA_2, which is hydrophobic, was best able to penetrate lipid monolayers, whereas several positively hydrophilic PLA_2 enzymes were not able to penetrate monoloayers. Hydrophilic activity, however, seemed to be a prerequisite for specific presynaptic neurotoxicity, which was associated with residues in the β-sheet region away from the active site. The results of these studies are in agreement with our conclusions that all properties of the PLA_2 molecule must be considered when attempting to evaluate its pharmacological properties; enzymatic activity alone is insufficient, and indeed for some pharmacological properties may be irrelevant.

References

Albuquerque, E. X. and Thesleff, S. (1968). Effects of phospholipase A and lysolecithin on some electrical properties of the muscle membrane. *Acta physiol. scand.* **72**, 248–52.

Alouf, J. E. (1977). Cell membranes and cytolytic bacterial toxins. In *The specificity and action of animal, bacterial and plant toxins* (ed. P. Cuatrecasas), pp. 219–70. Halsted Press, John Wiley, New York.

Ansell, G. B., Hawthorne, J. N., and Dawson, R. M. C. (1973). *Form and function of phospholipids* (2nd edn). Elsevier, Amsterdam.

Avigad, G. (1976). Microbial phospholipases. In *Mechanisms in bacterial toxinology* (ed. A. W. Bernheimer) pp. 99–167. John Wiley, New York.

Barrington, P. L., Yang, C. C., and Rosenberg, P. (1984a). Cardiotoxic effects of *Naja nigricollis* venom phospholipase A_2 are not due to phospholipid hydrolytic products. *Life Sci.* **35**, 987–95.

——, Condrea, E., Soons, K. R., Yang, C. C., and Rosenberg, P. (1984b). Effect of carboxylate group modification on enzymatic and cardiotoxic properties of snake venom phospholipases A_2. *Toxicon* **22**, 743–58.

Bartels, E. and Rosenberg, P. (1972). Correlation between electrical activity and splitting of phospholipids by snake venoms in the single electroplex. *J. Neurochem.* **19**, 1251–65.

Berridge, M. J. (1984). Inositol triphosphate and diacyglycerol as second messengers. *Biochem. J.* **220**, 345–60.

Billah, M. M. and Lapetina, E. G. (1983). Platelet-activating factor stimulates metabolism of phosphoinositides in horse platelets: possible relationship to Ca^{2+} mobilization during stimulation. *Proc. nat. Acad. Sci. USA* **80**, 965–8.

Boffa, M. C. and Boffa, G. A. (1976). A phospholipase A_2 with anticoagulant activity. II. Inhibition of the phospholipid activity in coagulation. *Biochim. biophys. Acta* **429**, 839–52.

——, Barbier, D., and de Angulo, M. (1983). Anticoagulant effect of cardiotoxins. *Thrombosis Res.* **32**, 635–40.

——, Delori, P., and Soulier, J. P. (1972). Anticoagulant factors from viperidae venoms. Platelet phospholipid inhibitors. *Thromb. Diath. haemorrh.* **28**, 509–23.

——, Verheij, H. M., and de Haas, G. H. (1982). Procoagulant phospholipid hydrolysis, penetration ability and anticoagulant activity of phospholipases A_2. *Thromb. Haemostas.* **47**, 299.

Bon, C., Changeux, J. P., Jeng, T. W., and Fraenkel-Conrat, H. (1979). Postsynaptic effects of crotoxin and of its isolated subunits. *Eur. J. Biochem.* **99**, 471.

Bosch, H. Van Den (1980). Intracellular phospholipases A. *Biochim. biophys. acta* **604**, 191–246.

Brazil, O. V., Excell, B. J., and De Sa, S. S. (1973). The importance of phospholipase A in the action of the crotoxin complex at the frog neuromuscular junction. *J. Physiol. Lond.* **234**, 63P–64P

Breithaupt, H. (1976). Neurotoxic and myotoxic effects of *Crotalus* phospholipase A and its complex with crotapotin. *Naunyn-Schmiedeberg's Arch. Pharmakol.* **292**, 271–8.

Breithaupt, H. and Habermann, E. (1973). Biochemistry and pharmacology of phospholipase A from *Crotalus terrificus* venom as influenced by crotopotin. In *Animal and plant toxins* (ed. E. Kaiser), pp. 83–8. Goldmann, Munich.

Chang, C. C. (1979). The action of snake venoms on nerve and muscle. In *Snake venoms* (ed. C. Y. Lee). *Handbook of experimental pharmacology* Vol. 52, pp. 159–212. Springer, New York.

—— and Su, M. J. (1980). Mutual potentiation, at nerve terminals, between toxins from snake venoms which contain phospholipase A activity: β-bungarotoxin, crotoxin, taipoxin. *Toxicon* **18**, 641–8.

——and ——(1982). Presynaptic toxicity of the histidine-modified phospholipase A_2-inactive, β-bungarotoxin, crotoxin and notexin. *Toxicon* **20**, 895–905.

Chi, E. Y., Henderson, W. R., and Klebanoff, S. J. (1982). Phospholipase A_2-induced rat mast cell secretion. Role of arachidonic acid metabolites. *Lab. Invest.* **47**, 579–85.

Condrea, E. (1974). Membrane-active polypeptides from snake venom: cardiotoxins and haemocytotoxins. *Experientia* **30**, 121–9.

—— (1979). Hemolytic effects of snake venom. In *Snake venoms* (ed. C. Y. Lee). *Handbook of experimental pharmacology*, Vol. 52, pp. 448–79. Springer, New York.

——, Rosenberg, P., and Dettbarn, W.-D. (1967). Demonstration of phospholipid splitting as the factor responsible for increased permeability and block of axonal conduction induced by snake venom. I. Study on lobster axons. *Biochim. biophys. acta.* **135**, 669–81.

——, Yang, C. C., and Rosenberg, P. (1980). Comparison of a relatively toxic phospholipase A_2 from *Naja nigricollis* snake venom with that of a relatively nontoxic phospholipase A_2 from *Hemachatus haemachatus* snake venom-I. Enzymatic activity on free and membrane bound substrates. *Biochem. Pharmacol.* **29**, 1555–63.

——, Fletcher, J. E., Rapuano, B. E., Yang, C. C., and Rosenberg, P. (1981a). Dissociation of enzymatic activity from lethality and pharmacological properties by carbamylation of lysines in *Naja nigricollis* and *Naja naja atra* snake venom phospholipases A_2. *Toxicon* **19**, 705–20.

——, Rapuano, B. E., Fletcher, J. E., Yang, C. C., and Rosenberg, P. (1981b). Effects of arginine modification of *Naja nigricollis* and *Naja naja atra* snake venom phospholipases A_2 on enzymatic activity, lethality, and anticoagulant action. *Toxicon* **19**, 721–5.

——, Fletcher, J. E., Rapuano, B. E., Yang, C. C., and Rosenberg, P. (1981c). Effect of modification properties of a toxic phospholipase A₂ from *Naja nigricollis* snake venom and less toxic phospholipase A₂ from *Hemachatus haemachatus* and *Naja naja atra* snake venoms. *Toxicon* **19**, 61–71.

——, ——, and —— (1981d). Lack of correlation between anticoagulant activity and phospholipid hydrolysis by snake venom phospholipase A₂. *Thromb. Haemostas.* **45**, 82–5.

——, ——, and —— (1982). Additional evidence for a lack of correlation between anticoagulant activity and phospholipid hydrolysis by snake venom phospholipases A₂. *Thromb. Haemostas.* **47**, 298.

——, Rapuano, B. E., Fletcher, J. E., Yang, C. C. and Rosenberg, P. (1983a). Ethoxyformylation and guanidination of snake venom phospholipases A₂: effects on enzymatic activity, lethality, and some pharmacological properties. *Toxicon* **21**, 209–18.

——, ——, Soons, K. R., Yang, C. C., and Rosenberg, P. (1983b). Effect of methylation of histidine 48 on some enzymatic and pharmacological activities of snake venom phospholipases A₂. *Life Sci.* **32**, 1455–61.

——, ——, and —— (1983c). Anticoagulant activity and plasma phosphatidylserine hydrolysis by snake venom phospholipases A₂. *Thromb. Haemostas.* **49**, 151.

——, Soons, K. R., Barrington, P. L., Yang, C. C., and Rosenberg, P. (1985). Effect of alkylation of tryptophan residues on the enzymatic and pharmacological properties of snake venom phospholipase A₂. *Can. J. Physiol. Pharmacol.* **63**, 331–9.

Deenen, L. L. M. Van (1981). Topology and dynamics of phospholipids in membranes. *FEBS Lett.* **123**, 3–15.

Dennis, E. A. (1983). Phospholipases. In *The enzymes* (ed. P. D. Boyer) Vol. 16, pp. 307–53, Academic Press, New York.

Dijkstra, B. W., Drenth, J., and Kalk, K. H. (1981). Structure and action of phospholipase A₂. In *Structural aspects of recognition and assembly in biological macromolecules* (eds. M. Balaban, J. L. Sussman, W. Traub, and A. Yonath) pp. 287–304. Balaban ISS, Philadelphia.

Doery, H. M. and Pearson, J. E. (1964). Phospholipase B in snake venom and bee venom. *Biochem. J.* **92**, 599–602.

Dowdall, M. J., Fohlman, J. P., and Watts, A. (1979). Presynaptic action of snake venom neurotoxins on cholinergic systems. In *Advances in cytopharmacology* (ed. B. Ceccarelli and F. Clementi), Vol. 3, pp. 63–76. Raven Press, New York.

Dufton, M. J. and Hider, R. C. (1983). Classification of phospholipases A₂ according to sequence. Evolutionary and pharmacological implications. *Eur. J. Biochem.* **137**, 545–51.

——, Eaker, D., and Hider, R. C. (1983). Conformational properties of phospholipases A₂. Secondary structure predictions, circular dichroism, and relative interface hydrophobicity. *Eur. J. Biochem.* **137**, 537–44.

Dumarey, C., Sket, D., Joseph, D., and Boquet, P. (1975). Basic phospholipase of *Naja nigricollis* venom. *C.R. Acad. Sci.* (*D*) (*Paris*) **280**, 1633–5.

Etemadi, A.-H. (1980). Membrane asymmetry, a survey and critical appraisal of the methodology. II Methods for assessing the unequal distribution of lipids. *Biochim. biophys. acta* **604**, 423–75.

Farese, R. V. (1983). The phosphatidate–phosphoinositide cycle: an intracellular messenger system in the action of hormones and neurotransmitters. *Metabolism* **32**, 628–41.

Fisher, S. K. and Agranoff, B. W. (1985). The biochemical basis and functional significance of enhanced phosphatidate and phosphoinositide turnover. In *Phospholipids in nervous tissue* (ed. J. Eichberg), pp. 241–95. John Wiley, New York.

Fletcher, J. E., Elliott, W. B., Ishay, J., and Rosenberg, P. (1979). Phospholipase A and B activities of reptile and hymenoptera venoms. *Toxicon* **17**, 591–9.

——, Yang, C. C., and Rosenberg, P. (1982). Basic phospholipase A₂ from *Naja nigricollis* snake venom. Phospholipid hydrolysis and effects on electrical and contractile activity of the rat heart. *Toxicol. appl. Pharmacol.* **66**, 39–54.

—— Rapuano, B. E., Condrea, E., Yang, C., and Rosenberg, P. (1981). Relationship between catalysis and toxicological properties of three phospholipase A₂ from elapid snake venoms. *Toxicol appl. Pharmacol.* **59**, 375–88.

——, ——, ——, —— C. C., Ryan, M., and Rosenberg, P. (1980). Comparison of a relatively toxic phospholipase A₂ from *Naja nigricollis* snake venom with that of a relatively non-toxic phospholipase A₂ from *Hemachatus haemachatus* snake venom — II. Pharmacological properties in relationship to enzymatic activity. *Biochem. Pharmacol.* **29**, 1565–74.

Fraenkel-Conrat, H. (1982–83). Snake venom neurotoxins related to phospholipase A₂. *J. Toxicol. toxin Rev.* **1**, 205–21.

Freitas, J. C. De, Blankemeier, L. A., and Jacobs, R. S. (1984) *In vitro* inactivation of the neurotoxic action of β-bungarotoxin by the marine natural product, manoalide. *Experientia* **40**, 864–5.

Giambalvo, C. and Rosenberg, P. (1976). The effect of phospholipases and proteases on the binding of γ-aminobutyric acid to junctional complexes of rat cerebellum. *Biochim. biophys. acta* **436**, 741–56.

Gopalakrishnakone, P., Dempster, D. W., Hawgood, B. J., and Elder, H. Y. (1984). Cellular and mitochondrial changes induced in the structure of murine skeletal muscle by crotoxin, a neurotoxic phospholipase A₂ complex. *Toxicon* **22**, 85–98.

Haest, C. W. and Deuticke, B. (1976). Possible relationship between membrane proteins and phospholipid asymmetry in the human erythrocyte membrane. *Biochim. biophys. acta* **436**, 353–65.

Halpert, J. (1979). Structure and function of neuro and myotoxic phospholipases: modification with ethoxyformic anhydride of notechis II-5 from the venom of the Australian tiger snake *Notechis scutatus scutatus*. In *Advances in cytopharmacology* (ed. B. Ceccarelli and F. Clementi), Vol. 3, pp. 45–62. Raven Press, New York.

—— and Eaker, D. (1975). Amino acid sequence of a presynaptic neurotoxin from the venom of *Notechis scutatus scutatus* (Australian tiger snake). *J. biol. Chem.* **250**, 6990–7.

——, Eaker, D., and Karlsson, E. (1976). The role of phospholipase activity in the action of a presynaptic neurotoxin from the venom of *Notechis scutatus scutatus* (Australian tiger snake). *FEBS Lett.* **61**, 72–6.

Harris, J. B. and Johnson, M. A. (1978). Further observations on the pathological responses of rat skeletal muscle to toxins isolated from the venom of the Australian tiger snake, *Notechis scutatus scutatus*. *Clin. exp. Pharmacol. Physiol.* **5**, 587–600.

—— and Maltin, C. A. (1982). Myotoxic activity of the crude venom and the principal neurotoxin, taipoxin, of the Australian Taipan, *Oxyuranus scutellatus*. *Br. J. Pharmacol.* **76**, 61–75.

——, Johnson, M. A., and Karlsson, E. (1975). Pathological responses of rat skeletal muscle to a single subcutaneous injection of a toxin isolated from the venom of the Australian tiger snake, *Notechis scutatus scutatus*. *Clin. exp. Pharmacol. Physiol.* **2**, 383–404.

Harvey, A. L. L., Hider, R. C., and Khader, F. (1983). Effect of phospholipase A on actions of cobra venom cardiotoxins on erythrocytes and skeletal muscle. *Biochim. biophys. acta* **728**, 215–21.

Hawley, M. R. and Emson, P. C. (1979). Neuronal degeneration induced by stereotoxic injection of β-bungarotoxin into rat brain. *Neurosci. Lett.* **11**, 143.

Hawthorne, J. N. (1983). Polyphosphoinositide metabolism in excitable membranes. *Biosci. Rep.* **3**, 887–904.

Heilbronn, E. (1969). The effect of phospholipases on the uptake of atropine and acetylcholine by slices of mouse brain cortex. *J. Neurochem.* **16**, 627–35.

Heinrikson, R. L. (1982). Structure–function relationships in phospholipases A_2. In *Proteins in biology and medicine* (ed. R. A. Bradshaw, R. L. Hill, J. Tang, L. Chih-chuan, T. Tien-chin, and T. Chen-lu), pp. 131–52. Academic Press, New York.

Hirasawa, K. and Nishizuka, Y. (1985). Phosphatidylinositol turnover in receptor mechanism and signal transduction. *Rev. Pharmacol. Toxicol.* **25**, 147–70.

Hirata, F. and Axelrod, J. (1980). Phospholipid methylation and biological signal transmission. *Science* **209**, 1082–90.

—— and —— (1982). Phospholipid methylation and biological signal transmission. In *Frontiers in cellular research*, pp. 55–58. PJD Publications, Westbury, New York.

Hokin, L. E. (1985). Receptors and phosphoinositide generated second messengers. *A. Rev. Biochem.* **54**, 205–35.

Hoskin, F. C. G. and Rosenberg, P. (1965). Penetration of sugars, steroids, amino acids and other compounds into the interior of the squid giant axon. *J. gen. Physiol.* **49**, 47–56.

Howard, B. D. (1982). Presynaptic polypeptide neurotoxins. *TIBS* April 1982, pp. 167–9.

—— and Gundersen, C. B. (1980). Effects and mechanisms of polypeptide neurotoxins that act presynaptically. *A. Rev. Pharmacol. Toxicol.* **20**, 307–36.

—— and Truog, R. (1977). Relationship between the neurotoxicity and phospholipase activity of β-bungarotoxin. *Biochemistry* **16**, 122.

Ikezawa, H., Taguchi, R., Asahi, Y., and Tomita, M. (1982–83). The physiological actions of bacterial phospholipases C on eucaryotic cells and their membranes. *J. Toxicol. toxin Rev.* **1**, 223–55.

Irvine, R. F. (1982). How is the level of free arachidonic acid controlled in mammalian cells? *Biochem. J.* **204**, 3–16.

Johansson, P. and Thesleff, S. (1968). A comparison of the effects of phospholipase C and tetrodotoxin on spike generation in muscle. *Eur. J. Pharmacol.* **4**, 347.

Joubert, F. J. (1975). *Hemachatus haemachatus* (Ringhals) venom. Purification, some properties and amino acid sequence of phospholipase A (fraction DE-1). *Eur. J. Biochem.* **52**, 539–45.

Karlsson, E. (1979). Chemistry of protein toxins in snake venoms. In *Snake venoms* (ed. C. Y. Lee). *Handbook of experimental pharmacology* Vol. 52. pp. 159–212. Springer, New York.

Kawaguchi, H. and Yasuda, H. (1984). Platelet-activating factor stimulates phospholipase in quiescent Swiss mouse 3T3 fibroblast. *FEBS Lett.* **176**, 93–6.

Kelly, R. B., von Wedel, R. J., and Strong, P. N. (1979). Phospholipase-dependent and phospholipase-independent inhibition of transmitter release by β-bungarotoxin. In *Advances in cytopharmacology* (ed. B. Ceccarelli and F. Clementi), pp. 77–85. Raven Press, New York.

Kirschmann, C., Ten-Ami, I., Smorodinski, I., and De Vries, A. (1971). Effect of phospholipase and trypsin on histidine uptake by mouse brain slices. *Biochem. biophys. acta.* **233**, 644–51.

Knickelbein, R. G. and Rosenberg, P. (1980). Differential phospholipid hydrolysis by phospholipase C in sarcolemma of muscles with calcium or sodium generated action potentials. *Toxicon* **18**, 71–86.

Kondo, K., Narita, K., and Lee, C. Y. (1978). Amino acid sequence of the two polypeptide chains in β₁ bungarotoxin from the venom of *Bungarus multicinctus*. *J. Biochem.* **83**, 101–15.

——, Toda, H. Narita, K., and Lee, C. Y. (1982). Amino acid sequence of β₂ bungarotoxin from *Bungarus multicinctus* venom. The amino acid substitutions in the B chains. *J. Biochem. (Tokyo)* **91**, 1519–29.

Krebs, J. J. R. (1982). The topology of phospholipids in artificial and biological membranes. *J. Bioenerg. Biomembr.* **14**, 141–57.

Lapetina, E. G. and Siess, W. (1983). The role of phospholipase C in platelet responses. *Life Sci.* **33**, 1011–18.

Lee, C. Y. and Chang, C. C. (1966). Modes of action of urified toxins from Elapid venoms on neuromuscular transmission. *Mem. Inst. Butantan* **33**, 555–72.

—— and Ho, C. L. (1982). The pharmacology of phospholipase A₂ isolated from snake venoms with particular reference to their effects on neuromuscular transmission. In *Advances in pharmacology and therapeutics II. Biochemical immunological pharmacology* (eds. H. Yoshida, Y. Hagihara, and S. Ebashi), Vol. 4, pp. 37–52. Pergamon Press, New York.

——, Chen, Y. M., and Karlsson, E. (1976). Postsynaptic and musculotrophic effects of notexin, a presynaptic neurotoxin from the venom of *Notechis scutatus scutatus* (Australian tiger snake). *Toxicon* **14**, 493–4.

——, Ho, C. L., and Eaker, D. (1977). Cardiotoxin-like action of a basic phospholipase A₂ isolated from *Naja nigricollis* venom. *Toxicon* **15**, 355–6.

McArdle, B., Thompson, R. H. S., and Webster, G. R. (1960). The action of lysolecithin and of snake venom on whole-cell preparations of brain, muscle and liver. *J. Neurochem.* **5**, 135–44.

Maraganore, J. M., Merutka, G., Cho, W., Welches, W., Kezdy, F. J., and Heinrikson, R. L. (1984). A new class of phospholipases A_2 with lysine in place of aspartate 49: functional consequences for calcium and substrate binding. *J. biol. Chem.* **259**, 13839–43.

Marlas, G. and Bon, C. (1982). Relationship between the pharmacological action of crotoxin and its phospholipase activity. *Eur. J. Biochem.* **125**, 157–65.

Martin, R. and Rosenberg, P. (1968). Fine structural alterations associated with venom action on squid giant nerve fibers. *J. cell Biol.* **36**, 341–53.

Martin, J. K., Luthra, M. G., Wells, M. A., Watts, R. P., and Hanahan, D. J. (1975). Phospholipase A_2 as a probe of phospholipid distribution in erythrocyte membranes. Factors influencing the apparent specificity of the reaction. *Biochemistry* **14**, 5400–8.

Mato, J. M. and Alemany, S. (1983). What is the function of phospholipid N-methylation? *Biochem. J.* **213**, 1–10.

Melchoir, W. B. and Fahrney, D. (1970). Ethoxyformylation of proteins. Reaction of ethoxyformic anhydride with α-chymotrypsin, papain and pancreatic ribonuclease at pH 4. *Biochemistry* **9**, 251.

Mohamed, A. H., Kamel, A., and Ayobe, M. H. (1969). Studies of phospholipase A and B activities of Egyptian snake venoms and a scorpion toxin. *Toxicon* **6**, 293–8.

Morrison, L. R. and Zamecnik, P. C. (1950). Experimental demyelination by means of enzymes, especially the alpha toxin of *Clostridium welchii*. *Arch. Neurol. Psychiatr.* **63**, 367–81.

Narahashi, T. (1974). Chemicals as tools in the study of excitable membranes. *Physiol. Rev.* **54**, 813–89.

Navran, S. S., Romstedt, T. C., Chang, J., Miller, D. D., Feller, D. R., and Akbar, H. (1984). Human platelet activation by bacterial phospholipase C is mediated by phosphatidylinositol hydrolysis but not generation of phosphatidic acid: inhibition by a selective inhibitor of phospholipase C. *Thromb. Res.* **33**, 499–510.

Ng, R. G. and Howard, B. D. (1978). Deenergization of nerve terminals by β-bungarotoxin. *Biochemistry* **17**, 4978.

—— and —— (1980). Mitochondria and sarcoplasmic reticulum as model targets for neurotoxic and myotoxic phospholipases A_2. *Proc. nat. Acad. Sci. USA* **77**, 1346.

Nishizuka, Y. (1983). Calcium, phospholipid turnover and transmembrane signalling. *Phil. Trans. R. Soc. Lond.* **B 302**, 101–12.

—— (1984). Turnover of inositol phospholipids and signal transduction. *Science* **225**, 1365–70.

Obidairo, T. K., Tampitag, S., and Eaker, D. (1976). Personal communication; also noted by Fohlman, J., Eaker, D., Karlsson, E., and Thesleff, S. Taipoxin an extremely potent presynaptic neurotoxin from the venom of the Australian snake taipan (*Oxyuranus s. scutellatus*). Isolation, characterization, quaternary structure and pharmacological properties. *Eur. J. Biochem.* **68**, 457.

Oliveira, C. R., Duarte, E. P., and Carvalho, A. P. (1984). Effect of phospholipase digestion and lysophosphatidylcholine on dopamine receptor binding. *J. Neurochem.* **43**, 455–65.

Pasternak, G. W. and Snyder, S. H. (1974). Opiate receptor binding: effects of enzymatic treatments. *Mol. Pharmacol.* **10**, 183–93.

Philipson, K. D., Frank, J. S., and Nishimoto, A. Y. (1983). Effects of phospholipase C on the Na^+ Ca^{2+} permeability of cardiac sarcolemmal vesicles. *J. biol. Chem.* **258**, 5905–10.

Prigent-Dachary, J., Boffa, M. C., Boisseau, M. R., and Dufourcq, J. (1980). Snake venom phospholipases A_2. A fluorescence study of their binding to phospholipid vesicles correlation with their anticoagulant activities. *J. biol. Chem.* **225**, 7734–9.

Puijk, W. D., Verheij, H. M., and de Haas, G. H. (1977). The primary structure of phospholipase A_2 from porcine pancreas: a reinvestigation. *Biochim. biophys. acta* **492**, 254–9.

Radvanyi, F. R. and Bon, C. (1984). Investigations on the mechanism of actions of crotoxin. *J. Physiol.* **79**, 327–33.

Randolph, A., Sakmar, T. P., and Heinrikson, R. L. (1980). Phospholipases A_2: structure, function and evolution. In *Frontiers in protein chemistry* (ed. T. Liu, G. Mamiya, and T. T. Yasunobu) pp. 297–322. Elsevier, Amsterdam.

Roelofsen, B. (1982). Phospholipases as tools to study the localization of phospholipids in biological membranes: a critical appraisal. *J. Toxicol. toxin Rev.* **1**, 87–197.

Rooijen, L. A. A., Van, Fisher, S. K., and Agranoff, B. W. (1985). Biochemical aspects of stimulated turnover of inositol lipids in the nervous system. In *Phospholipids in the nervous system* (ed. L. A. Horrocks, J. N. Kanfer, and G. Porcellati) Vol. 2, *Physiological roles*, pp. 31–38, Raven Press, New York.

Rosenberg, P. (1965). Effects of venoms on the squid giant axon. *Toxicon* **3**, 125–31.

—— (1966). Use of venoms in studies on nerve excitation. *Mem. Inst. Butantan* **33**, 477–508.

—— (1970). Function of phospholipids in axons: depletion of membrane phosphorus by treatment with phospholipase. C. *Toxicon* **8**, 235–43.

—— (1971). The use of snake venoms as pharmacological tools in studying nerve activity. In *Neuropoisons: their pathophysiological actions* (ed. L. L. Simpson), Vol. 1, Ch. 5, pp. 111–37. Plenum Press, New York.

—— (1972). Use of phospholipases in studying nerve structure and function. In *Toxins of animal and plant origin* (eds. A. DeVries and E. Kochva), pp. 449–61. Gordon and Breach, London.

—— (1973a). Venoms and enzymes: effects on permeability of isolated single electroplax. *Toxicon* **11**, 149–154.

—— (1973b). Effect of stimulation and acetylcholine on ^{32}P and ^{14}C incorporation into phospholipids of the eel electroplax. *J. pharm. Sci.* **62**, 1552–4.

—— (1976a). Bacterial and snake venom phospholipases: enzymatic problems in the study of structure and function in bioelectrically excitable tissues. In *Animal, plant and microbial toxins* (ed. A. Ohsaka, K. Hayashi, and Y. Sawai), Vol. II, pp. 229–61. Plenum Press, New York.

—— (1976b). Effect of phospholipases A_2 and C on structure and phospholipids of the electroplax. *Toxicon* **14**, 319–28.

—— (1979). Pharmacology of phospholipase A_2 from snake venoms. In *Snake venoms* (ed. C. Y. Lee). Springer, New York.

—— and Condrea, E. (1968). Maintenance of axonal conduction and membrane permeability in presence of extensive phospholipid splitting. *Biochem. Pharmacol.* **17**, 2033–44.

—— and Ehrenpreis, S. (1961). Reversible block of axonal conduction by curare after treatment with cobra venom. *Biochem. Pharmacol.* **8**, 192–206.

—— and Hoskin, F. C. G. (1963). Demonstration of increased permeability as a factor responsible for the effect of acetylcholine on the electrical activity of venom treated axons. *J. gen. Physiol.* **46**, 1065–73.

—— and Mautner, H. G. (1967). Acetylcholine receptor: similarity in axons and junctions. *Science* **155**, 1569–71.

—— and Ng, K. Y. (1963). Factors in venoms leading to block of axonal conduction by curare. *Biochim. biophys. acta* **75**, 116–28.

—— and Podleski, T. R. (1962). Block of conduction by acetylcholine and D-tubocurarine after treatment of squid axon with cottonmouth moccasin venom. *J. pharmacol. exp. Ther.* **137**, 249–62.

—— and Podleski, T. R. (1963). Ability of venoms to render squid axons sensitive to curare and acetylcholine. *Biochim. biophys. acta* **75**, 104–15.

——, Ishay, J., and Gitter, S. (1977). Phospholipases A and B activities of the oriental hornet (*Vespa orientalis*) venom and venom apparatus. *Toxicon* **15**, 141–56.

——, Condrea, E., Rapuano, B. E., Soons, K. R., and Yang, C. C. (1983a). Dissociation of pharmacological and enzymatic activities of snake venom phospholipases A_2 by modification of carboxylate groups. *Biochem. Pharmacol.* **32**, 3525–30.

——, ——, Fletcher, J. E., Rapuano, B. E., and Yang, C. C. (1983b). Dissociation between enzymatic activity and pharmacological properties of snake venom phospholipase A_2. *Toxicon Suppl.* **3**, 371–5.

Salach, J. I., Turini, P., Seng, R., Hauber, J., and Singer, T. P. (1971). Phospholipase A of snake venoms. Isolation and molecular properties of isoenzymes from *Naja naja* and *Vipera russellii* venoms. *J. biol. Chem.* **246**, 331–9.

Samuelsson, B. (1981). Prostaglandins, thromboxanes, and leukotrienes: formation and biological roles. *Harvey Lect.* **75**, 1–40.

Sen, I. and Cooper, J. R. (1975). Effect of β-bungarotoxin on the release of acetylcholine from brain synaptosomal preparations. *Biochem. Pharmacol.* **24**, 2107.

——, Grantham, P. A., and Cooper, J. R. (1976). Mechanism of action of β-bungarotoxin on synaptosomal preparations. *Proc. nat. Acad. Sci. USA.* **73**, 2664.

——, Baba, A., Schulz, R. A., and Cooper, J. R. (1978). Mechanism of action of notexin and notechic II-5 on synaptosomes. *J. neurochem.* **31**, 969–76.

Shen, B. W. and Lau, J. H. (1979). Phospholipases. In *The biochemistry of atherosclerosis* (ed. A. M. Scanu, R. W. Wissler, and G. S. Getz) pp. 275–91, Marcel Dekker, New York.

Shier, W. T. (1982). Cytolytic mechanisms: self destruction of mammalian cells by activation of endogenous hydrolytic enzymes. *J. Toxicol. toxin Rev.* **1**, 1–32.

Shiloah, J., Klibansky, C., and De Vries, A. (1973). Phospholipase isoenzymes from *Naja naja* venom. I. Purification and partial characterization. *Toxicon* **11**, 481–90.

Shukla, S. D. (1982). Phosphatidylinositol specific phospholipase C. *Life Sci.* **30**, 1323–35.

Siess, W., Weber, P. C., and Lapetina, E. G. (1984). Activation of phospholipase C is dissociated from arachidonate metabolism during platelet shape change induced by thrombin or platelet activating factor. *J. biol. Chem.* **259**, 8286–92.

Sket, D. and Gubensek, F. (1976). Pharmacological study of phospholipase A from *Vipera ammodytes* venom. *Toxicon* **14**, 393–6.

Slotta, K. H. and Fraenkel-Conrat, H. (1938). Schlangengifte III Mitt. Reiningung and Kristallisation des Klapper-schlangengiftes. *Ber. Dtsch. chem. Ges.* **71**, 1076–81.

Soons, K. R., Yang, C. C., and Rosenberg, P. (1984). Binding of phospholipase A_2 to isolated heart muscle. *Biochem. Pharmacol.* **33**, 3914–17.

Spande, T. F., Witkop, B., Degani, Y., and Patchornik, A. (1970). Selective cleavage and modification of peptides and proteins. *Adv. prot. Chem.* **24**, 97.

Strong, P. N., Goerke, J., Oberg, S. G., and Kelly, R. B. (1976). β-bungarotoxin, a pre-synaptic toxin with enzymatic activity. *Proc. nat. Acad. Wash.* **73**, 178–182.

Su, M. J. and Chang, C. C. (1984). Presynaptic effects of snake venom toxins which have phospholipase A_2 activity (β-bungarotoxin, taipoxin, crotoxin). *Toxicon* **22**, 631–40.

Sun, A. Y. (1974). The effect of phospholipases on the active uptake of norepinephrine by synaptosomes isolated from the cerebral cortex of guinea pig. *J. Neurochem.* **22**, 551–6.

Thudichum, J. L. W. (1884). *A treatise on the chemical constitution of the brain*. Ballière, Tindall, London.

Tobias, J. M. (1955). Effects of phospholipases, collagenase and chymotrypsin on impulse conduction and resting potential in the lobster axon with parallel experiments on frog muscle *J. Cell comp. Physiol.* **46**, 183–207.

Tobias, G. S., Donlon, M., Shain, W. and Catravas, G. (1976). β-bungarotoxin relationship of phospholipase activity to toxicity. *Fedn. Proc. Fedn. Am. Socs.exp. Biol.* **35**, 800.

Tsai, I. H., Wu, S. H., and Lo, T. B. (1981). Complete amino acid sequence of a phospholipase A_2 from the venom of *Naja naja atra* (Taiwan cobra). *Toxicon* **19**, 141–52.

Tu, A. T. (1977). *Venoms: chemistry and molecular biology*. John Wiley, New York.

Vapaatalo, H. and Parantainen, J. (1978). Prostaglandins: their biological and pharmacological role. *Med. Biol.* **56**, 163–83.

Verheij, H. M., Slotboom, A. F., and De Haas, G. H. (1981). Structure and function of phospholipase A_2. *Rev. Physiol. Biochem. Pharmacol.* **91**, 91–203.

——, Boffa, M. C., Rotnen, C., Bryckaert, M. C., Verger, R., and De Haas, G. H. (1980). Correlation of enzymatic activity and anticoagulant properties of phospholipases A_2. *Eur. J. Biochem.* **112**, 25–32.

Viljoen, C. C., Botes, D. P., and Kruger, H. (1982). Isolation and amino acid sequence of caudoxin, a presynaptic acting toxic phospholipase A_2 from the venom of the horned puff adder (Bitis caudalis). *Toxicon* **20**, 715–37.

Wagner, G. M., Mart, P. E., and Kelly, R. B. (1974). β-bungarotoxin inhibition of calcium accumulation by rat brain mitochondria. *Biochem. Biophys. res. Commun.* **58**, 475–481.

Wells, M. A. (1973). Spectral perturbations of *Crotalus adamanteus* phospholipase A_2 induced by divalent cation binding. *Biochemistry* **12**, 1080.

Wernicke, J. F., Oberjat, T., and Howard, B. D. (1974). β-neurotoxin reduces neurotransmitter storage in brain synapses. *J. Neurochem.* **22**, 781–8.

——, Vanker, A. D., and Howard, B. D. (1975). The mechanism of action of β-bungarotoxin. *J. Neurochem.* **25**, 483–96.

Zahler, P., Kasermann, D., and Reist, M. (1985). Membrane-bound phospholipases: properties and functions. In *Biomembranes, dynamics, and biology* (ed. R. M. Burton and F. C. Guerra), pp. 179–192, Plenum Press, New York.

Zan, Y. P., Condrea, E., Yang, C. C., and Rosenberg, P. (1983). Phospholipid hydrolysis in serum lipoproteins by a basic phospholipase A_2 from *Naja nigricollis* snake venom and an acidic phospholipase A_2 from *Naja naja atra* snake venom. *Toxicon* **21**, 481–90.

Zeller, E. A. (1951). Enzymes as essential components of bacterial and animal toxins. In *The enzymes* (ed. J. B. Sumner and K. Myrback), Vol. 1, Part 2, pp. 986–1013. Academic Press, New York.

10

Mechanisms of intoxication by protein toxins

Kirsten Sandvig and Sjur Olsnes

Introduction

A number of protein toxins exert their effect on cells in the following way: after binding to the cell surface, an enzymatically active part of the molecule passes through the cell membrane into the cytosol. Such toxins include the bacterial toxins diphtheria toxin, *Pseudomonas aeruginosa* toxin, *Shigella* toxin, cholera toxin, pertussis toxin, anthrax toxin, and the heat-labile toxin of *E. coli*, as well as the plant toxins abrin, ricin, modeccin, and viscumin (for review, see Olsnes and Sandvig 1983, 1985). Most of these toxins have been shown to consist of two distinct moieties. One polypeptide chain, designated the A-moiety, carries the enzymatic activity and is linked by a disulphide bond to the B-moiety that binds the toxin to cell surface receptors. The binding moiety consists of one or several polypeptides held together with non-covalent bonds.

The mechanism of protein transfer across biological membranes is still not known in detail. There is, however, evidence that many of these protein toxins enter the cytosol from intracellular compartments, which they reach after receptor-mediated endocytosis. Nevertheless, in spite of their structural similarities, the entry mechanisms of these toxins are not identical. The toxins have different requirements for entry and appear to enter the cytosol from different intracellular compartments.

Information about the entry of four of these toxins, the plant toxins abrin, ricin, modeccin, and the bacterial toxin diphtheria toxin, will be presented in this review.

Requirements for entry of abrin and ricin

Amines and ionophores, known to increase the pH of acidic cell compartments, do not protect cells against the plant toxins abrin and ricin. This indicates that these toxins do not require low pH at any stage of their entry. Indeed, NH$_4$Cl and low concentrations of monesin sensitize cells to abrin and ricin (Sandvig and Olsnes 1982a; Sandvig, Olsnes, and Pihl 1979). The low concentrations of monensin required for this sensitization are unlikely to affect endosome acidification. However, such low concentrations of monensin have been found to interfere with protein glycosylation in the Golgi apparatus. It was, therefore of interest to determine whether other compounds known to interfere with glycoprotein synthesis and processing sensitize cells to abrin and ricin. Tunicamycin, which inhibits addition of carbohydrate to asparagine (Elbein 1981), and swainsonine, which inhibits processing of carbohydrates on glycoproteins (Tulsiani, Harris, and Touster 1982), also sensitize the cells to ricin (Fig. 10.1).

It is possible that ricin competes with newly formed glycoproteins for modification by enzymes in the Golgi apparatus or for transport between the different Golgi elements. The effect of ricin on cells where protein synthesis had been blocked with cycloheximide or puromycin was, therefore, studied. These compounds were shown to sensitize the cells to ricin (Fig 10.1). Similar results were also obtained with abrin (data not shown). When the localization of ricin in the cells was studied by electron microscopy with ricin coupled to horseradish peroxidase, ricin was found in *trans* Golgi elements. However, at present it is not possible to conclude that transport of abrin and ricin to the Golgi apparatus is an obligatory step in the entry of these toxins into the cytosol.

In further attempts to characterize the entry process, the ion and pH requirements for toxin entry were studied. Transport of calcium ions appears to be required for entry of abrin, ricin, and modeccin into the cell. Thus, when Ca^{2+} entry was blocked with verapamil, the cells were protected against abrin (Table 10.1) and ricin as well as against modeccin. Control experiments showed that this protection was not due to reduced binding or

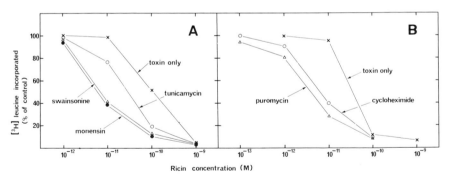

Fig. 10.1 Sensitization of Vero cells to ricin by tunicamycin, swainsonine, monensin, puromycin, and cycloheximide. Vero cells were preincubated for 30 min with and without tunicamycin and for 15 min with 1 μg ml⁻¹ swainsonine, 0.1 μM monensin, 1 mM puromycin and 10 μg ml⁻¹ cycloheximide; then increasing concentrations of ricin were added, and the incubation was continued at 37°C for 3 h. Finally, protein synthesis was measured over a 15-min period.

Table 10.1 Effect of various compounds and conditions on the sensitivity of Vero cells to abrin.

Condition A	Condition B	[a]ID_{50} for condition A ID_{50} for condition B
pH 7	pH 6	<0.01
2 mM Ca^{2+}	2 mM Co^{2+}	<0.01
0.1 mM Ca^{2+}	0.1 mM Ca^{2+} + 0.25 mM verapamil	<0.01
0.14 M NaCl, pH 7.2	0.14 M Na acetate, pH 7.2	<0.01
0.14 M NaCl, pH 7.2	0.14 M NaSCN, pH 7.2	<0.003

Increasing amounts of abrin were added to cells in a buffer containing 0.14 M NaCl, 20 mM Hepes (pH 7–7.2), and 2mM $CaCl_2$ except when otherwise indicated (condition A), or in a buffer that was identical except that one of the components was altered as indicated (condition B).

[a] Dose–response curves were constructed and the toxin concentration required to reduce protein synthesis to 50 per cent of the control value (ID_{50}) was measured.

endocytosis of the toxins. The calcium requirement appeared to be associated with the entry of fragment A. However, it is not known in which cellular compartment the required calcium transport takes place (Sandvig and Olsnes 1982b).

Neutral or slightly alkaline pH in the medium was also found to be required for entry of the plant toxins. The cells gradually became more protected when the pH was reduced from 7 to 6, but there was no corresponding reduction in the binding and endocytosis of the toxin at the low pH (Sandvig and Olsnes 1982a). The reason for the protection is not clear.

Addition of weak acids to the medium acidifies both the cytosol and intracellular compartments. Cells were protected when sodium acetate was substituted for NaCl (Table 10.2). Protection was also obtained at pH 7.2 when the toxins were added to cells in the presence of sodium thiocyanate (NaSCN) instead of NaCl (Sandvig and Olsnes 1985). NaSCN has been shown to decrease the pH close to the membrane and may, therefore, protect in a manner similar to low pH in the medium. In agreement with this hypothesis is the finding that the protection was overcome by increasing the pH in the medium from 7.2 to 7.6. Low pH had only a slight effect on the calcium transport into the cells. However, since little information is available about the various calcium transport systems that may operate in these cells, the possibility cannot be excluded that the uptake by one particular mechanism is affected more than the bulk uptake.

Structure–function relationship in diphtheria toxin

Diphtheria toxin is synthesized as a single polypeptide chain which is easily cleaved by trypsin-like proteases into two fragments linked by a disulphide bridge. Fragment A, which is the operative part of the molecule, is an enzyme that enters the cytosol and inhibits protein synthesis by an ADP-ribosylation that inactivates Elongation Factor 2. Fragment B is involved in the binding of the toxin to receptors at the cell surface and in addition plays a role in the entry of the A fragment (for review, see Olsnes and Sandvig 1983, 1985). An important feature of the B-fragment is that it contains a hydrophobic domain that is normally not exposed (Boquet, Silverman, Pappenheimer, and Vernon 1976). However, at acidic pH a conformational change takes place in the toxin as a result of which the hydrophobic domain is exposed. The toxin is then able to bind non-ionic detergents (Sandvig and Olsnes 1981). Experiments with artificial lipid bilayers have shown that the hydrophobic fragment is inserted into the lipid bilayer as a transmembrane protein. This insertion induces the formation of voltage-dependent ion-permeable channels across the bilayer (Kagan, Finkelstein, and Colombini 1981; Donovan, Simon, Draper, and Montal 1981). There is now good evidence that under normal conditions the transfer of the enzymatically active fragment across the membrane takes place in intracellular vesicles. A sufficiently low pH to expose the hydrophobic domain of the fragment B (pH < 5.4) is, under normal conditions, only found in intracellular vesicles. Furthermore, a number of compounds that increase the pH in intracellular acidic vesicles protect very efficiently against diphtheria toxin. However, it is possible to bypass the endocytic pathway if cells with surface-bound toxin are exposed to medium with low pH (Draper and Simon 1980; Sandvig and Olsnes 1980). Apparently, under these conditions the toxin inserts itself directly into the surface membrane, after which the enzymatically active fragment A is transferred to the cytosol. In the following experiments we have to a large extent taken advantage of this possibility, since it is much easier to control ion gradients and the electrical gradient across the surface membrane than across membranes of intracellular vesicles.

Requirements for the entry of diphtheria toxin at low pH

In attempts to elucidate the requirements for the transfer of fragment A across the membrane, we first determined whether a normal membrane potential is required. Since at low pH fragment A has a positive charge, it was conceivable that the negative interior of the cell might pull fragment A across the membrane. To test this possibility cells were incubated with pre-bound diphtheria toxin in a buffer containing isotonic KCl, which was shown to depolarize the cells, and the cells were then exposed to a low pH to induce toxin entry. The results showed that there was no difference in the extent of intoxication whether the cells were incubated in the presence of NaCl or KCl. It therefore appears that a normal membrane potential is not required for the transfer of fragment A across the membrane.

The pH of the cell interior is normally close to neutral. There is therefore a large pH gradient across the membrane when the cell exterior is exposed to low pH. This gradient could act as a driving force to induce entry of fragment A. To determine whether the pH gradient is indeed required for entry, the pH gradient in Vero cells was dissipated and an attempt was made to induce toxin entry by exposing the cells to medium with low pH.

For this purpose, cells were incubated with weak acids, such as acetic acid, which in their protonated form are able to penetrate the membrane. When the acids enter the cytosol they dissociate and thus decrease the internal pH. When the cytosol had been acidified in this way, entry of diphtheria toxin fragment A induced by exposure of the cells to medium with low pH was markedly reduced (Fig 10.2). Clearly it is not sufficient for toxin entry that the exterior of the cell is exposed to low pH; it appears that a pH gradient across the membrane is required for entry to occur. A number of conditions affect the binding of diphtheria toxin to cells. Thus, when cells were treated with low concentrations of tumour-promoting phorbol esters like TPA (12-*O*-tetradecanoyl-phorbol-13 acetate), the ability to bind diphtheria toxin was greatly reduced (Fig 10.3). Treatment with vanadate and fluoride

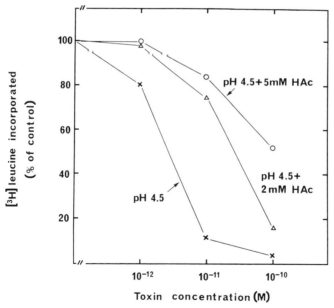

Fig. 10.2 Inhibition of diphtheria toxin entry by acetic acid. Vero cells were incubated for 10 min with and without the indicated concentrations of acetic acid in Hepes medium adjusted to pH 4.5. Increasing concentrations of diphtheria toxin were then added. After 20 min incubation the low-pH medium was removed and the cells were incubated overnight in growth medium containing diphtheria antitoxin. The incorporation of ³H-leucine over 15 min was then measured.

also greatly decreased the binding ability of the cells. To induce this reduction in binding ability, it was necessary to incubate the cells at physiological temperature. Reduction of binding did not occur in cells depleted of ATP. Since ATP activates protein kinase C (Nishizuka 1984) and since vanadate and fluoride inhibit dephosphorylation reactions (Carpenter 1981; Mumby and Traugh 1979), it is tempting to speculate that phosphorylation of the binding site for diphtheria toxin eliminates the binding capability of the cells.

For binding to occur it is also necessary that anions are present in the buffer. Thus, when cells were incubated with ^{125}I-labelled diphtheria toxin in a buffer osmotically balanced with mannitol, very little binding took place (Fig 10.3). On the other hand, if cells with pre-bound diphtheria toxin were exposed to medium containing no permeant anions, the major part of the bound toxin remained bound to the cells. In spite of this, we were unable to induce entry of fragment A into the cytosol at low pH if the medium did not contain permeant anions (Fig 10.4). This indicates that anions are required for the transport. Further support for this is provided by the fact that when cells with pre-bound toxin were exposed to inhibitors of anion transport like SITS (4-acetamido-4-isothiocyano-stilbene-2,2'-disulphonic acid) and piretanide, the cells were protected against intoxication even in the presence

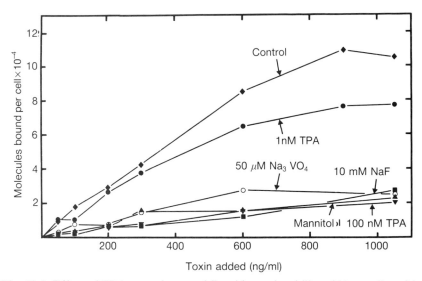

Fig. 10.3 Effect of TPA, vanadate, and fluoride on the ability of Vero cells to bind ^{125}I-diphtheria toxin. Vero cells were incubated for 1 h at 37°C in Hepes medium at pH 7, with the additions shown in the figure, and were then chilled to 24°C. In one case (▲) the incubation was in 260 mM mannitol, 1 mM Ca(OH)$_2$, 20 mM MES adjusted to pH 7 with Tris. Then increasing amounts of ^{125}I-diphtheria toxin were added and the ability of the cells to bind the toxin was measured.

of permeant anions. This indicates that it is not sufficient that permeant anions are present —anion entry must be allowed to take place (Fig 10.5).

When cells with pre-bound diphtheria toxin were exposed to low pH, the toxin was very efficiently inserted into the cell membrane. Thus, after such treatment the toxin became inaccessible to labelling with ^{125}I by the lactoperoxidase method. Furthermore, the ability of the cells to take up $^{35}SO_4^{2-}$ and $^{36}Cl^-$ by antiport was greatly reduced (Fig. 10.6). Thus, the J_{max} for Cl^- was reduced from 1.6×10^8 to 6.2×10^7 ions per cell per second, while the J_{max} for SO_4^{2-} was reduced from 3.1×10^6 to 3.7×10^5 ions per cell per second. On the other hand, the K_m for the ions remained the same before and after toxin treatment. This indicates that the inserted toxin in some way

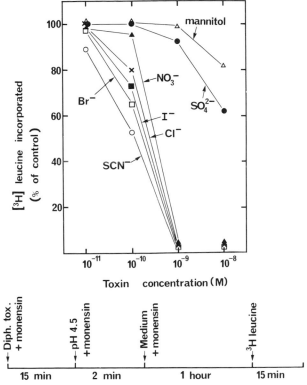

Fig. 10.4 Ability of different anions to support entry of diphtheria toxin at low pH. Vero cells were incubated for 15 min at 37°C with increasing concentrations of diphtheria toxin in Hepes medium containing 10 μM monensin. Then the medium was removed and a buffer containing 20 mM MES, adjusted to pH 4.5 with Tris, 10 μM monensin, 0.14 M of the sodium salt of the anion indicated or 260 mM mannitol was added to the cells. After 2 min at 37°C this buffer was removed and Hepes medium containing 10 μM monensin was added. One hour later the rate of protein synthesis was measured.

interferes with the anion antiporter in the cells. It is an interesting possibility
that the anion antiporter is identical with the diphtheria toxin receptor in
Vero cells.

Insertion of diphtheria toxin into the membrane at low pH took place
even in the absence of permeant anions, although transfer of fragment A to
the cytosol did not take place under these conditions. However, when the
cells were subsequently treated with low pH in the presence of permeant
anions, the cells were intoxicated (Fig 10.7).

It is therefore, apparently possible to separate the entry process into two
parts. It may be important that the entry during the second exposure to low
pH did not take place unless the cells had been exposed to medium with
neutral pH for a short interval between the two treatments with low pH. The
probable reason for this requirement is that the cytosol had been acidified
during the first exposure to low pH since the experiment was carried out in
the presence of monensin, and that entry requires that the pH in the cytosol
is neutral. The experiments, therefore, further support the view that a pH

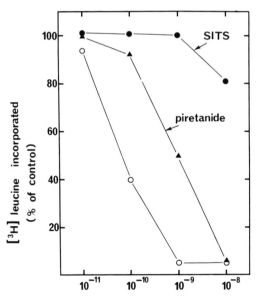

Fig. 10.5 Inhibition of entry of diphtheria toxin at low pH by piretanide and SITS.
Vero cells were incubated with 10 μM monensin and increasing concentrations of
diphtheria toxin for 15 min. Then the medium was removed and the cells were
incubated for 2 min with or without 2 mM piretanide or 0.1 mM SITS in a buffer
containing 20 mM MES, adjusted to pH 4.5 with Tris, 10 μM monensin, and 0.14 M
NaCl. The buffer was then removed, Hepes medium with 10 μM monensin was
added, and 1 h later the rate of protein synthesis was measured.

gradient across the membrane is necessary for toxin entry. Possibly, the pH gradient acts as a driving force for the translocation.

When diphtheria anti-toxin was added before the second exposure to low pH, intoxication was inhibited. This indicates that the toxin remains exposed to the surrounding medium after insertion of fragment B into the membrane at low pH in the absence of permeant anions.

Mechanisms involved in the entry of modeccin

As in the case of diphtheria toxin, the plant toxin modeccin also appears to require low pH for entry. Thus, cells are protected against modeccin by NH_4Cl, chloroquine and the protonophores FCCP (carbonylcyanide *p*-trifluoromethoxyphenylhydrazone) and CCCP (carbonylcyanide *m*-chlorophenylhydrazone) (Sandvig, Sundan, and Olsnes 1984), which all increase the pH of acidic vesicles in the cells. This further indicates that modeccin

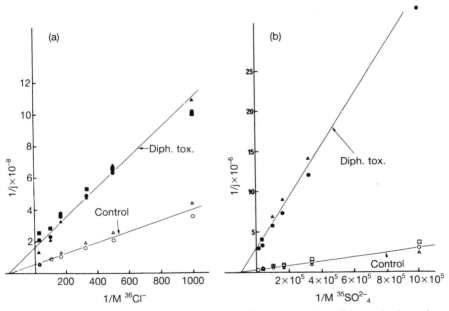

Fig. 10.6 Double reciprocal plots of chloride (a) and sulphate (b) uptake in toxin-treated and untreated cells. Vero cells were incubated for 20 min at 37°C in 0.3 ml Hepes medium, pH 7, with and without 3 μg ml⁻¹ diphtheria toxin and then treated for 5 min with Hepes medium, pH 4.5. The cells were washed twice with mannitol buffer, pH 6, and the uptake of ³⁶Cl⁻ (a) and ³⁵SO₄²⁻ (b) was measured at 24°C in the presence of increasing concentrations of the unlabelled anion. The initial rate of anion uptake was measured and the data were transformed to Lineweaver–Burk plots. Closed symbols: diphtheria toxin present. Open symbols, controls without diphtheria toxin.

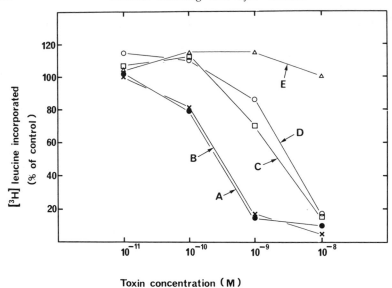

Fig. 10.7 Ability of toxin inserted into membranes in the absence of permeant anions to enter upon subsequent exposure to NaCl at low pH. Vero cells were incubated with increasing concentrations of diphtheria toxin for 15 min in Hepes medium, pH 7.5, containing 10 μM monensin. The medium was then removed and the cells were incubated in various buffers containing 10 μM monensin as described in Table 10.2. Finally the cells were incubated with ^{3}H-leucine and protein synthesis was measured over a period of 10 min.

Table 10.2 Flow diagram of medium changes and additions in Fig. 10.7

Sample	15 min	2 min	5 min	2 min	60 min
A	Toxin	260 mM mannitol, pH 4.5	medium, pH 7.2	0.14 M NaCl, pH 4.5	medium, pH 7.2
B	Toxin	260 mM mannitol, pH 7.0	medium, pH 7.2	0.14 M NaCl, pH 4.5	medium, pH 7.2
C	Toxin	260 mM mannitol, pH 4.5	medium, pH 7.2	medium, pH 7.2	medium, pH 7.2
D	Toxin	260 mM mannitol, pH 4.5	medium, pH 7.2 + antitoxin	0.14 M NaCl, pH 4.5 + antitoxin	medium, pH 7.2 + antitoxin
E	Toxin	260 mM mannitol, pH 7.0	medium, pH 7.2 + antitoxin	0.14 M NaCl, pH 4.5 + antitoxin	medium, pH 7.2 + antitoxin

must also be endocytosed before it can enter the cytosol. The entry mechanism for modeccin appears to be more complex than that described for diphtheria toxin. Thus, it has not been possible to induce rapid entry of modeccin from the cell surface into the cytosol by exposing cells with bound modeccin to medium with low pH. Furthermore, when modeccin is added to cells, protein synthesis begins to decline after a much longer period than in the case of diphtheria toxin (Fig 10.8). Since both binding and endocytosis of modeccin take place rapidly, it appears that it is the transport of modeccin from the endocytic vesicle into the cytosol, which is the most time-consuming process. This is supported by the finding that compounds known to raise the pH of endocytic vesicles are able to protect well against modeccin, even if they are added to the cells as much as 1 h after the addition of modeccin (Sandvig *et al.* 1984).

When Vero cells were incubated with modeccin and diphtheria toxin at 20°C rather than at 37°C, the toxic effect of modeccin was much more markedly reduced than that of diphtheria toxin. It has been demonstrated that both fusion of endocytic vesicles with lysosomes and transport within the Golgi apparatus are inhibited at low temperature (Dunn, Hubbard, and Aronson 1980; Saraste and Kuismanen 1984; Matlin and Simons 1983). The data therefore suggest that fusion of modeccin-containing vesicles with another cellular compartment is required for entry to take place. As

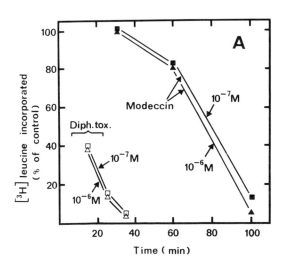

Fig. 10.8 Rate of protein synthesis inhibition by diphtheria toxin and modeccin. The indicated amounts of toxin were added to Vero cells and, after different periods of incubation at 37°C, the rate of protein synthesis over a 10 min period was measured. Indicated on the abscissa is the time from addition of toxin to the cells until 5 min after addition of ³H-leucine.

described above, the low concentrations of monensin that interfere with normal glycosylation and transport within the Golgi apparatus (Tartakoff 1983) strongly protect against modeccin (Sandvig and Olsnes 1982a). Possibly, modeccin must be transported to another cellular compartment, such as the Golgi apparatus, before it can enter the cytosol. We had found earlier that modeccin is much less effective in inhibiting cell-free protein synthesis than would be expected from its extreme toxicity for cells. This suggests that the molecule is altered after entry into the cells, a process that might take place in the Golgi apparatus.

Conclusions

Entry of diphtheria toxin into the cell involves binding of the toxin to cell surface receptors and the transfer of an enzymatically active fragment A across the membrane. The binding of toxin to the cells is reduced by several compounds known to increase the level of phosphorylation in the cells. Furthermore, permeable anions are required for optimal binding. Permeable anions are also required for the transport of fragment A across the membrane. Although insertion of fragment B into the membrane takes place in buffers osmotically balanced with mannitol, it is necessary to expose the cells to low pH and permeable anions simultaneously for entry of fragment A to take place.

Modeccin also seems to require low pH for entry. However, the entry mechanism differs from that of diphtheria toxin. It has not been possible to induce entry of modeccin from the cell surface into the cytosol by exposure of cells with surface-bound toxin to low pH.

Abrin and ricin also appear to enter the cytosol from intracellular vesicles, but they do not appear to require low pH for entry and these toxins enter most efficiently when the pH of the medium is slightly alkaline. The entry of these toxins appears to depend upon a Ca^{2+} flux and this is also the case with modeccin. Whereas binding to cell surface receptors and endocytosis is required for the normal entry of all toxins considered here, the toxins apparently utilize different mechanisms in their transfer across the cellular membrane to gain access to their target in the cytosol.

References

Boquet, P., Silverman, M. S., Pappenheimer, Jr., A. M., and Vernon, W. B. (1976). Binding of Triton X-100 to diphtheria toxin, crossreacting material 45, and their fragments. *Proc. nat. Acad. Sci. USA* **73**, 4449–53.

Carpenter, G. (1981). Vanadate, epidermal growth factor and the stimulation of DNA synthesis. *Biochem. Biophys. Res. Commun.* **102**, 1115–21.

Donovan, J. J., Simon, M. I., Draper, R. K., and Montal, M. (1981). Diphtheria toxin forms channels in planar lipid bilayers. *Proc. nat. Acad. Sci. USA* **78**, 172–6.

Draper, R. K. and Simon, M. I. (1980). The entry of diphtheria toxin into mammalian cell cytoplasm: evidence for lysosomal involvement. *J. cell Biol.* **87**, 849–54.

Dunn, W. A., Hubbard, A. L., and Aronson, Jr. N. N. (1980). Low temperature selectively inhibits fusion between pinocytic vesicles and lysosomes during heterophagy of ^{125}I-asialo fetuin by the perfused rat liver. *J. biol. Chem.* **255**, 5971–8.

Elbein, A. D. (1981). The tunicamycins — useful tools for studies on glycoproteins. *Trends. biochem. Sci.* **6**, 219–21.

Kagan, B. L., Finkelstein, A., and Colombini, M. (1981). Diphtheria toxin forms large pores in phospholipid bilayer membranes. *Proc. nat. Acad. Sci. USA* **78**, 4950–4.

Matlin, K. S. and Simons, K. (1983). Reduced temperature prevents transfer of a membrane glycoprotein to the cell surface but does not prevent terminal glycosylation. *Cell* **34**, 233–43.

Mumby, M. and Traugh, J. A. (1979). Dephosphorylation of translational initiation factors and 40S ribosomal subunits by phosphoprotein phosphatases from rabbit reticulocytes. *Biochemistry* **18**, 4548–56.

Nishizuka, Y. (1984). The role of protein kinase C in cell surface signal transduction and tumour promotion. *Nature* **308**, 693–8.

Olsnes, S. and Sandvig, K. (1983). Entry of toxic proteins into cells. In *Receptor-mediated endocytosis, receptors, and recognition* (ed. P. Cuatrecasas, and T. F. Roth), Series B, Vol. 15, pp. 189–236. Chapman and Hall, London.

—— and —— (1985). Entry of polypeptide toxins into animal cells. In *Endocytosis* (ed. I. Pastan and M. C. Willingham), pp. 195–234. Plenum, New York.

Sandvig, K. and Olsnes, S. (1980). Diphtheria toxin entry into cells is facilitated by low pH. *J. cell Biol.* **87**, 828–32.

—— and —— (1981). Rapid entry of nicked diphtheria toxin into cells at low pH. Characterization of the entry process and effects of low pH on the toxin molecule. *J. biol. Chem.* **256**, 9068–76.

—— and —— (1982a). Entry of the toxic proteins abrin, modeccin, ricin and diphtheria toxin into cells. II. Effect of pH, metabolic inhibitors, and ionophores and evidence for toxin penetration from endocytic vesicles. *J. biol. Chem.* **257**, 7504–13.

—— and —— (1982b). Entry of the toxic proteins abrin, modeccin, ricin and diphtheria toxin into cells. I. Requirement for calcium. *J. biol. Chem.* **257**, 7495–503.

—— and —— (1985). Effect of the chaotrophic anions thiocyanate and perchlorate on the entry of ricin into Vero cells. *Biochem. J.* **228**, 521–3.

——, ——, and Pihl, A. (1979). Inhibitory effect of ammoniumchloride and chloroquine on the entry of the toxic lectin modeccin into HeLa cells. *Biochem. Biophys. Res. Commun.* **90**, 648–55.

——, Sundan, A., and Olsnes, S. (1984). Evidence that diphtheria toxin and modeccin enter the cytosol from different vesicular compartments. *J. cell Biol.* **98**, 963–70.

Saraste, J. and Kuismanen, E. (1984). Pre- and post-Golgi vacuoles operate in the transport of Semliki Forest Virus membrane glycoproteins to the cell surface. *Cell* **38**, 535–49.

Tartakoff, A. M. (1983). Perturbation of vesicular traffic with the carboxylic ionophore monensin. *Cell* **32**, 1026–8.

Tulsiani, D. R. P., Harris, T. M., and Touster, O. (1982). Swainsonine inhibits the biosynthesis of complex glycoproteins by inhibition of Golgi mannosidase II. *J. biol. Chem.* **257**, 7936–9.

11

Membrane damage caused by bacterial toxins: recent advances and new challenges

J. H. Freer

Introduction

Space does not permit a comprehensive coverage of all membrane-damaging toxins produced by bacteria and the reader is referred to other sources for additional information on this topic (see Alouf and Geoffroy 1984; Middlebrook and Dorland 1984; Jeljaszewicz and Wadstrom 1978). Here, I have restricted discussion to selected toxins, where new information has clarified some of the earlier work on membrane-damaging activity, or to selected examples of toxins, which constitute new and challenging problems in terms of their modes of membrane damage. There are of course many toxins not mentioned in this review that otter further challenges to researchers in this field, and perhaps those I have offended by omitting their favourite toxins here, will be stimulated to correct the situation by writing a review of their own.

Bacterial toxins can generally be divided into two broad categories on the basis of their chemical composition and their modes of action. The first group consists of the endotoxins, structurally and functionally a very closely related group of lipopolysaccharides found exclusively as major components in the outer membrane of Gram-negative bacterial cell walls. While the endotoxins have profound and multiple effects in diseases caused by Gram-negative bacteria and are also capable of interacting with and modifying the properties of membranes of mammalian cells (for review see Wicken and Knox 1980), they are not usually recognized as belonging to the toxins responsible for direct membrane damage.

The second category of toxins found in bacteria constitute a much more heterogeneous group of high molecular weight protein or glycoprotein antigens of widely diverse structure and mechanisms of toxicity. All of these toxins interact in some way with cell membranes, either via highly specific receptor molecules (often consisting of glycoconjugates on the target cells, which mediate binding of the toxin prior to its active toxic phase, e.g. GM1 ganglioside receptor for cholera toxin) or via relatively non-specific receptors on the cell surface such as zwitterionic or acidic phospholipids, as for staphylococcal delta lysins.

Toxins that cause functional membrane damage (no detectable physical modification of membrane structure) to cells via initial membrane binding followed by internalization of the toxin or part of the toxin, are in most instances composed of two functionally distinct moieties. One is responsible for toxin binding to the target cell surface and is called the B or binding subunit, the other subunit is responsible for the active toxic reactions and is called the A or active subunit. The AB design for toxins is not restricted to bacterial toxins but is also found in plant toxins such as ricin and abrin, which also share with some bacterial toxins the same mode of toxicity.

The AB design principle is found in toxins, such as diphtheria toxin, that are synthesized as a single polypeptide chain, with distinct functional domains corresponding to the A and B moieties. Such domains are usually activated following proteolytic cleavage ('nicking'), although the two fragments are often still covalently linked via a thiol bridge, which subsequently undergoes reductive cleavage to release the active fragment. In other instances, the A and B subunits are synthesized as distinct polypeptides, which are later assembled at the bacterial surface into a complex holotoxin containing a single A subunit and multiple B subunits (e.g. cholera toxin, shiga toxin, pertussis toxin) before release from the bacterial cell.

One of the most germane topics presently being addressed is the mechanism(s) of internalization of the A subunits in intoxicated cells and the part played by the B subunits in transmembrane passage of the active moiety (see Sandvig, this volume). It is beyond doubt that the A subunit in such toxins as cholera toxin (CT) and the closely related heat-labile toxin (LT) of *Escherichia coli* cause functional membrane damage by elevating the activity of the membrane-bound multi-component adenylate cyclase complex. Thus, by directly modifying a regulatory component (G protein) of the cyclase — an integral membrane enzyme complex — the toxin causes an elevation of intracellular cAMP, which in turn alters the normal ion transport properties of the cell membrane (functional membrane damage). The consequent malabsorption of sodium ions and hypersecretion of water, chloride, and bicarbonate ions results in fluid accumulation in the lumen of the gut and promotes a massive diarrhoea.

However, what is not clear and still offers a challenging area for research is the exact manner in which the A subunit gains access to its target membrane protein. This same question also applies to other toxins with different intracellular targets, such as shiga toxin, diphtheria toxin, and several others.

Even more fascinating questions relate to the mechanisms of transmembrane passage of the clostridial neurotoxins which, in order to reach their targets in the central nervous system (tetanus toxin) or at the neuromuscular junction (botulinum toxin), must cross multiple membranes without loss of activity.

Structural damage to membranes can be induced by a variety of mechanisms, including enzymic hydrolysis of membrane components, insertion of surface active peptides resulting in membrane 'solubilization', partial insertion of proteins into the hydrophobic domain, or insertion of proteins across the membrane with the subsequent formation of transmembrane channels or pores. All of these mechanisms are found as part of the spectrum of activity of the so-called membrane-damaging bacterial toxins.

Pore-forming toxins and toxin fragments

Streptolysin O and other SH-activated toxins

Four genera of Gram-positive bacteria, namely *Bacillus*, *Clostridium*, *Streptococcus*, and *Listeria*, contain numerous species that produce extracellular cytolytic protein toxins with remarkably similar properties. In addition, *Streptococcus pneumoniae* produces an intracellular toxin in this category. These common properties include the following (Alouf and Geoffroy 1984):

   (a) lethal (cardiotoxic) to animals;
   (b) cytolytic to eukaryotic cells;
   (c) require prior reduction for biological activity;
   (d) inactivated by oxidation or SH-group reagents;
   (e) antigenically related and stimulate cross-reacting precipitating and neutralizing antibodies;
   (f) inactivated by cholesterol and related 3-β-hydroxy-sterols;
   (g) thought to damage cell membranes by interacting with sterols.

All of these toxins (see Table 11.1) probably consist of single polypeptide chains with a molecular weight within the range 48–68 kdalton depending on the producing species and the method of estimation. Recent evidence

Table 11.1 Examples of SH-activated toxins with selected physical properties.

Name of lysin	Producer species	m.w. (k dalton)[a]	pI[a]
Perfringolysin O	*C. perfringens*	59–64	5.8–6.9
Tetanolysin	*C. tetani*	48–53	5.6–6.1
Cereolysin	*B. cereus*	55	6.6
Thuringiolysin	*B. thuringiensis*	55	nd
Alveolysin	*B. alvei*	63	5.1
Streptolysin O	*S. pyogenes*	68	7.8
Pneumolysin	*S. pneumoniae*	60	4.9

[a]Data from Alouf (1984).

indicates that some of the variation in reported values for molecular weight for the same toxin may be due to more than one active form of the toxin. For example, Bhakdi, Tranum-Jensen, and Sziegoleit (1985) recently reported isolating two forms of streptolysin O (SLO) with molecular weights of 69 kdalton and 57 kdalton. Both forms were actively haemolytic although differing in pI (6–6.4 and 7–7.5, respectively). Also, Chakraborty, Gilmore, Hacker, Huhle, Kathareou, Knapp, Kreft, Müller, Leimeister, Parrisius, Wagner, and Goebel (1986) recently cloned a second cereolysin (cereolysin B) that differs entirely from the classic SH-activated toxin and consists of two components, one of which appears to function as the receptor for the other. Neither of the two proteins cross-react with anti-SLO antibodies.

The pI values vary depending upon the toxin, but the majority of the lysins are slightly acidic at neutral pH (Table 11.1). The relatively wide variation in the range of both pI values and molecular weights is in keeping with findings of wide differences in amino acid composition for different SH-activated toxins. Such indications of fundamental differences in composition and structure of toxins within this group contrast with their similarities, indicated by the antigenic cross-reactivity and similar modes of action. It seems very likely that there are highly conserved functional domains in these molecules, which serve as epitopes and are involved in the lytic activity. These domains must, however, represent relatively small regions of the molecules, since in a recent genetic study Kehoe and Timmis (1984) used the cloned SLO gene as a probe to investigate inter-relatedness between eight SH-activated toxins and found no hybridization with the SLO probe at 80 per cent stringency.

The most well-studied member of this group of about 15 toxins is streptolysin O, although cereolysin, tetanolysin, perfringolysin, pneumolysin, listeriolysin, thuringiolysin, and alveolysin have also been purified to homogeneity. One of the characteristic features of the membrane lesions produced by these lysins is the presence of ring- and arc-shaped structures 35–38 nm in diameter, found both associated with the membranes and also free in the surrounding medium (Fig 11.1). For many years there was speculation that these represented complexes of toxin and cholesterol sequestered from the membrane, and that this removal of sterol resulted, by some unknown mechanism, in membrane destabilization and eventual lysis (Bernheimer 1974; Duncan and Schlegel 1975). However, the significance of the observation of ring and arc structures in purified perfringolysin preparation (Smyth, Freer, and Arbuthnott 1975) in the absence of membrane or cholesterol was clarified by the more recent observations of Rottem, Cole, Habig, Barile, and Hardegree (1982), who showed that the appearance of rings and arcs in purified tetanolysin was a function of protein concentration and that the rings and arcs almost certainly represented polymerized toxin alone. In support of the earlier suggestion of Smyth *et al.*

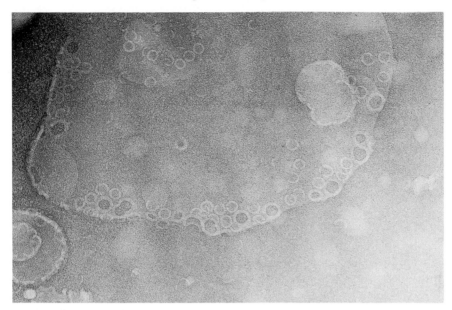

Fig. 11.1 Electronmicrograph of a negatively stained preparation showing lesions bordered by ring- and arc-shaped toxin polymers after interaction of perfringolysin with liposomes (cholesterol: sphingomyelin: ovolecithin: phosphatidylethanolamine, molar ratio 1.8:2.1:1.3:1.0). Magnification = 170 000

(1975), it is now generally agreed that the ring and arc structures seen after toxin–membrane interactions most probably represent toxin polymer, the formation of which is induced by favourable orientation of toxin at the membrane surface due to its affinity for sterol.

The presence of rings and arcs in purified preparations of tetanolysin and perfringolysin as well as the complete absence of detectable sterol in rings and arcs derived from membrane lesions (Bhakdi *et al.* 1985) provide convincing evidence that the lesions seen at the membrane surface are toxin polymers and not toxin–sterol complexes as originally thought.

Earlier suggestions that the rings seen on the surface of toxin-damaged membranes represented transmembrane pores fell out of favour when Cowell, Kim, and Bernheimer (1978) concluded from a freeze-fracture study of cereolysin-induced damaged erythrocytes that the lesions did not represent pores that spanned the full width of the membrane. However, more recent data from a comprehensive ultrastructural study of the interaction of SLO with both erythrocyte and liposome membranes by Bhakdi *et al.* (1985) provides compelling evidence that, at least at relatively high toxin concentrations, the lesions induced by this toxin are indeed transmembrane pores, which are lined with the polymerized toxin. A single lesion would be sufficient to result in lysis of the erythrocyte. The relatively large diameter of the lesions induced by this group of toxins (estimated pore diameter c. 15 nm) differentiates the mode of lysis from the colloid osmotic mechanisms involved in lysis induced by toxins such as staphylococcal alpha toxin (see below). The estimated size of the lesion produced in the membrane by SLO is in keeping with a non-colloidal osmotic lysis mechanism, as was indicated by earlier observations of concurrent release of both $^{86}Rb^{+}$ and haemoglobin in SLO-treated erythrocytes (Duncan 1974).

Calculations based on the size of the lesion, assuming values of 0.73 for partial specific volume and 69 000 for molecular weight of the monomer, suggest that each pore might be lined by a toxin polymer consisting of 70–80 monomers. This figure for the number of monomers in a single lesion compares well with the earlier estimate of 114 molecules necessary for lysis of an erythrocyte by SLO (Alouf and Raynaud, 1968). Additional evidence for the penetration of the membrane interior by alveolysin was gained from labelling of membrane-bound toxin with the amphiphilic glycolipid photoreactive probe, 12-(4-azido-2-nitrophenoxy)stearoyl-(1-^{14}C)-glucosamine (12-APS-GlcN). This molecule spontaneously inserts into membranes and when subjected to u.v. irradiation, covalently radiolabels adjacent proteins in the hydrophobic domain of the membrane at a depth of 1.3 nm from the membrane surface (Jolivet-Reynaud, Geoffroy, Igolen, and Alouf 1982).

The high specificity of the SH-activated toxins for membranes which contain 3-β-hydroxysterols is well recognized (Smyth and Duncan 1978) and it is clearly documented that membranes lacking sterols are resistant to lysis by these agents (Bernheimer and Davidson 1965). It might seem inconsistent therefore that oligomeric rings isolated from toxin-treated membranes bind tightly to phosphatidyl choline liposomes lacking cholesterol (Bhakdi *et al*. 1985). However, current evidence suggests that the specificity of the monomer–cholesterol interaction leads to toxin orientation at the cholesterol-containing membrane surface, which favours toxin polymerization to form the highly ordered ring structures. These, once formed, are extremely stable and appear to have a lipophilic convex face and a hydrophilic concave face, favouring tight association with membranes or liposomes independent of sterol. Their initial formation on the membrane however, appears to be critically dependent upon specific interaction with sterol in the membrane. The earlier model proposed by Alouf (1977) for SLO, which involved two distinct topological active sites on the molecule, the so-called f or fixation site and the l or lytic site, is not incompatible with this concept. The f site corresponds to the high affinity site for sterol, the favourable orientation of which is promoted by the presence of phospholipids. However, the l site may represent not a lytic site in the sense of a site that is directly involved in penetration of the membrane, but a site that is involved in toxin–toxin interaction, leading to polymer formation.

Subsequent to this step, the polymer initiates the active membrane-damaging event. However, it is possible that other toxins in this group differ in their mode of lysis (see Blumenthal and Habig 1984).

Staphylococcal alpha toxin

Pathogenic strains of *Staphylococcus aureus* produce an exceptional range of toxins and virulence factors. There are four well-recognized membrane-damaging toxins (sometimes referred to as lysins, haemolysins, or cytolysins) produced by this species, the alpha, beta, gamma, and delta toxins. The relative amount of each toxin produced depends upon the producer strain as well as the conditions of cultivation of the organism. The toxins of this species have been extensively reviewed recently (Freer and Arbuthnott 1983) and in this discussion, only data relating to membrane-damaging activity will be emphasized.

The alpha toxin gene of *S. aureus* Wood 46, the strain most widely used for alpha toxin purification, has recently been cloned and sequenced (Gray and Kehoe 1984). The sequence data confirm earlier estimates of molecular weight of about 33 000 (Freer and Arbuthnott 1983) and reports that the toxin is secreted via the classic signal sequence mechanism (Tweten, Christianson, and Iandolo 1983).

Ultrastructural and biochemical studies in the 1960s by Freer, Arbuthnott, and Bernheimer (reviewed by Freer and Arbuthnott 1983) established that the monomeric toxin, a basic protein (pI = 8.5) with a sedimentation coefficient of 3.0 S (alpha 3 S toxin) aggregated on contact with membranes, lipid dispersions, or lipid monolayers to a higher molecular weight form consisting of six monomers arranged in a circular manner (alpha 12 S toxin) with an outside diameter of approximately 10 nm and a central hole of approximately 2–3 nm diameter (Freer, Arbuthnott, and Bernheimer 1968). Although polymerization was accompanied by loss of haemolytic activity, this activity could be partially restored by treatment of the inactive 12 S polymer and 8 M urea followed by dialysis against neutral buffer. In freshly purified toxin preparations, an equilibrium exists where about 10 per cent of the protein is in the 12 S form and 90 per cent in the active 3 S form (Arbuthnott, Freer, and Bernheimer 1967). Interaction of the monomeric toxin with cell membranes or lipid monolayers and bilayers was not only accompanied by the formation of membrane-bound 12 S toxin rings (Fig 11.2) but was also coincident with loss of membrane integrity, as evidenced by leakage of sequestered marker molecules from liposomes and colloid osmotic lysis of erythrocytes. In the case of toxin interacting with the mixed lipid monolayer compressed to 10 mN m^{-1}, appearance of 12 S toxin in the monolayer was accompanied by an increase in surface pressure of about 10 mN m^{-1} and an increase in surface potential. These increases were indicative of the relatively high surface activity of the toxin, which resulted

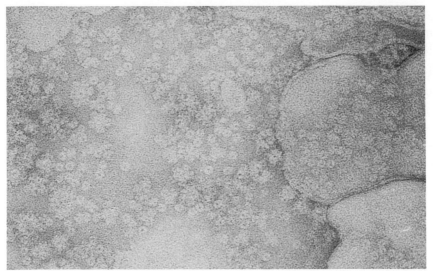

Fig. 11.2 Electron micrograph showing a negatively stained lecithin dispersion after treatment with staphylococcal alpha toxin; note the polymeric form of the toxin (12 S toxin) both free and associated with the lipid bilayers. Magnification = 360 000.

in monolayer penetration. The relatively high surface activity of the alpha toxin has since been confirmed in a number of studies (see Colacicco and Buckelew, 1971; Freer, Arbuthnott, and Billcliffe 1973).

While the toxin is active in terms of membrane disruption or induction of permeability changes on a wide variety of cells, including both erythrocytes and various mammalian cell lines, rabbit erythrocytes display a markedly higher sensitivity to haemolysis than those of other species. This provides a sensitive and convenient assay for the toxin, but unwarranted effort has been expended in attempts to elucidate the basis for the increased sensitivity of rabbit erythrocytes, which in all likelihood has no significance in terms of the activity of this toxin in staphyolococcal disease. Nevertheless, the exact mechanism of membrane modification by the agent has eluded clarification until very recently.

Freer *et al.* (1973) demonstrated profound changes consistent with protein penetration in the hydrophobic fracture plane of erythrocyte membranes after treatment with relatively high concentrations of alpha toxin and suggested that membrane disruption was a result of penetration of the membrane by toxic protein, which in turn resulted in loss of selective ion permeability (Freer 1982). This would then lead to cell disruption by colloid osmotic lysis in the case of erythrocytes, which lack effective repair systems. More recently, Thelestam, Jolivet-Reynaud, and Alouf (1983) labelled alpha-toxin-treated erythrocytes with the amphiphilic glycolipid photoreactive probe, 12-APS-GlcN (see above). This study confirmed the earlier data of Freer *et al.* (1968, 1973), showing penetration of toxin into the hydro-phobic domain of the membrane. In a recent series of elegant studies combining ultrastructural and biochemical data (reviewed in Bhakdi and Tranum-Jensen, 1983), Bhakdi and his co-workers confirmed the earlier observations relating to lipid-induced polymerization of toxin (Freer and Arbuthnott 1983) and considerably extended the studies to include the isolation of membrane-bound polymeric ring forms of toxin. These are water insoluble, and can be induced to form by reaction of monomeric toxin with deoxycholate micelles. These rings will bind lipid or detergent and will reincorporate into liposomes. When generated on the membrane of resealed erythrocyte ghosts, they will induce the formation of trans-membrane pores with an exclusion limit which corresponds to markers of about 3 nm effective diameter. This is in excellent agreement with the size of the central hole seen in the hexameric form of the toxin and provides strong circumstantial evidence in favour of a mechanism of toxin-induced mem-brane damage which involves the formation of transmembrane pores.

Whether or not specific receptor molecules are involved in toxin binding to membranes is not yet clear, although they are certainly not necessary for toxin induced damage to occur in liposomes. Earlier results from binding studies with rabbit and human erythrocytes suggested that rabbit erythrocytes carried 10^5 high affinity toxin receptors per cell, whereas human erythrocytes lacked these receptors but were nonetheless sensitive to higher doses of toxin (Cassidy and Harshman 1976; Harshman 1979). More recently Bhakdi, Muhly, and Fussle (1984a) showed that the sensitivity of human erythrocytes to alpha-toxin haemolysis could be increased relative to that of rabbit erythrocytes by reducing the pH value of the erythrocyte suspension to about 5.0. In all instances, toxin binding and effective haemolysis was accompanied by the appearance of polymeric ring forms of the toxin on the membranes, adding further support to the pore theory of membrane disruption. High affinity toxin receptors similar to those found on rabbit erythrocytes appear to be present on the myelin of rabbit vagus nerve (Harshman, personal communication). As little as 0.2 µg ml^{-1} of alpha toxin causes dramatic destabilization of the lamellae of the myelin sheath of rabbit vagus nerve *in vitro*, with extensive vesicularization occur-ring within 20 min. Similar changes can also be seen in the central nervous system in the mouse where the cortical myelinated trunks show similar vesiculation of myelin 10 min after i.c. injection of 1 µg of toxin (Harshman 1979). Preliminary evidence suggests that the toxin binds to a proteolipopro-tein receptor on myelin similar to the receptor found on the rabbit erythrocyte membrane.

From data reported and discussed very briefly above, the likely sequence of events involved in the process of alpha toxin-induced damage to cell membranes is as follows;

Toxin monomers bind to the cell membrane and partially insert into the lipid domain. Following binding is a temperature sensitive step which probably corresponds to lipid-dependent lateral diffusion or reorientation of monomer or monomer/receptor complex with the formation of a polymeric toxin complex and the induction of a transmembrane pore or channel. The efflux of small ions such as potassium is followed in the erythrocyte by influx of water, osmotic swelling, and eventual lysis with release of haemoglobin. The osmotic swelling stage can be largely prevented or at least considerably delayed by the presence of osmotic stabilizers such as sucrose (Cooper, Madoff, and Weinstein 1964), and initial release of K^+ can be delayed by low temperature ($0°C$), which prevents membrane damage but does not inhibit toxin binding (Freer 1982). Toxin binding can be prevented by Zn^{2+} ions (Avigad and Bernheimer 1978) whereas Ca^{2+} ions largely protect against alpha-toxin-induced haemolysis by preventing the early release of small ions. The postulated mechanism of protection is by prevention of the formation of the hexameric toxin complex on the membrane through a direct effect of the divalent ion on membrane stability and structure rather than on toxin binding or levels of intracellular calcium *per se* (Harshman and Sugg 1985). The stiffening effect on the membrane bilayer that results from the interaction of Ca^{2+} ions with the head groups of acidic phospholipids is well recognized.

The protective effect of divalent cations such as calcium and magnesium on erythrocytes or lymphoma cells treated with potentially lytic doses of alpha toxin was also noted by Bashford, Adler, Patel, and Pasternak (1984) who in addition showed the general applicability of divalent cation protection against membrane damage caused by other membrane permeabilizing agents such as Sendai virus and complement. They concluded that, in the case of alpha toxin, the calcium effect was a non-specific one that was probably mediated through field neutralization in the electrical double layer rather than from specific cation binding site interactions at the cell surface.

Very recent data (Menestrina, 1986) shows that alpha toxin does indeed display pronounced pore-forming ability when allowed to interact with planar bilayer membranes of either neutral or acidic phospholipids and forms gated ion-selective channels that display voltage-dependent closure in the presence of divalent cations such as calcium. This interesting new data should stimulate research aimed at a more precise characterization of toxin-induced channels responsible for the early changes in ion permeability in eukaryotic cells.

Diphtheria toxin fragment B

Extracellular diphtheria toxin is a single polypeptide of m.w.$=58\ 390$, produced by cotranslational secretion and released as an inactive protoxin which is subsequently activated by proteolytic cleavage giving two fragments joined by a disulphide bridge. The N-terminal A fragment contains ADP-ribosyl transferase activity, whereas the C-terminal B fragment, is responsible for the binding of holotoxin to specific protein receptors on sensitive cells and subsequently mediating transport of the A fragment across the membrane of the receptosome (endocytotic vesicle containing membrane bound toxin–receptor complex) into the target cell cytoplasm, a step thought to be induced by acidic conditions in the vesicle. Here, the A fragment inactivates the cell's protein sythesising machinery by catalysing the transfer of an ADP-ribose moiety from endogenous NAD to Elongation Factor 2 (for review see Middlebrook and Dorland 1985).

The way in which the B fragment or part of it mediates the transfer of the A fragment across the endosome membrane has been the focus of research in a number of laboratories (Middlebrook and Dorland 1985). The amino acid sequence of fragment B derived from cleavage peptides correlates well with the sequence predicted from the nucleotide sequence of the cloned toxin gene. Functional domains on cleavage peptides of the B fragment have been identified and their tertiary structure predicted from sequence data (Falmagne, Capiau, Cabiaux, Deleers, and Ruysschaert 1984). The B fragment (342 amino acid residues; m.w. = 37 240) contains three such domains. The N-terminal surface lipid-associating domain (residues 1–77), which is hydrophilic is thought to be responsible for binding of the B fragment to the surface of phospholipid bilayers by ionic interactions. The central transverse lipid-associating domain (residues 78–178) is highly hydrophobic and contains two alpha helical amphiphilic regions. This fragment contains the regions which are responsible for the induction of strong, voltage-dependent increases in ion conductance in lipid bilayers and, at low pH, forms channels in planar bilayer membranes similar to the channel-forming activity of the whole toxin. The third domain, which corresponds to the C-terminal region of the B fragment (residues 179–342), is responsible for specific binding of the toxin to its receptors on the target cell surface, but is also thought to be involved in the initial events of membrane penetration and anchoring which are a prelude to the formation of a membrane channel at low pH. It is via this channel that the A fragment may be transported into the cytoplasm (Falmagne, *et al.* 1984). In an independent study, Kagan, Finkelstein, and Colombini (1981) showed that an N-terminal peptide (B45) of fragment B, which includes the N-terminal and central fragments described by Falmagne *et al.* (1984), formed voltage-dependent channels in planar lipid bilayers.

Tetanus toxin fragment B
Tetanus toxin, like diphtheria toxin, is composed of two chains. The intact molecule as synthesized by the bacterial cell is a single polypeptide of m.w.

= 150 000, which is nicked by extracellular proteases to yield a light or alpha chain (m.w. = 50 000) and a heavy or beta chain (m.w. = 100 000) still linked to each other by a disulphide bridge (Fig 11.3). The B chain can be split by papain to yield a carboxy terminal fragment (C fragment) and the remainder of the B chain still linked by a disulphide bridge to the A chain (the so-called B fragment).

Boquet and Duflot (1984) noted the strikingly similar structural design of diphtheria toxin and tetanus toxin and reasoned that this may imply similar mechanisms in both toxins for promoting the passage of the active fragment across membrane barriers to intracellular targets. They further showed that under similar acidic conditions (pH values below 5.0) the N-terminal fragment of the heavy chain of tetanus toxin, like the similar region of diphtheria toxin fragment B, showed a pronounced increase in its capacity to bind detergent and also acquired the ability to form ion-permeable channels in bilayer vesicles and planar lipid bilayers. These activities were strictly pH-dependent and only associated with the N-terminal region of the heavy chain. No increases in detergent binding or in channel-forming activity were associated with the alpha chain or with fragment C.

In these cases of channel formation, it is apparent that toxin fragments have the ability to damage membranes by inducing changes in selective ion permeability, but that the formation of these channels is induced by pH-dependent conformational changes in the fragments that occur only in the low pH environment of endocytotic vesicles or endolysosomal fusion vesicles. The resulting channel in some way facilitates the passage of the active fragment through the membrane and in so doing delivers the toxic moiety to its target.

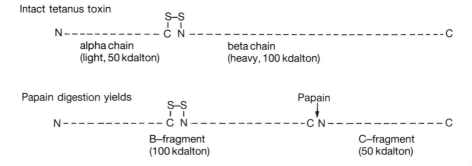

Fig. 11.3 Structure of tetanus toxin.

Surface-active toxins

Staphylococcal delta-lysin

Staphylococcal delta-lysin (delta-toxin) consists of an extracellular, 26 amino acid residue, highly surface-active polypeptide, which displays lytic activity against a wide range of cell types and membrane-bounded structures (for review see Freer and Arbuthnott 1983). It has many unusual properties which include high thermostability (no loss of activity after 1 h at 80°C), inhibition by phospholipids and serum, and solubility in aqueous solutions and in chloroform:methanol (2:1 v/v)) (Freer and Arbuthnott 1976). The striking similarity in structure and properties between this toxin and melittin, the major lytic peptide of bee venom has frequently been noted and is discussed in a number of recent reviews (see Freer and Arbuthnott 1983; Freer, Birkbeck, and Bhakoo 1984).

The similarities between these two lytic peptides do not, however, extend to their amino acid sequences (see Fig 11.4), which differ considerably in charge distribution. The charge distribution of delta toxin appears to be highly conserved in the variant forms of the toxin isolated from canine strains of *Staphylococcus aureus* (Turner 1978), where most, but not all of the changes in sequence from that found in the toxin derived from human strains can be accounted for by single base substitutions.

The sequence of polar or charged and non-polar residues in the delta toxin molecule led Freer and Birkbeck (1982) to propose that the molecule might adopt an alpha-helical configuration, which would result in a laterally amphipathic rod with distinct hydrophobic and hydrophilic faces along the

Delta toxin (human strains)

H₃N–M–A–Q–D–I–I–S–T–I–G–D–L–V–K–W–I–I–D–T–V–N–K–F–T–K–K–COO
+   –   –   +   –   +   + +   –

Delta toxin (canine strains)

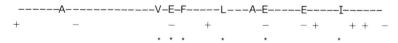

*=substitution equivalent to one base change

Melittin

H₃N–G–I–G–A–V–L–K–V–L–T–T–G–L–P–A–L–I–S–W–I–K–R–K–R–Q–Q–CONH₂
+   +   + + + +

Fig. 11.4 Sequences and charge distribution of delta toxins and melittin.

long axis. The rod would be of sufficient length to span a lipid bilayer membrane and the lateral association of multimers of such rods, with hydrophobic faces associating with hydrocarbon regions of the bilayer, may lead to the formation of transmembrane pores that would account for the lytic activity of the toxin.

Evidence showing the formation of ion-selective transmembrane pores in black lipid membranes by melittin has been presented by Tosteson and Tosteson (1981), who concluded from melittin-induced changes in electrical properties of the bilayer that tetrameric complexes were formed in the membrane.

The wide range of target structures affected by the delta toxin and its relatively low specific activity are also in keeping with a surface–active mechanism of lysis. Bhakoo, Birkbeck, and Freer (1982, 1985) and Freer *et al.* (1984) investigated the specificity of the interaction of delta toxin with lipids by assessing the ability of the toxin to penetrate lipid monolayers of different composition and surface pressure. They confirmed earlier observations of Colaccico, Basu, Buckelew, and Bernheimer (1977) that the toxin had unusually high surface activity, and went on to define the influence of lipid head group, and length and degree of saturation of the hydrocarbon chain on the ability of the toxin to penetrate the monolayer. Their data showed that delta lysin had relatively low specificity for lipid head group, and penetrated films of either neutral or acidic lipids with equal vigour. This contrasted with melittin, which showed a distinct preference for films of acidic phospholipids (Bougis, Rochat, Pieroni, and Verger (1981).

Bhakoo *et al.* (1982, 1985) extended their comparative study to include toxin-induced leakage of ATP from large unilamellar vesicles of defined lipid composition. The sensitivity to toxin-induced leakage was increased by decreasing hydrocarbon chain length or increasing *cis* unsaturation, both of which would promote fluidity in the hydrocarbon chains. At relatively high concentrations, delta toxin causes fragmentation of lipid bilayer vesicles with the formation of small disc-like structures about 50 nm in diameter. These were interpreted as consisting of fragments of bilayer stabilized and rendered 'soluble' by a boundary of toxin monomers arranged such that their hydrophobic faces associated with the hydrocarbon region of the bilayer and their hydrophilic faces associated with the surrounding aqueous phase. The toxin molecules could thus form a continuous boundary layer around the fragment rendering it stable in the bilayer conformation. This fragmentation, which occurs at relatively high concentrations of toxin, would be likely to occur when toxin in the transmembrane configuration reached a concentration sufficient to allow coalescence of toxin and fragmentation of the bilayer.

Earlier determinations of molecular weight suggested that delta toxin exists in aqueous dispersions as a high molecular weight aggregate

(>100 kdalton) dissociated by low concentrations of Tween 80 to an aggregate of about 21 000 dalton, which may correspond to a hexamer (Kantor, Temples, and Shaw 1972). In contrast, X-ray crystallographic data shows that melittin exists as a tetramer in aqueous suspension (Terwilliger, Weissman, and Eisenberg 1982).

Recent physical studies on delta toxin have shown clear differences in its behaviour in solution when compared to melittin. By monitoring the intrinsic fluorescence of Trp 15 in the delta toxin molecule, Dufourcq and associates (Dufourcq, Dufourc, Faucon, Birkbeck, and Freer, unpublished observations), showed that decreasing the dielectric constant of the suspending medium of the toxin resulted in fluorescence changes which suggested the dissociation of the toxin aggregates into monomers. Very similar effects on the fluorescence spectrum could be achieved by reducing the concentration of toxin to below 1 μM in water at pH 7.5. Thus at neutral pH in aqueous solutions, the toxin can exist as a highly associated form or, at lower concentrations more likely to be relevant in lytic situations in nature, as a much smaller toxin species. Dissociation of the multimeric toxin would also be promoted at the surface of the target membrane since the dielectric constant decreases markedly at the membrance surface (Dawson, Drake, Helliwell, and Hider 1978).

This contrasts with the behaviour of melittin, which shows a lower stability in its highly associated form. The increased stability of delta lysin complexes could result from ion pairing of lys–asp residues in addition to the hydrophobic interactions. Similar but more complex changes in fluorescence of Trp 15 occur when the toxin interacts with lysophosphatidyl choline (lysoPC), irrespective of the state of association of the toxin or the molecular arrangement of the lysoPC (monomeric or micellar form) (Dufourcq *et al.*, unpublished results).

Clostridium perfringens *delta toxin*

A recently purified cytolytic toxin from *C. perfringens* is the delta toxin, which is haemolytic for the erythrocytes of even-toed ungulates (Alouf and Jolivet-Reynaud 1981). Although the data on the precise mode of membrane damage induced by this toxin is still fragmentary, several interesting features of its activity merit discussion. Its cytolytic activity is not restricted to erythrocytes but extends to other cell types including rabbit, human, and guinea pig platelets and the toxin is lethal to some types of rabbit leucocyte. It appears that its haemolytic spectrum and specific cytotoxicity for certain subpopulations of rabbit leucocytes reflect the presence of a cell surface GM2 ganglioside-containing toxin receptor (Jolivet-Reynaud and Alouf 1982). Binding of radio-iodinated toxin to sheep erythrocytes was specific, tight, rapid, saturable and practically irreversible (Jolivet-Reynaud and Alouf 1983). The erythrocytes contained an estimated 7000 sites per cell.

This compares with an estimated 5000 high affinity sites per rabbit erythrocyte for staphylococcal alpha toxin (Cassidy and Harshman 1976). Bound toxin could be removed from the cell by extraction with chaotropic agents in contrast to SH-activated toxins, which resist such extraction, probably due to their insertion in the lipid bilayer and strong hydrophobic associations with membrance lipids. Also, 12 APS GlcN does not label the membrane-associated clostridial delta toxin, whereas it does label both membrane-associated forms of SH-activated toxins and staphylococcal alpha toxin (see above).

Toxin-induced haemolysis by delta toxin is characterized by a rapid binding phase (which occurs at 0°C but is faster at 37°C, followed by a markedly temperature-dependent process leading to irreversible loss of selective permeability. This is similar to the sequence of events for a number of cytolytic toxins (e.g. staphylococcal alpha toxin) but different from the lysis induced by detergents or staphylococcal delta toxin, where there is no lag between binding and loss of selective permeability, and no temperature dependent phase (Kreger, Kim, Zaboretsky, and Bernheimer 1971).

Haemolysins of aeromonads and vibrios

Aeromonas hydrophila *alpha and beta haemolysins*

Aeromonas hydrophila is an aquatic Gram-negative motile bacterium classically recognized as a pathogen of cold-blooded animals. In recent years however, this same organism has been implicated in a wide variety of infections in humans. It produces a range of extracellular virulence factors, among which are the alpha and the beta haemolysins.

The alpha haemolysin is an acidic protein with pI = 4.8 and m.w. = 65 000. Rat erythrocytes are most sensitive to haemolysis whereas sheep erythrocytes are the most resistant. In the human embryonic lung fibroblast assay system, which sizes the functional 'holes' produced by cytolytic agents (Thelestam and Mollby 1979), the alpha haemolysins behaved like surface active agents, including staphylococcal delta toxin, in that all three different sized markers (amino-isobutyric acid, m.w. = 103; nucleotide, m.w. = 1000; RNA, m.w. = >200 000) were released concurrently, indicating that the functional holes were large. However, unlike delta toxin, cytotoxicity was not induced at 0°C and the morphological changes induced in the fibroblasts were different (Thelestam and Ljungh 1981). The formation of the membrane lesion was dependent on temperature, as was the binding of the toxin, and cells previously exposed to toxin could be rescued by resuspension in fresh medium. Ljungh and Wadstrom (1983) concluded from these results that the lysis mechanism could be enzymic, although no definitive evidence is yet available.

Ljungh and Wadstrom (1983) also found the beta haemolysin as an extracellular heat-labile acidic protein of m.w. = 50–51 000 with two components separable on the basis of charge. These probably represent charge isomers with pI = 4.2 and 5.5. The beta toxin is probably similar to the toxin originally described by Bernheimer, Avigad, and Avigad (1975) as aerolysin, although the lysin described by him had phospholipase activity which was not evident in the preparation described by Ljungh and Wadstrom (1983). Like the alpha lysin, the beta haemolysin preferentially lysed erythrocytes of rat whereas those of sheep were the most resistant tested. Sensitivity to lysis correlated with the toxin-binding capacity of erythrocytes, and binding could be reduced by prior treatment of the erythrocyte with proteases or phospholipase C (Bernheimer *et al.* 1975). More recent data by Howard and Buckley (1982) indicated that the receptor for beta haemolysin on rat and mouse erythrocytes was a membrane glycoprotein. Like several other cytolysins already described, binding of beta haemolysin to target cells was temperature independent, but subsequent membrane damage was not evident until the temperature was raised above 20°C. Like the alpha haemolysin, beta haemolysin was cytotoxic for fibroblasts and a variety of other cultured mammalian cell lines, but the cytopathic effects differed from each other. While alpha haemolysin caused rounding of fibroblasts and fading of the nuclei, the beta haemolysin caused the cytoplasm to become extensively vacuolated before the cells eventually burst. Once exposed to the beta toxin, the cytotoxicity was irreversible (cf. alpha haemolysin).

Ljungh and Wadstrom (1983) observed partial immunological cross-reactivity between the alpha and beta haemolysins by gel diffusion analysis. Also, alpha haemolysin was partially neutralized by anti beta-haemolysin serum. While this observation might suggest interrelationship between the two toxins, the possible presence of minor cross-contamination in the purified antigens must be considered. The resolution of the question of possible relatedness between these and other haemolysins in this group must await a more detailed genetic analysis of toxigenic strains.

Haemolysins of halophilic vibrios
Vibrio parahaemolyticus, a common cause of food poisoning associated with consumption of marine shellfish, can produce up to four different haemolysins, but details of their mode of membrane damage are lacking. The most well defined one is the extracellular thermostable direct haemolysin (TDH or Kanagawa phenomenon-associated haemolysin), which is produced by most clinical isolates but rarely by environmental isolates (Kaper, Campen, Seidler, Baldini, and Falkow 1984). TDH (reviewed by Ljungh and Wadstrom 1983) is an acidic protein (pI = 4.2 or 4.9) and consists of two identical subunits, the molecular weight of the dimer

being 42–44 kdalton. Like the haemolysins of *Aeromonas* described above, the erythrocyte most susceptible to lysis by TDH is that of the rat. Also, binding is temperature independent, but elevated temperature is required for induction of membrane damage, which is maximal at 37°C. Toxin binding is enhanced by the presence of the divalent cations Ca^{2+}, Mg^{2+}, and Mn^{2+}, but unaffected by Zn^{2+}. Like many of the other haemolysins already described, haemolysis appears to follow a similar pattern of a temperature-independent binding step followed by a temperature-dependent membrane alteration that leads to a change in permeability properties. The similarity in physical and biological properties between TDH and the beta haemolysin of *Aeromonas hydrophila* has been noted previously by Ljungh and Wadstrom (1983), although its genetic and taxonomic significance is not clear.

Recently, haemolysins in several other pathogenic halophilic vibrios have been reported. *V. damsela*, *V. vulnificus*, and *V. fluvialis* all produce lethal toxins with potent haemolytic activity, which is maximal against mouse and rat erythrocytes, as was found for the haemolysins of *Aeromonas*.

The *V. damsela* mouse erythrocyte haemolysin described by Kreger (1984) and Kothary and Kreger (1985) is a heat-labile extracellular protein with m.w. = 69 000 and pI = 5.6. The haemolysin is very active against erythrocytes of rat, mouse, rabbit, and damselfish, is cytotolytic for CHO cells, and lethal for mice. It differs in its properties from the haemolysins produced by *V. cholerae* El Tor (Honda and Finkelstein 1979), the non–01 *V. cholerae* (Yamamoto, Al-Omani, Honda, Takeda, and Miwatani 1984), and *V. vulnificus*. It also differs from the DTH of *V. parahaemolyticus* (see above), and it may differ from the haemolytic factors produced by *V. vulnificus* and described by Clarridge and Zigelboim-Daum (1985). One of these haemolysins protected sheep erythrocytes from the haemolytic action of staphylococcal beta toxin, which is a sphingomyelinase C. Such activities strongly suggest that this haemolysin may have phopholipase D activity, although this has not been investigated to date.

The haemolysin of *V. vulnificus* (Gray and Kreger 1985) also shows haemolytic activity against rabbit erythrocytes, although only 40 per cent of that shown against mouse erythrocytes. This haemolysin has been partially characterized and has m.w. = 56 000 and pI = 7.1. The lysin is almost totally inactivated by cholesterol at levels 100-fold greater than those required to inactivate SH-activated toxins, and lysis appears to be a multihit rather than a single-hit process, following the two-stage process outlined above.

Initial characterization of the cytotoxic factors produced by clinical isolates of *V. fluvialis* (Wall, Kreger, and Richardson 1984) included a component of m.w. = 34.5 kdalton, with pI = 4.4–4.5. This had both haemolytic activity against mouse erythrocytes and phospholipase A2 activity. Whether or not these reflect two different components must await further investigation.

Future challenges

From the small selection of toxins discussed in this article, it is apparent that there still remain considerable areas of ignorance about the precise ways in which cytolytic toxins bring about membrane disruption. By studying the interaction of toxin and membrane at the molecular level, utilizing biophysical techniques and artificial membranes, important new information has been gained concerning the behaviour of membrane-active toxins and membrane structure. The extensive biophysical studies with melittin and pure lipid systems exemplify this approach.

However, this may be a somewhat misleading approach to the problems of intoxication of living systems. Many cytolytic toxins have very subtle effects on cells at concentrations far below those required for cell lysis, for example effects on the membranes of the cells of the immune system associated with changes in adhesiveness, or responsiveness to chemotactic or mitogenic agents (Alouf 1985). Also, we know that many toxins can act synergistically as well as possibly blocking receptors shared with other pharmacologically reactive compounds *in vivo*. It is important to better define these activities of toxins.

It is clear that the newly described haemolysins of the halophilic vibrios and related species are important virulence factors, and that they share several features in common, and may have similar receptor specificities. The degree of interrelatedness in terms of structural homology and mode of action offers another fascinating challenge for the toxinologist.

Much precise information is now becoming available on the structure of a wide variety of toxins as a result of advances in gene cloning technology. The next important phase of research must involve the prediction of tertiary structure and how this relates to biological activity.

References

Alouf, J. E. (1977). Cell membranes and cytolytic bacterial toxins. In *Specificity and action of animal, bacterial and plant toxins*. (ed. P. Cuatrecasas), pp. 221–700 Chapman and Hall, London.

—— (1985). Interaction of bacterial protein toxins with host defense mechanisms. In *Bacterial protein toxins* (ed. P. Falmagne, J. E. Alouf, F. J. Fehrenbach, M. Thelestam, and J. Jeljaszewicz), pp. 121–30. *Zbl. Bakt.* Suppl. 5. Gustav Fischer, Stuttgart.

—— and Geoffroy, C. (1984). Structure–activity relationships in sulfhydryl-activated toxins. In *Bacterial protein toxins* (ed. J. E. Alouf, F. J. Fehrenbach, J. H. Freer, and J. Jeljaszewicz), pp. 165–72. Academic Press, London.

—— and Jolivet-Reynaud, C. (1981). Purification and characterisation of *Clostridium perfringens* delta toxin, *Infect. Immunol.* **31**, 536–46.

—— and Raynaud, M. (1968). Action de la streptolysine O sur les membranes cellulaires. 1. Fixation sur la membrane erythrocytaire. *Ann. Inst. Pasteur Paris* **114**, 812–27.

Arbuthnott, J. P., Freer, J. H., and Bernheimer, A. W. (1967). Physical states of staphylococcal alpha toxin. *J. Bacteriol.* **94**, 1170–7.

Avigad, L. S. and Bernheimer, A. W. (1978). Inhibition of hemolysins by zinc and its reversal by histidine. *Infect. Immunol.* **19**, 1101–3.

Bashford, C. L., Adler, G. M., Patel, K, and Pasternak, C. A. (1984). Common action of certain viruses, toxins, and activated complement: pore formation and its prevention by extracellular Ca. *Biosc. Rep.* **4**, 797–805.

Bernheimer A. W. (1974). Interaction between membranes and cytolytic bacterial toxins. *Biochim. biophys. acta* **344**, 27–50.

—— and Davidson, M. (1965). Lysis of pleuropneumonia-like organisms by staphylococcal and streptococcal toxins. *Science* **148**, 1229–31.

——, Avigad, L. S., and Avigad, G. (1975). Interactions between aerolysin, erythrocytes, and erythrocyte membranes. *Infect. Immunol.* **11**, 1312–18.

Bhakdi, S. and Tranum-Jensen, J. (1983). Membrane damage by channel-forming proteins. *Trans Biochem. Sci.* (April), 134–6

——, Muhly, M., and Fussle, R. (1984a). Correlation between toxin binding and hemolytic activity in membrane damage by staphylococcal alpha toxin. *Infect. Immunol*, **46**, 318–23.

——, Tranum-Jensen, J., and Sziegoleit, A. (1985). Mechanism of membrane damage by streptolysin O. *Infect. Immunol.* **47**, 62–70.

——, Roth, M., Sziegoleit, A., and Tranum-Jensen, J. (1984b). Isolation and identification of two haemolytic forms of streptolysin O. *Infect. Immunol.* **46**, 394–400.

Bhakoo, M., Birkbeck, T. H., and Freer, J. H. (1982). Interaction of *Staphylococcus aureus* delta lysin with phospholipid monolayers. *Biochemistry* **21**, 6879–83.

——, ——, and —— (1985). Phospholipid-dependent changes in membrane permeability induced by staphylococcal delta lysin and bee venom melittin. *Can. J. Biochem. Cell Biol.* **63**, 1–6.

Blumenthal, R., and Habig, W. H. (1984). Mechanism of tetanolysin-induced membrane damage: studies with black lipid membranes. *J. Bacteriol.* **157**, 321–3.

Boquet, P. and Duflot, E. (1984). Fragment B of tetanus toxin forms channels in lipid vesicles at low pH. In *Bacterial protein toxins* (ed. J. E. Alouf, F. J. Fehrenbach, J. H. Freer, and J. Jeljaszewicz), pp. 421–6. Academic Press, London.

Bougis, P., Rochat, H., Pieroni, G., and Verger, R. (1981). Penetration of phospholipid monolayers by cardiotoxins. *Biochemistry* **20**, 4915–20.

Cassidy, P. and Harshman, S. (1976). Studies on the binding of staphylococcal ^{125}I-labelled alpha toxin to rabbit erythrocytes. *Biochemistry* **15**, 2348–55.

Chakrabory, T., Gilmore, M., Hacker, J., Huhle, B., Kathareou, S., Knapp, S., Kreft, J., Müller, B., Leimeister, M., Parrisius, J., Wagner, W., and Goebel, W. (1986). Genetic approaches to the study of haemolytic toxins in bacteria. In *Bacterial protein toxins* (ed. P. Falmagne, J. E. Alouf, F. J. Fehrenbach, M. Thelestam, and J. Jeljaszeiwicz), pp. 241–52. *Zbl Bakt.* Suppl. 15. Gustav Fischer, Stuttgart.

Clarridge, J. E. and Zigelboim-Daum, S. (1985). Isolation and characterization of two hemolytic phenotypes of *Vibrio damsela* associated with a fatal wound infection. *J. clin. Microbiol.* **21**, 302–6.

Colacicco, G. and Buckelew, R. (1971). Lipid monolayers: influence of lipid film and urea on the surface activity of staphylococcal alpha toxin. *Lipids* **6**, 546–553.

——, Basu, M. K., Buckelew, A. R., and Bernheimer, A. W. (1977). Surface properties of membrane systems. Transport of staphylococcal delta toxin from aqueous to membrane phase. *Biochim. biophys. acta* **465**, 378–90.

Cooper, L. Z., Madoff, M. A., and Weinstein, L. (1964). Heat stability and species range of purified staphylococcal alpha toxin. *J. Bacteriol.* **91**, 1686–92.

Cowell, J. L., Kim, K. S., and Bernheimer, A. W. (1978). Alteration by cereolysin of the structure of cholesterol-containing membranes. *Biochim. biophys. acta* **507**, 230–41.

Dawson, C. R., Drake, A. F., Helliwell, J., and Hider, R. C. (1978). The interaction of bee venom melittin with lipid bilayer membranes. *Biochim. biophys. acta* **510**, 75–86.

Duncan, J. L. (1974). Characteristics of Streptolysin O hemolysis: kinetics of hemoglobin and [86]Rubidium release. *Infect. Immunol.* **9**, 1022–7.

Duncan, J. L. and Schlegel, R. (1975). Effect of streptolysin O on erythrocyte membranes, liposomes, and lipid dispersions. A protein–cholesterol interaction. *J. cell Biol.* **67**, 160–73.

Falmagne, P., Capiau, C., Cabiaux, V., Deleers, M., and Ruysschaert, J -M. (1984). Fragment B of diphtheria toxin: correlation between amino-acid sequence and lipid binding properties. In *Bacterial protein toxins* (ed. J. E. Alouf, F. J. Fehrenbach, J. H. Freer, and J. Jeljaszewicz), pp. 139–46. Academic Press, London.

Fitton, J. E., Dell, A., and Shaw, W. V. (1980). The amino acid sequence of the delta haemolysin of *Staphylococcus aureus*. *FEBS Lett.* **115**, 209–12.

——, Hunt, D. F., Marasco, J., Shabanowitz, J., Winston, S., and Dell, A. (1984). The amino acid sequence of delta haemolysin purified from a canine isolate of *Staphylococcus aureus*. *FEBS Lett.* **169**, 25–29.

Freer, J. H. (1982). Cytolytic toxins and surface activity. *Toxicon* **20**, 217–22.

—— and Arbuthnott, J. P. (1976). Biochemical and morphologic alterations of membranes by bacterial toxins. In *Mechanisms in bacterial toxinology* (ed. A. W. Bernheimer), pp. 169–94. John Wiley, New York.

—— and —— (1983). Toxins of *Staphylococcus aureus*. *Pharmacol. Ther.* **19**, 55–101.

—— and Birkbeck, T. H. (1982). Possible conformation of delta lysin, a membrane-damaging peptide from Staphylococcus aureus. *J. theor. Biol.* **94**, 535–40.

——, Arbuthnott, J. P., and Bernheimer, A. W. (1968). Interaction of staphylococcal alpha toxin with artificial and natural membranes. *J. Bacteriol.* **95**, 1153–68.

——, ——, and Billcliffe, B. (1973). Effects of staphylococcal alpha toxin on the structure of erythrocyte membranes: a biochemical and freeze-etching study. *J. gen. Microbiol.* **75**, 321–32.

——, Birkbeck, T. H., and Bhakoo, M. (1984). Interaction of staphylococcal delta lysin with phospholipid monolayers and bilayers — a short review. In *Bacterial protein toxins* (ed. J. E. Alouf, F. J. Fehrenbach, J. H. Freer, and J. Jeljaszewicz), pp. 181–90. Academic Press, London.

Gray, G. S. and Kehoe, M. (1984). Primary sequence of the alpha toxin gene from *Staphylococcus aureus* Wood 46. *Infect. Immunol.* **46**, 615–18.

Gray, L. D., and Kreger, A. S. (1985). Purification and characterization of an extracellular cytolysin produced by *Vibrio vulnificus*. *Infect. Immunol.* **48**, 62–72.

Harshman, S. (1979). Action of staphylococcal alpha toxin on membranes: some recent advances. *Mol. cell. Biochem.* **23**, 143–52.

—— and Sugg, N. (1985). Effect of Ca ions on staphylococcal alpha toxin-induced hemolysis of rabbit erythrocytes. *Infect. Immunol.* **47**, 37–40.

Honda, T., and Finkelstein, R. A. (1979). Purification and characterization of a hemolysin produced by *Vibrio cholerae* biotype El Tor: another toxic substance produced by cholera vibrios. *Infect. Immunol.* **26**, 1020–7.

Howard, S. P. and Buckley, J. T. (1982). Membrane glycoprotein receptor and hole-forming properties of a cytolytic protein toxin. *Biochemistry* **21**, 1662–7.

Jeljaszewicz, J. and Wadstrom, T. (ed.) *Bacterial protein toxins and cell membranes*. Academic Press, London (1978).

Jolivet-Reynaud, C. and Alouf, J. E. (1983). Binding of *Clostridium perfringens* ^{125}I-labelled delta toxin to erythrocytes. *J. biol. Chem.* **258**, 1871–7.

——, Geoffroy, C., Igolen, J., and Alouf, J. E. (1982). Study of membrane-bacterial cytolysins interaction using photoreactive probe and chaotropic agents. *Toxicon* **20**, 260–1.

Kagan, B. L., Finkelstein, A. L., and Colombini, M. (1981). Diphtheria toxin fragment forms large pores in phospholipid bilayer membranes. *Proc. nat. Acad. Sci. USA* **78**, 4950–4.

Kantor, H. S., Temples, B., and Shaw, W. V. (1972). Staphylococcal delta hemolysin: purification and characterisation. *Archs. Biochem. Biophys.* **151**, 142–56.

Kaper, J. B., Campen, R. K., Seidler, R. J., Baldini, M. M., and Falkow, S. (1984). Cloning of the thermostable direct or Kanagawa phenomenon associated hemolysin of *Vibrio parahemolyticus*. *Infect. Immunol.* **45**, 290–2.

Kehoe, M. and Timmis, K. N. (1984). Cloning and expression in *Escherichia coli* of streptolysin O determinant from *Streptococcus pyogenes*: characterization of the cloned streptolysin O determinant and demonstration of the absence of substantial homology with determinants of other thiol-activated toxins. *Infect. Immunol.* **43**, 804-10.

Kothary, M. H. and Kreger, A. S. (1985). Purification and characterization of an extracellular cytolysin produced by *Vibrio damsela*. *Infect. Immunol.* **49**, 25–31.

Kreger, A. S. (1984). Cytolytic activity and virulence of *Vibrio damsela*. *Infect. Immunol.* **44**, 326–31.

——, Kim, K. S., Zaboretsky, F., and Bernheimer, A. W. (1971). Purification and properties of staphylococcal delta hemolysin. *Infect. Immunol.* **3**, 449–65.

Ljungh, A. and Wadstrom, T. (1983). Toxins of *Vibrio parahaemolyticus* and *Aeromonas hydrophila*. *J. Toxicol. toxin Rev.* **1**(2), 257–307.

Menestrina, G. (1986). Ionic channels formed by *Staphylococcus aureus* alpha-toxin: voltage dependent inhibition by di- and tri-valent cations *J. Membrane Biol.* **90**, 177–90.

Middlebrook, J. L. and Dorland, R. B. (1984). Bacterial toxins: cellular mechanisms of action. *Microbiol. Rev.* **48**, 181–98.

Rottem, S., Cole, R. M., Habig, W. H., Barile, M. F., and Hardegree, M. C. (1982). Structural characteristics of tetanolysin and its binding to lipid vesicles. *J. Bacteriol.* **152**, 888–92.

Smyth, C. J., and Duncan, J. L. (1978). Thiol-activated (oxygen-labile) cytolysins. In *Bacterial toxins and cell membranes* (ed. J. Jeljaszewicz and T. Wadstrom), pp. 130–78. Academic Press, London.

Smyth, C. J., Freer, J. H., and Arbuthnott. (1975). Interaction of *Clostridium perfringens* θ-haemolysin, a contaminant of commercial phospholipase C, with erythrocyte ghost membranes and lipid dispersions. *Biochim. biophys. acta* **382**, 479–93.

Terwilliger, T. C., Weissman, L., and Eisenberg, D. (1982). The structure of melittin in the form 1 crystals and its implication for melittin's lytic and surface activity. *Biophys. J.* **37**, 353–61.

Thelestam, M., and Ljungh, A. (1981). Membrane-damaging and cytotoxic effects on human fibroblasts of alpha- and beta-hemolysin from *Aeromonas hydrophila*. *Infect. Immunol.* **34**, 949–55.

Thelestam, M., and Mollby, R. (1979). Classification of microbial, plant and animal cytolysins on their membrane-damaging effect on human fibroblasts. *Biochim. biophys. acta* **557**, 156–69.

Thelestam, M., Jolivet-Reynaud, C., and Alouf, J. E. (1983). Photolabelling of staphylococcal alpha toxin from within rabbit erythrocyte membranes. *Biochem. Biophys. Res. Commun.* **111**, 444–9

Tosteson, M. T., and Tosteson, D. C. (1981). The sting — melittin forms channels in lipid bilayers. *Biophys. J.* **36**, 109–16.

Turner, W. H. (1978). Purification and characterization of an immunologically distinct delta haemolysin from a canine strain of *Staphylococcus aureus*. *Infect. Immunol.* **20**, 485–94.

Tweten, R. K., Christianson, K. K., and Iandolo, J. J. (1983). Transport and processing of staphylococcal alpha toxin. *J. Bacteriol.* **156**, 524–8.

Wicken, A. J., and Knox, K. W. (1980). Bacterial cell surface amphiphiles. *Biochim. biophys. acta.* **604**, 1–26.

Wall, V. W., Kreger, A. S., and Richardson, S. H. (1984). Production and partial characterization of a *Vibrio fluvialis* cytotoxin. *Infect. Immunol.* **46**, 773–7.

Yamamoto, K., Al-Omani, M., Honda, T., Takeda, Y., and Miwatani, T. (1984). Non-01 *Vibrio cholerae* hemolysin: purification, partial characterization, and immunological relatedness to El-Tor hemolysin. *Infect. Immunol.* **45**, 192–6.

12

Bacterial toxins and their effect on the gut

Nigel Evans

Introduction

In the developing world diarrhoea due to communicable infectious agents is a major cause of morbidity and mortality, especially in children and particularly when complicated by malnutrition. It has been estimated that children under the age of five suffer between 2.2 and 3 diarrhoeal illnesses per year with a total mortality of 7 per cent (Snyder and Merson 1982), rising to 20 per cent in the poorest geographical areas. In Africa, Asia, and Latin America there are between 5 and 10 million deaths from diarrhoea per annum (Walsh and Warren 1979). In the industrial world life-threatening infections still occur in the young and in institutions, although the majority of these infectious are mild and little more than inconvenient. Collectively, however, diarrhoeal illness is an important cause of lost production and morbidity. Calf, lamb, and piglet diarrhoea is also associated with a high mortality and is consequently of major economic importance.

Pathogenesis of bacterial diarrhoea

Infectious diarrhoea, in animals and humans, may be caused by bacterial pathogens acting through a variety of mechanisms (Table 12.1). Organisms are ingested in food or water, or transmitted by direct faecal–oral contamination; occasionally toxins are ingested preformed. A relatively small bacterial inoculum (10^1–10^4) may be required to initiate *Salmonella* and *Shigella* infections. In the case of *Vibrio cholerae* and toxin producing *Escherichia coli* a far larger inoculum (10^9) is required to enable sufficient organisms to survive passage through the stomach (Gangarosa 1978). These infections are consequently uncommon in hygienic environments, unless there is a common source outbreak.

Certain bacteria (Table 12.2) elaborate enterotoxins which are exotoxins active within the intestine. The capacity to produce enterotoxins is usually genetically controlled by plasmid DNA and is transferable. The enterotoxins induce diarrhoea by augmenting secretion or by decreasing normal

212

Table 12.1 Pathogenesis of bacterial diarrhoea.

	Primary site of action	Enterotoxin production	Cytotoxin production	Histological damage	Inflammatory reaction
Enterotoxin-producing bacteria	[a]SI	+ +	−	−	−
Toxins ingested	SI	+	+	±	−
Effacement of brush border	SI	−	±	±	−
Enteroinvasive bacteria	Colon Ileum	+	+ +	+ +	+ +

[a] SI = small intestine.

absorption without causing histological damage. The diarrhoea is copious and watery and there may be abdominal distension. The virulence of entero-toxigenic bacteria is enhanced by ability of the organism to adhere to the small intestinal mucosa. Adherent organisms possess fimbrial appendages which are antigenic, plasmid mediated, and transferable. Such organisms are protected from the peristaltic flow and are able to colonize the small intestine.

In certain circumstances toxins may be elaborated during the growth of *Staphylococcus aureus* in food. These toxins are then ingested and within a few hours precipitate the diarrhoea, vomiting, and abdominal cramps of food poisoning.

The classical enteropathogenic *E. coli* (EPEC) adhere to and efface the brush border of the small intestine where it is postulated they inhibit normal absorption. EPEC do not produce enterotoxins detectable in the standard bioassay systems, but some may produce *Shiga*-like cytotoxin (O'Brien, LaVeck, Thompson, and Formal 1982; Cleary, Mathewson, Faris, and

Table 12.2 Bacteria that produce enterotoxins.

Aeromonas hydrophila	Non-cholera vibrios
Bacillus cereus	*Pseudomonas* spp.
Campylobacter jejuni	*Salmonella* spp.
Clostridium spp.	*Serratia* spp.
Edwardsiella tarda	*Shigella* spp.
Enterobacter cloacae	*Staphylococcus aureus*
Escherichia coli	*Vibrio cholerae*
Klebsiella pneumoniae	

Pickering 1985), which destroys the apical cytoplasm of the enterocyte, thus potentiating the diarrhoeal effect (Ulshen and Rollo 1980).

Invasive organisms (Table 12.3) primarily infect the colon or ileum, where they cause marked inflammation and ulceration which produces dysenteric diarrhoea with tenesmus, abdominal cramps, and fever.

The stools typically contain blood, mucus, and white cells. Organisms in this category produce cytotoxins that inhibit protein synthesis and disrupt the structural integrity of the host cell. This in turn aids the invasive process and causes more inflammation with an infiltration of polymorphonuclear neutrophils. Some organisms in this group produce enterotoxins. Moreover, the products of inflammation potentiate diarrhoea by stimulating the local production of prostaglandins and other secretagogues. The mechanism of invasion involves local brush border destruction followed by invagination of the cell membrane. The bacteria are engulfed within vacuoles and further invasion and cytotoxic damage of adjacent cells produces the typical ulceration. In shigellosis the organisms penetrate and proliferate intraepithelially but *Salmonella*, *Campylobacter*, and *Yersinia* species proliferate in the lamina propria and mesenteric lymph nodes, while further invasion by *Salmonella typhi* in susceptible hosts leads to systemic infection and enteric fever.

Absorption and secretion in the gut

In health there is a striking bidirectional movement of electrolytes and water across the intestinal mucosa with the balance in favour of net absorption. Our knowledge of the mechanisms that control these complex secretory and absorptive pathways has been greatly enhanced by studies of cholera toxin and the heat-labile (LT) and heat-stable (STa, STb) toxins of *E. coli*. As we shall see, cholera toxin and LT bind to monosialoganglioside receptors on the apical membrane and, after a time lag, ADP-ribosylate a regulatory portion of the enzyme adenylate cyclase (Field 1980). This results in prolonged stimulation of intracellular cyclic AMP (Table 12.4). In contrast heat-stable toxins bind promptly to protein receptors and activate guanylate cyclase, which results in the formation of intracellular cyclic GMP. Both cyclic AMP, cyclic GMP, and intracellular Ca^{2+} (the 'second messengers')

Table 12.3 Enteroinvasive bacteria.

Campylobacter jejuni
Escherichia coli
Salmonella spp.
Shigella spp.
Yersinia enterocolitica

Table 12.4 Primary intestinal secretory mechanisms.

Extracellular stimulus	Toxin receptor	Second messenger	Third messenger	Secretory mechanism
Cholera toxin	Ganglioside	cAMP	A kinase	
E. coli LT	Ganglioside	cAMP	A kinase	Cl⁻ secretion ↑
ªVIP, prostaglandins	—	cAMP	A kinase	Na⁺ absorption ↓ ? mediated by Ca²⁺
E. coli STa	Protein	cGMP	G kinase	
A23187, serotonin, acetylcholine	—	Ca²⁺	C kinase	
E. coli STb	?	?	?	HCO₃⁻ secretion

ª VIP = vasoactive intestinal peptide.

cause intestinal secretion by activation of specific protein kinases, which are thought to phosphorylate membrane proteins, thereby altering epithelial transport and causing net secretion.

Villus absorption and crypt secretion

Electrolyte absorption and secretion in the small and large intestine are separate processes that take place in different cells. Na^+ is the principal ion to be actively absorbed, while Cl^- mediates secretion (Fig. 12.1). Absorption occurs through mature cells at the tip of the villus, whereas secretion occurs through crypt cells. Water merely follows the osmotic gradients induced by the active transport of electrolytes and other metabolites. Bacterial toxins that stimulate production of the cyclic nucleotides cause diarrhoea by stimulating electrogenic Cl^- secretion in the crypts and by impairing Na^+ absorption in the villi. Thus, selective destruction of the villus tip by hypertonic saline does not block cholera-induced secretion (Roggin, Banwell, Yardley, and Hendrix 1972), and an increased level of cyclic AMP in flounder intestine (which has no crypts) causes reduced absorption, but no secretion (Field, Karnaky, Smith, Bolton, and Kinter 1978b; Frizzell, Smith, Vosburgh, and Field 1979). Fluid droplets have also been observed to form under oil-covered guinea pig jejunal and rabbit colonic mucosa, where there are crypts (Nasset and Ju 1973; Welsh, Smith, Fromm and Frizzell 1982).

Until recently it was assumed that toxins diffuse into the crypts to stimulate the cells through specific apical membrane receptors. This concept was supported by the observation that rat intestine exposed to cholera toxin for 5 min exhibited reduced absorption and activation only of villus tip adenylate cyclase, whereas a 30 min exposure also activated adenylate cyclase in

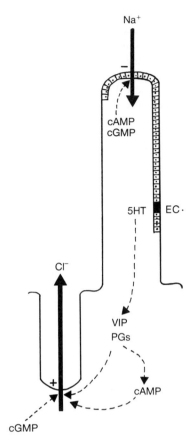

Fig. 12.1 Villus absorption and crypt secretion. Na$^+$ is the principal ion absorbed through mature villous cells, while Cl$^-$ is secreted through crypt cells. The cyclic nucleotides induced by enterotoxins stimulate secretion and inhibit absorption. The crypts may be stimulated through serotonin (5HT) released from enterochromaffin cells (EC). Serotonin excites vasoactive intestinal peptide (VIP) release via the enteric nervous system and stimulates the production of prostaglandins (PGs).

the crypts and elicited net secretion (De Jonge 1975). An alternative mechanism of crypt stimulation by the enteric nervous system has also been proposed. Cassuto, Jodal, Sjövall, and Lundgren (1981) have suggested that bacterial toxins stimulate enterochromaffin cells in the villus epithelium with release of serotonin into the *lamina propria*. They postulated that serotonin excites non-cholinergic, non-adrenergic neurones with the release of vasoactive intestinal peptide (VIP) serosally onto the crypt enterocyte. Further work is required to confirm this hypothesis, but:

(a) cholera toxin-induced secretion can be inhibited by drugs that block neurotransmission (tetrodotoxin, lidocaine and hexamethonium), and

(b) Cassuto *et al.* (1981) have shown that cholera toxin releases serotonin and VIP, both of which are known to stimulate secretion of electrolytes and water. The activity of VIP is mediated by cyclic AMP and serotonin by Ca^{2+}.

Ion transport, Na^+ absorption, and Cl^- secretion

Absorption takes place as a two-stage process. Na^+ enters the cell from the gut lumen and is then actively transported across the basolateral membrane by the activity of Na–K ATPase (Fig. 12.2). This sodium pump generates a chemical and an electrical gradient, that favour passive Na^+ absorption. The electrical gradient, in which the cytoplasm is negative, relative to the extracellular medium, is created by an exchange mechanism by which two K^+ ions enter the cell in exchange for three Na^+ ions leaving. The extrusion of Na^+ into the lateral intercellular spaces or through the basal membrane results in the osmotic absorption of water. Na^+ may also be absorbed in combination with a carrier protein that translocates glucose or amino acids. This process is electrogenic and results in 'solvent drag', whereby additional Na^+ and Cl^- are absorbed in the bulk flow of water through and between the cells via the tight junctions. This glucose-mediated enhancement of Na^+ and water absorption is exploited in oral rehydration therapy.

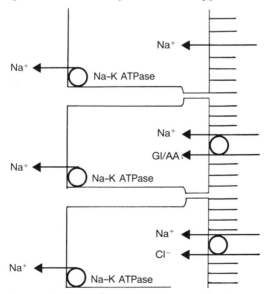

Fig. 12.2 Villus absorption. Na^+ absorbed (i) passively down an electrochemical gradient maintained by Na–K ATPase, (ii) coupled to glucose or amino acid or (iii) coupled to Cl^-.

Enterotoxins and the cyclic nucleotides alter neither Na–K ATPase activity nor the Na–glucose, Na–amino acid carrier. It is possible that an electrically neutral coupled mechanism for NaCl entry is susceptible to the action of bacterial toxins. Turnberg, Bieberdorf, Morawski, and Fordtran (1970) proposed a pair of parallel ion exchanges (Fig. 12.3), in which Na$^+$ is absorbed in exchange for H$^+$, and Cl$^-$ is absorbed in exchange for HCO$_3^-$. These two exchanges act as an NaCl absorption pump, with the secreted H$^+$ and HCO$_3^-$ reacting in the lumen to form carbon dioxide and water, which simply diffuses out. There is preliminary evidence that Ca^{2+} has an inhibitory effect on the anion exchange component (Fan, Faust, and Powell 1983), but as yet no direct proof of a cyclic nucleotide effect. Gunther and Wright (1983) were unable to demonstrate an inhibitory effect of cyclic AMP on the Na$^+$: H$^+$ exchange in rabbit jejunal brush border membrane vesicles.

In the Cl$^-$ secretory cell, cyclic nucleotides or Ca^{2+} increase the permeability of the apical membrane to Cl$^-$, which then passes from cell to lumen down an electrochemical gradient (Fig. 12.4). The latter is created by an NaCl entry process located on the basolateral membrane of the crypt enterocytes. The Na$^+$ entering with Cl$^-$ is recycled across the basolateral membrane by Na–K ATPase and the Cl$^-$ accumulates within the cell. The Na$^+$ in the lateral intracellular space then diffuses into the lumen and the movement of Cl$^-$ and Na$^+$ creates a flow of water from blood to lumen.

Rabbit ileum and porcine colon exposed to cyclic nucleotide stimulation also exhibit secretion of HCO$_3^-$ (Hubel 1974; Argenzio and Whipp 1981). It is not known whether this takes place through parallel ion exchanges in the villi or through electrogenic transport in the crypts.

Intracellular and extracellular messengers, cyclic nucleotides, Ca^{2+}, and neurohormones

Ca^{2+} and its regulatory protein calmodulin play a central role in the intracellular regulation of electrolyte movements (Donowitz 1983). When intracellular Ca^{2+} in rabbit ileum is increased by means of the calcium ionophore A23187, intestinal secretion occurs without affecting the levels of

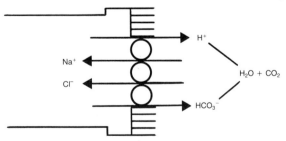

Fig. 12.3 Dual ion exchangers. Na$^+$ is absorbed in exchange for H$^+$ and Cl$^-$ is absorbed in exchange for HCO$_3^-$.

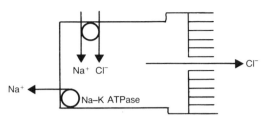

Fig. 12.4 Crypt secretion. The permeability of the apical membrane to Cl⁻ is increased by cyclic nucleotides or Ca^{2+}. Na Cl enters the cell through the basolateral membranes and the Na^+ is recycled by Na–K ATPase.

the cyclic nucleotides. Lowering intracellular Ca^{2+} by exposing the ileum to bathing solutions containing low concentrations of Ca^{2+} or to calcium channel blockers such as verapamil, increases active absorption. The extracellular signals that regulate intracellular Ca^{2+}, may be provided by some of the neurohumoral agents known to be present in the gut, including acetylcholine, VIP, serotonin, substance P, neurotensin, and prostaglandins (Fig. 12.5). Serotonin, substance P, neurotensin and carbachol (a cholinergic analogue) can all be shown to decrease NaCl absorption or increase

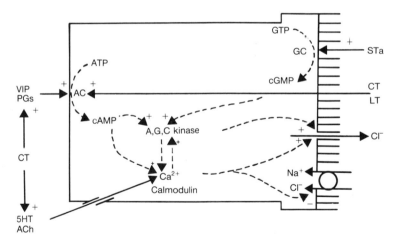

Fig. 12.5 Possible role of toxins, cyclic nucleotides, neurohormones, and Ca^{2+}. Cholera toxin (CT) or *E. coli* LT stimulate the production of cyclic AMP via adenylate cyclase (AC). *E. coli* STa stimulates production of cyclic GMP via guanylate cyclase (GC). The cyclic nucleotides cause secretion by stimulating specific kinases (A and G kinase) and/or by releasing Ca^{2+} from endoplasmic stores. Ca^{2+} or calmodulin may stimulate a Ca^{2+}-dependent protein kinase (C kinase). Acetyl choline (ACh), serotonin (5HT), and other neurohormones may raise intracellular Ca^{2+} levels and induce secretion by Ca^{2+} gating. Na Cl absorption is inhibited by Ca^{2+} and/or by the cyclic nucleotides.

Cl⁻ secretion by Ca^{2+} dependent mechanisms (Keusch and Donowitz 1983). By contrast, dopamine stimulates NaCl absorption by decreasing basolateral Ca^{2+} absorption. The neurohormones are believed to activate hydrolysis of membrane-based phospholipids, particularly phosphatidyl inositol. This hydrolysis, which is itself Ca^{2+}-dependent and involves phospholipase C, is accompanied by Ca^{2+} gating across the basolateral membranes. Intracellular Ca^{2+} levels are also increased as the products of the hydrolysis (diacylglycerol and inositol triphosphate) stimulate Ca^{2+}-dependent kinase (C kinase) and release Ca^{2+} from intracellular stores in the endoplasmic reticulum (Berridge 1981).

The activity of Ca^{2+}, calmodulin, and the cyclic nucleotides are closely linked. Physiological concentrations of Ca^{2+} and calmodulin stimulate adenylate cyclase in the enterocyte (Amiranoff, Laburthe, Rouyer-Fessard, Demaille, and Rosselin 1983; Lazo, Rivaya, and Velasco 1984), although a similar effect upon guanylate cyclase is not so clear. Intestinal calmodulin may also activate the hydrolysis of cyclic AMP and cyclic GMP by phosphodiesterase. Cyclic nucleotides themselves release calcium from intracellular stores (Frizzel 1977), so that it has been suggested that Ca^{2+} rather than cyclic AMP or cyclic GMP is finally responsible for the anti-absorptive or secretory effects of various secretagogues, including the enterotoxins.

The evidence that Ca^{2+} has a role in toxin-induced secretion in animal models is confused. STa-induced secretion in suckling mice can be inhibited by Ca^{2+} channel blockers such as nifedipine, diltiazem, and disodium cromoglycate (Thomas and Knoop 1982), although the removal of Ca^{2+} from the luminal bathing medium did not inhibit the effect of STa on rabbit ileal mucosa (Field, Graf, Laird, and Smith 1978a). Agents such as lanthanum and trifluoperazine, which are known to interfere with Ca^{2+}-mediated processes, interfere with cholera toxin and ST-stimulated secretion as well as secretion stimulated by cyclic AMP and GMP (Leitch and Amer 1975; Greenberg, Murad, and Guerrant 1982; Thomas and Knoop 1982; Holmgren, Lange, and Lönnroth 1978). Cyclic GMP production was not, however, inhibited in rabbit ileal mucosa (Smith and Field 1980). Chlorpromazine, another potent inhibitor of Ca^{2+} calmodulin action, blocks STa and cyclic GMP-induced secretion in the infant mouse model (Greenberg and Guerrant 1981). Chlorpromazine also delays the time course of STa-induced secretion, so that Takeda, Honda, Takeda, and Miwatani (1981a) were unable to show an effect of chlorpromazine on STa-induced secretion with increasing time. High concentrations of the phenothiazines (trifluoperazine and chlorpromazine) are required in all models to inhibit cyclic nucleotide-induced secretion. This suggests that their effect is non-specific and not primarily related to intracellular Ca^{2+}. The importance of the various links between the cyclic nucleotides and Ca^{2+} and the role of Ca^{2+} in enterotoxin-induced secretion remains unclear (Fig. 12.5).

On the basis of present evidence it seems likely that Ca^{2+} is not directly involved in the stimulation of adenylate cyclase or guanylate cyclase by enterotoxins, although there may be a role for Ca^{2+}–calmodulin at a step distal to cyclic nucleotide production. Calcium released by the action of cyclic AMP or cyclic GMP may activate C kinase in a manner analagous to the activation of A and G kinases by cyclic AMP and cyclic GMP. The activity of the kinases and their effect on the phosphorylation of membrane proteins and membrane transport systems has recently been reviewed by De Jonge and Lohmann (1985) and will not be considered further.

Although no bacterial enterotoxin has been proven to stimulate secretion through a Ca^{2+}-dependent/cyclic nucleotide-independent mechanism, McGowan, Guerina, Wicks, and Donowitz (1985) have reported that *Entamoeba histolytica* induces a unique Ca^{2+}-dependent intestinal secretion. They suggested that serotonin released directly from amoebae invading the *lamina propria* is responsible for the watery diarrhoea seen in amoebiasis. Crude lysates of *E. histolytica* are known to have cytotoxic and enterotoxic activity (Lushbaugh, Kairalla, Cantey, Hofbauer, and Pittman 1978) and have recently been studied in Ussing chambers with rabbit ileum and rat colon. Addition of the lysate to the mucosal surface produced no effect on electrolyte transport but addition to the serosal surface caused an increase in short-circuit current (SCC) with inhibition of active Na^+ and Cl^- absorption and stimulation of Cl^- secretion. The SCC is the external current applied to neutralize the spontaneous potential difference of the tissue and is equivalent to the net active ion transport across it. The spontaneous potential difference is the difference in charge between serosal and mucosal surfaces and reflects the fact that normal Na^+ absorption makes the serosal surface positive with respect to the mucosal surface. The effect was dependent on serosal Ca^{2+}, was inhibited by verapamil, and was associated with reversible desensitization. These characteristics were similar to those observed with the neurohumoral agents acetylcholine, serotonin, substance P, and neurotensin. The last three were shown by radioimmunoassay to be present in the amoebic lysates. It was concluded that serotonin was the agent responsible for the intestinal secretion since bufotenine, an inhibitor of serotonin and anti-serotonin antibody, inhibited the ionic transport induced by amoebic lysates. Prostaglandins also appear to be involved because indomethacin and prior treatment with PGE_2 inhibited the effect.

Phospholipid hydrolysis and arachidonic acid metabolites
We have seen how certain neurohumoral agents activate phospholipase C hydrolysis of membrane-based phospholipids and how the products of hydrolysis, diacylglycerol, and inositol triphosphate increase intracellular Ca^{2+}. Arachidonic acid may be formed by additional lipase hydrolysis of diacylglycerol and by the action of phospholipase A2 (Ca^{2+}-dependent) on

other membrane phospholipids (phosphatidyl inositol, phosphatidyl choline, or phosphatidyl ethanolamine; Fig. 12.6). Arachidonic acid is in turn metabolized to various prostaglandins and leukotrienes by the cyclo-oxygenase and lipo-oxygenase pathways. PGE_2, and to a lesser extent other prostaglandins, stimulates intestinal secretion, at least in pharmacological doses, through the adenylate cyclase pathway. The lipo-oxygenase metabolites 5-hydroperoxyeicosatetraenoic acid (5HPETE) and 5-hydroxy-eicosatetraenoic acid (5HETE) have been shown to stimulate colonic secretion in the rabbit (Musch, Miller, Field, and Siegel 1982). This secretion is Ca^{2+} and cyclic nucleotide-independent.

The importance of these products of arachidonic acid metabolism and phospholipid hydrolysis as intracellular messengers in toxin-induced diarrhoea await clarification. They may be more important in invasive diarrhoea when vasoactive kinins, which can initiate phospholipid hydrolysis, are released as a result of tissue damage and inflammation. It is not known whether the resulting intestinal secretion is mediated through bradykinin receptors on the basolateral membrane of the enterocyte (Manning, Snyder, Kachur, Miller, and Field 1982) or through indirect stimulation by prostaglandins released from the lamina propria.

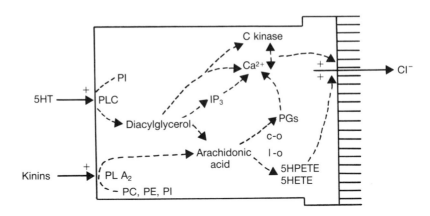

Fig. 12.6 Possible role of neurohormones, kinins, metabolites of phospholipid hydrolysis, and the arachidonic acid cascade. Hydrolysis of membrane-based phospholipids (phosphatidyl inositol, PI, phosphatidyl choline, PC, and phosphatidyl ethanolomine, PE) by serotonin (5HT) or by kinins released during inflammatory reactions produce:

(i) diacylglycerol and inositol triphosphate (IP_3), which stimulate C kinase and release Ca^{2+} from intracellular stores; and

(ii) arachidonic acid, which is further metabolized to prostaglandins by the cyclo-oxygenase (c-o) pathway or to 5HPETE and 5HETE by lipo-oxygenase (l-o).
(PLC = phospholipase C; PL A_2 = phospholipase A_2).

Enterotoxins: toxins that impair absorption or augment secretion

Toxins that activate adenylate cyclase, cholera toxin, and labile toxin (LT) of E. coli

Most of the work in this field has been undertaken with cholera toxin since its purification by Finkelstein and LoSpalutto (1970), although it is now clear that LT is structurally (Gill, Clements, Robertson, and Finkelstein 1981) and functionally similar (Table 12.5). Cholera toxin consists of two types of subunit, one large subunit A (m.w. 28 000) and five smaller B subunits (each of m.w. 11 000). The five B subunits are attached in a ring in which A lies loosely cradled. The B subunits bind to the intestinal epithelium via a membrane receptor that has been identified as GM1 ganglioside (Holmgren, Lönnroth, and Svennerholm 1973). After binding, the toxin–ganglioside complex is probably transported into the cell by endocytosis. The A subunit then dissociates into two further subunits, A1 and A2, by proteolytic cleavage of a disulphide bond. A2 probably stabilizes the toxin molecule, while A1 catalyses the transfer of an ADP-ribosyl group from NAD in the cytosol to an arginine residue of the alpha peptide of the regulatory component of adenylate cyclase (Moss, Garrison, Oppenheimer, and Richardson 1979). The ADP-ribosylation prevents inactivation of the cyclase, so that after an initial lag for the entry of A1, cyclic AMP will continue to be made for days after all extracellular toxin has been removed. For this reason recovery from cholera depends on replacement of stimulated

Table 12.5 The heat-labile (LT) and heat-stable (STa and STb) toxins of *E. coli*.

	LT	STa	STb
Heat lability	Labile	Stable	Stable
Molecular weight	102 000	2000	5000
Antigenicity	Antigenic	Poorly antigenic	?
Receptor	GM1 ganglioside	Protein	?
Cyclic nucleotide	Activates cAMP	Activates cGMP	Does not activate cAMP or cGMP
Activity	Delayed	No delay	No delay
Response	Prolonged	Reversible	Partially reversible
Method of assay	Tissue culture, ELISA, secretion in rabbit loops at 18 h	Secretion in infant mouse or rabbit loops at 4–6 h	Secretion in weaned piglet loops at 5 h
Specificity	Not tissue specific	Tissue specific	Species specific

cells by new cells migrating from the crypts to the villi or the turnover of protein to replace activated adenylate cyclase.

The ability of certain toxigenic *E. coli* to produce LT or ST is due to the presence of transmissible extrachromosomal plasmid DNA, whereas toxin production by *V. cholerae* is controlled by the chromosome. The amino acid sequence of cholera B subunits and LT B subunits has been determined and there is 79 per cent homology. Antitoxins against cholera toxin and LT cross-neutralize. The close chemical and immunological relationship between LT and cholera toxin extends to both A and B subunits. Indeed, hybrid toxins have been manufactured from cholera toxin A and LT B subunits, and *vice versa* (Takeda, Honda, Taga, and Miwatani 1981b).

LT and cholera toxin may be assayed in tissue culture models with Chinese hamster ovary (CHO) cells and Y1 adrenal cells, by enzyme-linked immunosorbent assays (ELISA), or in rabbit intestinal loops after 18 h.

Toxins that activate guanylate cyclase: heat-stable toxins

Various enteropathogenic bacteria, including *E. coli*, *Yersinia entercolitica* (Rao, Guandalini, Laird, and Field 1979) *Klebsiella pneumoniae* (Klipstein, Engert, and Houghton 1983), and *Enterobacter* spp. elaborate low molecular weight heat-stable enterotoxins known as ST. *E. coli* toxins have been studied in detail, but others appear similar in structure and mechanism of action. The *E. coli* STs are themselves a heterogeneous group that can be further subdivided (Table 12.5). STa is methanol-soluble and may be assayed by the suckling mouse bioassay. It stimulates intracellular guanylate cyclase activity and consequently increases cyclic GMP concentration. There is no effect on cyclic AMP or on phosphodiesterase activity (Field *et al.* 1978a). In contrast STb molecules are methanol-insoluble and elicit fluid secretion in weaned pigs but not in suckling mice. They have no effect on the cyclic nucleotides and will be discussed below. The genes encoding for STa and STb have been characterized (So and McCarthy 1980; Picken, Mazaitis, Maas, Rey, and Heynecker 1983). STa has been purified and its amino acid sequence determined (Chan and Gianella 1981; Aimoto, Takao, Shimonishi, Takeda, Takeda, and Miwatani 1982). All STa molecules that have been studied show a much shorter sequence of 18 amino acid residues, compared with that predicted by gene cloning studies, indicating that post-translational modification occurs during their elaboration. STa molecules have a high content of cysteine residues and disulphide linkages, which are probably responsible for their physical characteristics.

The effects of STa, in contrast to those of cholera toxin and LT, are rapid, without time lag, reversible, and tissue-specific. STa fails to stimulate guanylate cyclase in brain, heart, lungs, liver, pancreas, or gastric mucosa, but is active in the small and large intestine (Rao, Guandalini, Smith, and Field 1980; Guerrant, Hughes, Chang, Robertson, and Murad 1980).

Recently STa has been shown to stimulate cyclic GMP in rat basophilic leukaemia cells (Knoop and Thomas 1983) but this reaction is very different from that on the intestine; there is a detectable lag and the rise in cyclic GMP is only twofold compared with the tenfold increase in intestinal cells. The specificity of STa for intestine appears to be due to the presence of unique receptors (Gianella, Luttrell, and Thompson 1983; Frantz, Jaso-Friedman, and Robertson, 1984). The rabbit distal colon does not respond to STa, possibly because of the absence of the cyclic GMP-dependent phosphorylation system (G kinase; Rao, Nash, and Palfrey 1982). STa stimulates particulate but not soluble guanylate cyclase. Particulate cyclase is present mainly in the brush border of enterocytes with a steep ascending gradient of activity from crypt to villus tip. There is a parallel gradient of G kinase activity, so that ST is primarily anti-absorptive whereas LT and cholera toxin are also secretory.

Specific saturable binding sites for the toxin have been identified on rat enterocytes and basophilic leukaemia cells with radio-labelled STa. The binding sites are membrane-associated and proteinaceous. It is possible that the receptor is part of the cyclase molecule itself. Free radicals, nitroso compounds, and metabolites of arachidonic acid are important stimulators of guanylate cyclase activity in other tissues, but seem unimportant in the stimulation of intestinal particulate guanylate cyclase. Guerrant *et al.* (1980) observed that the free radical scavenger butylated hydroxyanisole inhibited both basal and STa-stimulated activity non-specifically. Dreyfus, Jaso-Friedman, and Robertson (1984) have shown that molecular oxygen is not required for guanylate cyclase activity. De Jonge (1984) observed a low response of rat intestine to nitroso compounds and Dreyfus *et al.* (1984) observed that STa did not alter the conversion of arachidonic acid to its metabolites; in particular no increase in the level of PGE_2, $PGE_2\alpha$ or thromboxane in rat jejunal cells was seen. Conversely, indomethacin, a cyclo-oxygenase inhibitor, prevents STa-induced but not cyclic GMP-induced fluid secretion in the suckling mouse assay (Madsen and Knoop 1978). This suggests that prostaglandins may be involved in the activation of guanylate cyclase by STa, but not in the induction of secretion by cyclic GMP.

STb toxin of E. coli, *an enterotoxin without effect on cyclic nucleotides or calcium ions*

The STb toxin, in contrast to STa, does not cause an increase in cyclic GMP in ligated intestinal loops of piglets, rats, or rabbits (Kennedy, Greenberg, Dunn, Abernathy, Ryerse, and Guerrant, 1984). In ligated porcine jejunal loop assays, crude toxin preparations of STb induce fluid secretion within 30 min, with a maximal response between 3 and 6 h. There is an immediate rise in SCC (see p. 221) after exposure of stripped porcine jejunal mucosa to

STb in the Ussing chamber. This is maximal at 15 min and paralleled by an increase in potential difference (Weikel and Guerrant 1985). These findings in conjunction with the *in vivo* experiments indicate a net secretory anion flux. Weikel and Guerrant (1985) suggest that this anion is HCO_3^-; in any case there was no change in Cl^- or Na^+ fluxes as judged by the use of labelled ^{22}Na and ^{36}Cl. The removal of Ca^{2+} and the addition of lanthanum does not inhibit secretion due to STb, suggesting that this secretion is calcium independent. The mediators of this unique secretion await clarification.

Toxins of Aeromonas and Campylobacter

Aeromonas hydrophila is an ubiquitous aquatic organism incriminated as a cause of gastroenteritis (Burke, Gracey, Robinson, Peck, Beaman, and Bundell 1983) and known to produce at least one enterotoxin. A heat-labile toxin causing fluid accumulation in rabbit intestinal loops has been partially purified. Like cholera toxin and LT it induces steroidogenesis and increases the cyclic AMP content in Y1 adrenal cells. However, it is not neutralized by antisera to cholera toxin and LT, nor does it bind to GM1 ganglioside (Ljungh, Eneroth, and Wadström 1982). It is probably not composed of A and B subunits. Cytotoxins are also produced that do not induce fluid secretion in rabbit intestinal loops, although they damage the mucosa (Ljungh and Kronevi 1982).

 Campylobacter jejuni may produce a cholera-like heat-labile toxin that elongates CHO cells, an effect that can be neutralized by cholera antitoxin (Ruiz-Palacios, Torres, Escamilla, Ruiz-Palacios, and Tamayo, 1983). Some strains produce a cytotoxin (Pennie, O'Brien, and Guerrant 1984) that is not neutralized by shigella antitoxin.

Cytotoxins: toxins that alter structure

Shigella toxin and shigellosis

Shigella toxin is produced by *Shigella dysenteriae* type 1 and other species of the genus as well as by some strains of *E. coli* (Cleary *et al.* 1985). Recently, it has been purified (Donohue-Rolfe, Keusch, Edson, Thorley-Lawson, and Jacewicz 1984) and found to be a protein composed of two polypeptide subunits. As with cholera and LT the larger active peptide (m.w. 32 000) is termed A and the smaller B (m.w. 6500). Five B subunits associate with one A to form the holotoxin which is transported from the cell surface to the interior by endocytosis. The use of subunit antisera has shown that B mediates the binding of toxin to cell membrane receptors. The surface receptor in HeLa cells is an asparagine-linked glycoprotein. Subunit A can be separated into A1 (m.w. 28 000–29 000) and A2 (m.w. 3000) (Reisbig, Olsnes, and Eiklid 1981); the former inhibits protein synthesis and has diverse effects in various physiological and experimental situations including cytotoxicity, enterotoxicity, and neurotoxicity. These biological activities co-purify and antibodies against one activity cross-neutralize the other activities. Shigella toxin does not interfere with peptide bond formation but probably inhibits peptide chain elongation by catalytic inactivation of the 60 S ribosomal subunit (Reisbig *et al.* 1981).

The colon is resistant to exogenous shigella toxin (Donowitz and Binder 1976) but the cytotoxin released from invading organisms results in protein synthesis inhibition and cell death. The ensuing ulcerative, inflammatory colitis is responsible for the dysenteric syndrome of fever, abdominal cramps, tenesmus, and bloody stools. In shigellosis, these symptoms are typically preceded by a period of watery diarrhoea. This initial phase of the illness in the rhesus monkey is associated with non-invasive colonization of the jejunum by the organism. Shigella toxin induces fluid secretion without tissue damage in rabbit proximal small intestine and has been shown to bind to specific receptors on rabbit microvillous membranes (Fuchs, Donohue-Rolfe, Montgomery, Keusch, and Grand 1984). It has been postulated that the organisms colonize the small intestine of humans without invasion and release an enterotoxin, which binds to a receptor and stimulates secretion. Colonization of the small bowel in humans, however, has not been proven. There is also controversy as to whether the adenylate cyclase–cyclic AMP system is activated or not (Charney, Gots, Formal, and Giannella 1976; Keusch, Donohue-Rolfe, and Jacewicz 1981).

Salmonellosis

The pathogenesis of salmonellosis is also unclear. Studies in the rhesus monkey (Rout, Formal, Dammin, and Giannella 1974) showed the jejunum in a secretory state without bacterial colonization, invasion, or histological damage. The ileum and colon were colonized and invaded by the organisms and there was evidence of inflammation with a marked polymorphonuclear cell infiltration and net colonic secretion. Jejunal biopsy studies in humans (Giannella, Broitman, and Zamcheck 1971) parallel the negative proximal histology and lack of luminal colonization in the monkey. Strains of *S. typhimurium* produce an enterotoxin active in the rabbit ileal loop with little or no histological damage and watery rather than haemorrhagic secretion. Salmonella toxin has been partially purified and there is evidence (reviewed by Stephen, Wallis, Starkey, Candy, Osborne, and Haddon 1985) that it bears some resemblance to cholera toxin.

In rabbit jejunal loops invading organisms cause a secretory response in 6–8 h, coinciding with a polymorphonuclear response. It is suggested that the inflammatory reaction releases prostaglandins (? kinin-mediated), which are responsible for the secretion. Gots, Formal, and Giannella (1974) showed that indomethacin (a prostaglandin inhibitor) abolished the secretion induced by *S. typhimurium* in rabbit loops but only partially inhibited the secretion produced by *V. cholerae* and *Shigella flexneri* type 2a. By 14 h, rabbit jejunal loops show blunting of villus tips, although the crypt histology remains intact. It is suggested that this damage inhibits absorption and adds to the net secretion. It is not known whether a cytotoxin is responsible for this effect, although Kétyi, Pásca, Emödy, Vertényi, Kocsis, and Kuch (1979) have shown that certain *Salmonella* species produce a toxin that cross neutralizes with shiga toxin, and Koo and Peterson (1983) and Koo, Peterson, Houston, and Molina (1984) have demonstrated that a crude *S. typhimurium* toxin inhibits protein synthesis in Vero cells and rabbit ileal epithelial cells.

Thus, prostaglandins released in response to inflammation, villus tip damage, cholera-like enterotoxin, and Shiga-like cytotoxin are possible mechanisms by which *Salmonella* spp. causes diarrhoea. In human salmonellosis it is not known when toxins or secretagogues are produced in relation to bacterial colonization and invasion, nor where they are active.

Staphylococcal toxins

There are at least seven antigenically distinct staphylococcal enterotoxins that cause vomiting and diarrhoea in staphylococcal food poisoning in humans. They induce emesis in monkeys by stimulating neural receptors in the gut rather than by stimulating the vomiting centre in the medulla (Elwell, Liu, Spertzel, and Beisel 1975). They are mostly heat-stable and resistant to trypsin, chymotrypsin, renin, and papain, with molecular weights in the range 25 000–35 000. The pathogenesis of the diarrhoea is less clear. In dogs net secretion of water, Na^+, K^+, and Cl^- has been observed in the small intestine (Elias and Shields 1976). No changes were observed in transmural potential difference or SCC in response to one of the enterotoxins suggesting non-electrogenic secretory mechanisms (Sullivan and Asano 1971). Mucosal damage due to cytotoxic activity has also been recorded (Merrill and Sprinz 1968).

Delta toxin, one of the four haemolysins of *Staphylococcus aureus*, is also an enterotoxin. It has recently been purified (Fitton, Dell, and Shaw 1980) and its amino acid sequence and molecular weight (m.w. 2977) established. At extremes of pH in aqueous solution it exists as a tetramer. Once the toxin binds to cell membranes it cannot be detected in the standard haemolytic assay, it is not therefore known whether delta toxin is produced in the host. In rabbit or guinea pig ileal segments it inhibits water absorption without a discernable lag (Kapral, O'Brien, Ruff, and Drugan 1976) and in guinea pig ileum an elevation of cyclic AMP has been recorded but only after a lag of 1 h (O'Brien and Kapral 1976). Delta toxin was shown to be cytotoxic in HeLa cell tissue culture and in the guinea pig ileum, where it causes swelling and shortening of the villi with destruction of the villus tips. In the Ussing chamber delta toxin caused an immediate increase in transmural potential difference and SCC. The conductance of the guinea pig ileum was increased and there was an increase in both absorption and secretion of Na^+ and Cl^-, but with net Na^+ and possibly Cl^- secretion (O'Brien, McClung, and Kapral 1978). The delay in the cyclic AMP response makes it unlikely these changes are mediated by cyclic nucleotides.

Clostridial toxins

Clostridium difficile is associated with pseudomembranous or antibiotic colitis in humans, necrotizing enterocolitis in sick neonates and caecitis in hamsters. Organisms produce two toxins, an enterotoxin (toxin A) and a cytotoxin (toxin B), both of which appear important in the disease process (Libby, Jortner, and Wilkins 1982). Paradoxically the toxins may also be present in the faeces of asymptomatic patients. Both toxins appear to be very large (m.w. 300 000) and are probably composed of multiple subunits. Preliminary evidence suggests that toxin A binds to a glycoprotein receptor on hamster brush border membranes. A study of crude *C. difficile* toxin (presumably containing A and B) in Ussing chambers revealed a secretory response from rabbit ileal mucosa (Hughes, Warhurst, Turnberg, Higgs, Giugliano, and Drasar 1983). There was delayed secretion of Cl^- and inhibition of Na^+ absorption, without tissue damage. No alteration in cyclic AMP or cyclic GMP was recorded but the response depended on the presence of Ca^{2+} in the bathing media. Stephen, Redmond, Mitchell, Ketley, Candy, Burdon, and Daniel (1984) reported experiments with purified toxin A in Ussing chambers when ion fluxes in rabbit ileal mucosa were seen only when there was damage to villus tips.

   C. spiroforme produces a fatal caecitis in rabbits mediated by a toxin that can be neutralized by antitoxin to *C. perfringens* Type E (iota toxin). Strains of *C. perfringens* Type A cause food poisoning when heat-resistant spores are ingested with inadequately heated food. The subsequent release of enterotoxin (Hauschild and Hilsheimer 1971) in the small intestine is responsible for the vomiting and diarrhoea. Type C strains of *C. perfringens* cause a necrotizing enteritis mediated by beta toxin (Sakurai and Duncan 1978). Many other clostridial species are known to produce toxins, but their importance in human and animal disease is unknown.

Implications for the future

In 1959, De demonstrated that a crude bacteria-free toxin preparation of *V. cholerae* induced fluid secretion in an isolated loop of rabbit ileum. Since then, as we have seen, our understanding of the pathogenesis of cholera and other bacterial diarrhoeas has greatly increased, together with our knowledge of absorptive and secretory mechanisms in the intestine. There have also been modest therapeutic advances. Oral rehydration with sugar-containing electrolyte solutions is both cheap and effective. Vaccines against *E. coli* adhesive antigens or LT given to domesticated pregnant animals protects the naturally fed offspring from *E. coli* diarrhoea. Various opiates, anti-inflammatory agents, Ca^{2+}, and calmodulin inhibitors and neurotransmitters have also had limited success in clinical trials in gastroenteritis. The provision of clean water, basic sanitation, and improved nutrition, where resources allow, has greatly reduced the local incidence of diarrhoea. Yet gastrointestinal infection is still responsible for human suffering on an immense scale. It is to be hoped that the next decade will see the development of oral vaccines against *E. coli* and cholera with antibacterial, antitoxin, or antiadhesive activity. It should also be possible to develop new, more specific antisecretory drugs as working knowledge of intestinal electrolyte transport is refined. If such therapeutic advances were accompanied by improvements in nutrition and sanitation the mortality and morbidity of infectious diarrhoea could be dramatically reduced.

Acknowledgements — I wish to thank Judy Lehmann and her staff for an excellent library service.

References

Aimoto, S., Takao, T., Shimonishi, Y., Takeda, T., Takeda, Y., and Miwatani, T. (1982). Amino acid sequences of heat-stable enterotoxin produced by human enterotoxigenic *Escherichia coli*. *Eur. J. Biochem.* **129**, 257–63.

Amiranoff, B. M., Laburthe, M. C., Rouyer-Fessard, C. M., Demaille, J. G., and Rosselin, G. E. (1983). Calmodulin stimulation of adenylate cyclase of intestinal epithelium. *Eur. J. Biochem.* **130**, 33–7.

Argenzio, R. A. and Whipp, S. C. (1981). Effects of *Escherichia coli* heat-stable enterotoxin, cholera toxin and theophylline on ion transport in porcine colon. *J. Physiol. (Lond.)* **320**, 469–87.

Berridge, M. J. (1981). Phosphatidylinositol hydrolysis: a multifunctional transducing mechanism. *Mol. cell. Endocrinol.* **24**, 115–40.

Burke, V., Gracey, M., Robinson, J., Peck, D., Beaman, J., and Bundell, C. (1983). The microbiology of childhood gastroenteritis: *Aeromonas* species and other infective agents. *J. infect. Dis.* **148**, 68–74.

Cassuto, J., Jodal, M., Sjövall, H., and Lundgren, O. (1981). Nervous control of intestinal secretion. *Clin. Res. Rev.* **1** (Suppl. 1), 11–21.

Chan, S. K. and Giannella, R. A. (1981). Amino acid sequence of heat-stable enterotoxin produced by *E. coli* pathogenic for man. *J. biol. Chem.* **256**, 7744–6.

Charney, A. N., Gots, R. E., Formal, S. B., and Giannella, R. A. (1976). Activation of intestinal mucosal adenylate cyclase by *Shigella dysenteriae* 1 enterotoxin. *Gastroenterology* **70**, 1085–90.

Cleary, T. G., Mathewson, J. J., Faris, E., and Pickering, L. K. (1985). Shiga-like cytotoxin production by enteropathogenic *Escherichia coli* serogroups. *Infect. Immunol.* **47**, 335–7.

De, S. N. (1959). Enterotoxicity of bacteria-free culture filtrates of *Vibrio cholerae*. *Nature. Lond.* **183**, 1533–4.

De Jonge, H. R. (1975). The response of small intestinal villus and crypt epithelium to cholera toxin in rat and guinea-pig. Evidence against a specific role of the crypt cells in cholera-induced secretion. *Biochim. biophys. acta* **381**, 128–43.

—— (1984). The mechanism of action of *Escherichia coli* heat-stable toxin. *Biochim. Soc. Trans.* **12**, 180–4.

—— and Lohmann, S. M. (1985). Mechanisms by which cyclic nucleotides and other intracellular mediators regulate secretion. In *Microbial toxins and diarrhoeal disease*. Ciba Foundation Symposium Vol. 112, pp. 116–38.

Donohue-Rolfe, A., Keusch, G. T., Edson, C., Thorley-Lawson, D., and Jacewicz, M. (1984). Pathogenesis of Shigella diarrhoea ix. Simplified high yield purification of Shigella toxin and characterization of subunit composition and functions by the use of subunit specific monoclonal and polyclonal antibodies. *J. exp. Med.* **160**, 1767–81.

Donowitz, M. (1983). Ca^{2+} in the control of active intestinal Na and Cl transport: involvement in neurohumoral action. *Am. J. Physiol.* **245**, G165–77.

—— and Binder, H. J. (1976). Effects of enterotoxins of *Vibrio cholerae*, *Escherichia coli* and *Shigella dysenteriae* Type 1 on fluid secretion and electrolyte transport in the colon. *J. infect. Dis.* **134**, 135–43.

Dreyfus, L. A., Jaso-Friedman, L., and Robertson, D. C. (1984). Characterisation of the mechanism of action of *Escherichia coli* heat-stable enterotoxin. *Infect. Immunol.* **44**, 493–501.

Elias, J. and Shields, R. (1976). Influence of staphylococcal enterotoxin on water and electrolyte transport in the small intestine. *Gut* **17**, 527–35.

Elwell, M. H., Liu, C. T., Spertzel, R. O., and Biesel, W. R. (1975). Mechanisms of oral staphylococcal enterotoxin B — induced emesis in the monkey. *Proc. Soc. Eur. Biol. Med.* **148**, 424–7.

Fan, C. C., Faust, R. G., and Powell, D. W. (1983). Coupled sodium–chloride transport by rabbit ileal brush border membrane vesicles. *Am. J. Physiol.* **244**, G375–85.

Field, M. (1980). Role of cyclic nucleotides in enterotoxic diarrhoea. In *Advances in cyclic nucleotide research* (ed. P. Hamet and H. Sands), Vol. 12, pp. 267–77. Raven Press, New York.

——, Graf, L. H., Laird, W. J., and Smith, P. Z. (1978a). Heat-stable enterotoxin of *Escherichia coli*: *in vitro* effects on guanylate cyclase activity, cGMP concentration and ion transport in small intestine. *Proc. nat. Acad. Sci. USA* **75**, 2800–4.

——, Karnaky, K. J., Smith, P. L., Bolton, J. E., and Kinter, W. B. (1978b). Ion transport across the isolated intestinal mucosa of the winter flounder, *Pseudopleuronectes Americanus* 1. Functional and structural properties of cellular and paracellular pathways for Na and Cl. *J. membr. Biol.* **41**, 265–93.

Finkelstein, R. A. and LoSpalutto, J. J. (1970). Production of highly purified choleragen and choleragenoid. *J. infect. Dis.* **121** (Suppl. 121), 63–72.

Fitton, J. E., Dell, A., and Shaw, W. V. (1980). The amino acid sequence of the delta haemolysin of *Staphylococcus aureus*. *FEBS Lett.* **115**, 209–12.

Frantz, J. C., Jaso-Friedman, L., and Robertson, D. C. (1984). Binding of *Escherichia coli* heat-stable enterotoxin to rat intestinal cells and brush border membranes. *Infect. Immunol.* **43**, 622–30.

Frizzel, R. A. (1977). Active chloride secretion by rabbit colon: calcium-dependent stimulation by ionophore A23187. *J. membr. Biol.* **35**, 175–87.

——, Smith, P. L., Vosburgh, E., and Field, M. (1979). Coupled sodium–chloride influx across brush border of flounder intestine. *J. membr. Biol.* **46**, 27–39.

Fuchs, G. T., Donohue-Rolfe, A., Montgomery, R. K., Keusch, G. T., and Grand, R. J. (1984). Evidence of a receptor for shigella toxin on rabbit intestinal microvillus membranes. *Gastroenterology* **86**, 1083.

Gangarosa, E. J. (1978). Epidemiology of *Escherichia coli* in the United States. *J. infect. Dis.* **137**, 634–8.

Giannella, R. A., Broitman, S. A., and Zamcheck, N. (1971). Salmonella enteritis 11. Fulminant diarrhoea in and effects on the small intestine. *Dig. Dis. Sci.* **16**, 1007–13.

——, Luttrell, M., and Thompson, M. (1983). Binding of *Escherichia coli* heat-stable enterotoxin to receptors on rat intestinal cells. *Am. J. Physiol.* **245**, G492–8.

Gill, D. M., Clements, J. D., Robertson, D. D., and Finkelstein, R. A. (1981). Subunit number and arrangement in *Escherichia coli* heat-labile enterotoxin. *Infect. Immunol.* **33**, 677–82.

Gots, R. E., Formal, S. B., and Giannella, R. A. (1974). Indomethacin inhibition of *Salmonella typhimurium*, *Shigella flexneri*, and cholera-mediated rabbit ileal secretion. *J. infect. Dis.* **130**, 280–4.

Greenberg, R. N. and Guerrant, R. L. (1981). *E. coli* heat-stable enterotoxin. *Pharmacol. Ther.* **13**, 507–31.

——, Murad, F., and Guerrant, R. L. (1982). Lanthanum chloride inhibition of the secretory response to *Escherichia coli* heat-stable enterotoxin. *Infect. Immunol.* **35**, 483–8.

Guerrant, R. L., Hughes, T. M., Chang, B., Robertson, D. C., and Murad, F. (1980). Activation of intestinal guanylate cyclase activity by heat-stable enterotoxin of *E. coli*: studies of tissue specificity, potential receptors and intermediates. *J. infect. Dis.* **142**, 220–8.

Gunther, R. D. and Wright, E. M. (1983). Na^+, Li^+ and Cl^- transport by brush border membranes from rabbit jejunum. *J. membr. Biol.* **74**, 85–94.

Hauschild, A. H. W. and Hilsheimer, R. (1971). Purification and characteristics of the enterotoxin of *Clostridium perfringens* type A. *Can. J. Microbiol.* **17**, 1425–33.

Holmgren, T., Lange, S., and Lönnroth, I. (1978). Reversal of cyclic AMP-mediated intestinal secretion in mice by chlorpromazine. *Gastroenterology* **75**, 1103–8.

Holmgren, J., Lönnroth, I., and Svennerholm, L. (1973). Fixation and inactivation of cholera toxin by GM1 gangliosides. *Scan. J. infect. Dis.* **5**, 77–8.

Hubel, K. A. (1974). The mechanism of bicarbonate secretion in rabbit ileum exposed to choleragen. *J. clin. Invest.* **53**, 964–70.

Hughes, S., Warhurst, G., Turnberg, L. A., Higgs, N. B., Giugliano, L. G., and Drasar, B. S. (1983). *Clostridium difficile* toxin-induced intestinal secretion in rabbit ileum *in vitro. Gut* **24**, 94–8.

Kapral, F. A., O'Brien, A. D., Ruff, P. D., and Drugan, W. J. (1976). Inhibition of water absorption in the intestine by *Staphylococcus aureus* delta-toxin. *Infect. Immunol.* **13**, 140–5.

Kennedy, D. J., Greenberg, R. N., Dunn, J. A., Abernathy, R., Ryerse, J. J., and Guerrant, R. L. (1984). Effects of *Escherichia coli* heat-stable enterotoxin STb on intestine of mice, rats, rabbits, and piglets. *Infect. Immunol.* **46**, 639–45.

Kétyi, I., Pásca, S., Emödy, L., Vertényi, A., Kocsis, B., and Kuch, B. (1979). *Shigella dysenteriae* 1-like cytotoxic enterotoxins produced by salmonella strains. *Acta. microbiol. Hung.* **26**, 217–23.

Keusch, G. T., Donohue-Rolfe, A., and Jacewicz, M. (1981). Shigella toxin(s): description and role in diarrhoea and dysentry. *Pharmacol. Ther.* **15**, 403–38.

—— and Donowitz, M. (1983). Pathophysiological mechanisms of diarrhoeal disease: diverse aetiologies and common mechanisms. *Scan. J. Gastroenterol.* **18**, (Suppl. 84), 33–43.

Klipstein, F. A., Engert, R. F., and Houghton, R. A. (1983). Immunological properties of purified *Klebsiella pneumoniae* heat stable enterotoxin. *Infect. Immunol.* **42**, 838–41.

Knoop, F. C. and Thomas, D. D. (1983). Stimulation of calcium uptake and cyclic GMP synthesis in rat basophilic cells by *Escherichia coli* heat stable enterotoxin. *Infect. Immunol.* **41**, 971–7.

Koo, F. C. W. and Peterson, J. W. (1983). Cell-free extracts of salmonella inhibit protein synthesis and cause cytotoxicity in eukaryotic cells. *Toxicon* **21**, 309–20.

——, ——, Houston, C. W., and Molina, N. C. (1984). Pathogenesis of experimental salmonellosis: inhibition of protein synthesis by cytotoxin. *Infect. Immunol.* **43**, 93–100.

Lazo, P. S., Rivaya, A., and Velasco, G. (1984). Regulation by calcium and calmodulin of adenylate cyclase from rabbit intestinal epithelium. *Biochim. biophys. acta* **798**, 361–7.

Leitch, S. J. and Amer, M. A. (1975). Lanthanum inhibition of *Vibrio cholerae* and *Escherichia coli* enterotoxin induced enterosorption and its effects on intestinal mucosal cyclic adenosine 3′, 5′ — monophosphate and cyclic guanosine 3′, 5′ — monophosphate levels. *Infect. Immunol.* **11**, 1038–44.

Libby, J. M., Jortner, B. S., and Wilkins, T. D. (1982). Effects of the two toxins of *Clostridium difficile* in antibiotic-associated caecitis in hamsters. *Infect. Immunol.* **36**, 822–9.

Ljungh, Å., Eneroth, P., and Wadström, T. (1982). Cytotonic enterotoxin from *Aeromonas hydrophila. Toxicon* **20**, 787–94.

—— and Kronevi, T. (1982). *Aeromonas hydrophila* toxins–intestinal fluid accumulation and mucosal injury in animal models. *Toxicon* **20**, 397–407.

Lushbaugh, W. B., Kairalla, A. B., Cantey, J. R., Hofbauer, A. F. and

Pittman, F. E. (1978). Isolation of a cytotoxin-enterotoxin from *Entamoeba histolytica. J. infect. Dis.* **139**, 9–17.

McGowan, K., Guerina, V., Wicks, J., and Donowitz, M. (1985). Secretory hormones of *Entamoeba histolytica*. In *Microbial toxins and diarrhoeal disease*. Ciba Foundation Symposium 112, pp. 139–154.

Madsen, G. L. and Knoop, F. C. (1978). Inhibition of the secretory activity of *Escherichia coli* heat-stable enterotoxin by indomethacin. *Infect. Immunol.* **22**, 143–7.

Manning, D. C., Snyder, S. H., Kachur, J. F., Miller, R. J., and Field, M. (1982). Bradykinin receptor-mediated chloride secretion in intestinal function. *Nature (Lond.)* **299**, 256–9.

Merrill, T. G. and Sprinz, H. (1968). The effect of Staphylococcal enterotoxin on the fine structure of the monkey jejunum. *Lab. Invest.* **18**, 114–23.

Moss, J., Garrison, S., Oppenheimer, N. J., and Richardson, S. H. (1979). NAD-dependent ADP-ribosylation of arginine and proteins by *Escherichia coli* heat labile enterotoxin. *J. biol. Chem.* **254**, 6270–2.

Musch, M. W., Miller, R. J., Field, M., and Siegel, M. I. (1982). Stimulation of colonic secretion by lipoxygenase metabolites of arachidonic acid. *Science* **217**, 1255–6.

Nasset, E. S. and Ju, J. S. (1973). Micropipette collection of succus entericus at crypt ostia of guinea pig jejunum. *Digestion* **9**, 205–11.

O'Brien, A. D. and Kapral, F. A. (1976). Increased cyclic 3′, 5′ — monophosphate content in guinea pig ileum after exposure to *Staphylococcus aureus* delta toxin. *Infect. Immunol.* **13**, 152–62.

——, McClung, H. J., and Kapral, F. A. (1978). Increased tissue conductance and ion transport in guinea pig ileum after exposure to *Staphylococcus aureus* delta-toxin *in vitro*. *Infect. Immunol.* **21**, 102–13.

——, LaVeck, G. D., Thompson, M. R., and Formal, S. B. (1982). Production of *Shigella dysenteriae* Type 1-like cytotoxin by *Escherichia coli. J. infect. Dis.* **146**, 763–9.

Pennie, R. A., O'Brien, A. D., and Guerrant, R. L. (1984). A derivative of *Campylobacter jejuni* is cytotoxic for HeLa cells. *Clin. Res.* **32**, 379A.

Picken, R. N., Mazaitis, A. J., Maas, W. K., Rey, M., and Heynecker, H. (1983). Nucleotide sequences of the gene for heat-stable enterotoxin 11 of *Escherichia coli. Infect. Immunol.* **42**, 269–75.

Rao, M. C., Guandalini, S., Laird, W. J., and Field, M. (1979). Effects of heat stable enterotoxin of *Yersinia enterocolitica* on ion transport and cyclic guanosine 3′, 5′ — monophosphate metabolism in rabbit ileum. *Infect. Immunol.* **26**, 875–8.

——, ——, Smith, P. L., and Field, M. (1980). Mode of action of heat-stable *E. coli* enterotoxin: tissue and subcellular specificities and role of cyclic GMP. *Biochim. biophys. acta* **632**, 35–46.

——, Nash, N. T., and Palfrey, H. C. (1982). Ca, calmodulin and cyclic nucleotide dependent phosphorylation of epithelial cells. *J. cell. Biol.* **95**, 254A.

Reisbig, R., Olsnes, S., and Eiklid, K. (1981). The cytotoxic activity of shigella toxin: evidence for catalytic inactivation of the 60 S ribosomal subunit. *J. biol. Chem.* **256**, 8739–44.

Roggin, G. M., Banwell, J. G., Yardley, J. H., and Hendrix, T. H. (1972). Unimpaired response of rabbit jejunum to cholera toxin after selective damage to villus epithelium. *Gastroenterology* **63**, 981–9.

Rout, W. R., Formal, S. B., Dammin, G. J., and Giannella, R. A. (1974). Pathophysiology of salmonella diarrhoea in the rhesus monkey: intestinal transport, morphological and bacteriological studies. *Gastroenterology* **67**, 59–70.

Ruiz-Palacios, G. M., Torres, N. I., Escamilla, E., Ruiz-Palacios, B., and Tamayo, J. (1983). Cholera-like enterotoxin produced by *Campylobacter* jejuni: characterisation and clinical significance. *Lancet* **2**, 250–2.

Sakurai, J. and Duncan, C. L. (1978). Some properties of beta-toxin produced by *Clostridium perfringens* Type C. *Infect. Immunol.* **21**, 678–80.

Smith, P. L. and Field, M. (1980). *In vitro* antisecretory effects of trifluoperazine and other neuroleptics in rabbit and human small intestine. *Gastroenterology* **78**, 1545–53.

Snyder, J. D. and Merson, M. H. (1982). The magnitude of the global problem of acute diarrhoeal disease: a review of acute surveillance data. *Bull. WHO* **60**, 605–13.

So, M. and McCarthy, B. J. (1980). Nucleotide sequence of bacterial transposon Tn 1681 encoding a heat-stable toxin (ST) and its identification in enterotoxigenic *Escherichia coli* strains. *Proc. nat. Acad. Sci. USA* **77**, 4011–15.

Stephen, J., Wallis, T. S., Starkey, W. G., Candy, D. C. A., Osborne, M. P., and Haddon, S. (1985). Salmonellosis: in retrospect and prospect. In *Microbial toxins and diarrhoeal disease*. Ciba Foundation Symposium Vol. 112, pp. 175–92.

——, Redmond, S. C., Mitchell, T. J., Ketley, J., Candy, D. C. A., Burdon, D. W., and Daniel, R. (1984). *Clostridium difficile* enterotoxin (toxin A): new results. *Biochem. Soc. Trans.* **12**, 194–5.

Sullivan, R. and Asano, T. (1971). Effects of staphylococcal enterotoxin B on intestinal transport in the rat. *Am. J. Physiol.* **220**, 1793–7.

Takeda, T., Honda, T., Takeda, Y., and Miwatani, T. (1981a). Failure of chlorpromazine to inhibit fluid accumulation caused by *Escherichia coli* heat-stable enterotoxin in suckling mice. *Infect. Immunol.* **32**, 480–3.

——, Honda, T., Taga, S., and Miwatani, T., (1981b). *In vitro* formation of hybrid toxins between subunits of *Escherichia coli* heat-labile enterotoxin and those of cholera enterotoxin. *Infect. Immunol.* **34**, 341–6.

Thomas, D. D. and Knoop, F. C. (1982). The effect of calcium and prostaglandin inhibitors on the intestinal fluid response to heat stable enterotoxin of *Escherichia coli*. *J. infect. Dis.* **145**, 141–7.

Turnberg, L. A., Bieberdorf, F. A., Morawski, S. G., and Fordtran, J. S. (1970). Interrelationship of chloride, bicarbonate, sodium and hydrogen transport in the human ileum. *J. clin. Invest.* **49**, 557–67.

Ulshen, M. H. and Rollo, J. L. (1980). Pathogenesis of *Escherichia coli* gastroenteritis in man — another mechanism. *New Eng. J. Med.* **302**, 99–101.

Walsh, J. A. and Warren, K. S. (1979). Selective primary health care. *New Engl. J. Med.* **301**, 967–74.

Weikel, C. S., and Guerrant, R. L. (1985). STb enterotoxin of *Escherichia coli*:

cyclic nucleotide-independent secretion. In *Microbial toxins and diarroheal disease*. Ciba Foundation Symposium Vol. 112, pp. 94–115.

Welsh, M. J., Smith, P. L., Fromm, M., and Frizzell, R. A. (1982). Crypts are the site of intestinal fluid and electrolyte secretion. *Science* **218**, 1219–21.

13

Novel roles of neural acceptors for inhibitory and facilitatory toxins

J. O. Dolly, J. D. Black, A. R. Black,
A. Pelchen-Matthews, and J. V. Halliwell

Neurotoxins as probes for membrane components concerned with communication in the nervous system.

Little information is available about the molecular properties of the macro-molecules in presynaptic nerve membranes that are responsible for neurotransmitter release and the control of cell excitability. Such functional components are difficult to identify and characterize biochemically because of their sparseness and problems inherent in monitoring such complex biological activities in broken cell preparations. Hence it is obligatory to use specific probes to label these elusive neural constituents. In the case of nicotinic acetylcholine receptors (reviewed by Dolly and Barnard 1984), voltage-sensitive Na^+ (Catterall 1984) and Ca^{2+} (*cf.* Miller 1984) channels, and one type of Ca^{2+}-dependent K^+ channel (Schmid-Antomarchi, Hugues, Norman, Ellory, Borsotto, and Lazdunski 1984), naturally occurring toxins have been instrumental in allowing extensive and elegant studies of these important proteins. Similarly, neurotoxins such as α-latrotoxin (Scheer and Meldolesi 1985) α-glycerotoxin (Bon, Saliou, Thieffry, and Manaranche 1985) and β-bungarotoxin (Othman, Spokes and Dolly 1982; Halliwell and Dolly 1982), which affect neurotransmitter release in very selective fashions, are useful for deciphering the steps in this process. Indeed, the unique functional specificities of several such neurotoxin probes (cf. Tauc 1984) ensure that elucidation of their molecular action will reveal physiologically relevant components or novel processes in the nervous system. In this contribution the effectiveness of such a strategy is illustrated by the use of toxins that inhibit (botulinum neurotoxins, BoNT) or facilitate (dendrotoxin, DTX) neurotransmitter release. Our recent studies have shown that BoNT is selectively targetted to cholinergic nerve terminals via acceptors that mediate endocytosis, while the potent convulsant DTX labels nerve membrane proteins associated with certain voltage-dependent

K$^+$-channels, which contribute to the regulation of neuron excitability and transmitter release.

BoNT as a marker for cholinergic neurons and as a tool for studying acceptor-mediated endocytosis at motor nerve terminals

Action of BoNT in the peripheral nervous system: selective inhibition of acetyl choline release

About eight different types (A,B,C,C$_1$,D,E,F, and G) of BoNT are produced by *Clostridium botulinum* (Sugiyama 1980). They are large proteins (m.w. *c*.150 000) that in the fully activated ('nicked') form consist of two disulphide-linked polypeptides (*c*.95 000 and *c*.55 000). Although their gross structures are similar and each causes pseudo-irreversible inhibition of acetyl choline release from peripheral nerves (reviewed by Simpson 1981), there are definite differences between the patterns of neuroparalysis they induce (Sellin, Thesleff, and Das Gupta 1983b; Sellin, Kauffman, and Das Gupta 1983a). For example, when injected in sublethal doses into rat leg, BoNT(B) is markedly less potent than BoNT(A) and gives rise to a smaller reduction in both spontaneous and evoked release of acetyl choline, as measured in the extensor digitorum longus muscle. These effects of BoNT types B and E are shorter-lasting than the changes induced by BoNT(A). Furthermore, 3,4-diaminopyridine is much less effective in reversing the inhibitory actions of BoNT(B) than in reversing BoNT(A) actions both on spontaneous and evoked quantal release of acetyl choline. In the case of preparations intoxicated with BoNT(B), treatment with 3,4-diaminopyridine resulted in asynchronous release after nerve stimulation. This abnormality was also seen on high-frequency stimulation of motor nerves poisoned with BoNT(D) (Harris and Miledi 1971) or tetanus toxin (Dreyer and Schmitt 1981). Despite these subtle differences between the two toxin types, both virtually eradicate nerve-evoked release of acetyl choline (quantal content reduced to <1 per cent of control level) and neither has any effect on a small population of miniature endplate potentials in skeletal muscle (Sellin *et al.* 1983b). In fact, BoNT has facilitated the characterization of these miniatures, which have slow rise-times and a skewed amplitude distribution. They apparently represent a population (Dolly, Lande, and Wray 1985) distinct from those that contribute to endplate potentials (Thesleff 1984). The reported abilities of β-bungarotoxin (Tse, Dolly, Hambleton, Wray, and Melling 1982; Tse, Wray, Melling, and Dolly 1986) or α-dinitrophenol (Sellin *et al.* 1983b) to induce synaptic potentials with normal rise times in BoNT-treated muscle suggest that their extended time to peak is not due to acetyl choline release at sites distant from the active zones (Thesleff 1982).

The transmitter specificity of BoNT in the peripheral nervous system has been examined in only one study, where a single, purified preparation of BoNT(A) was used (MacKenzie, Burnstock, and Dolly 1982). The findings indicated a selectivity for cholinergic (nicotinic or muscarinic) nerve terminals. Co-release of transmitters was invoked to explain the sensitivity to the toxin of non-adrenergic, non-cholinergic, excitatory responses recorded in guinea pig bladder after nerve stimulation. The much-reduced effectiveness of BoNT at non-cholinergic peripheral nerves will be explained below. To summarize the electrophysiological investigations, BoNT-induced inhibition of acetyl choline release seems to arise from a reduction in the Ca^{2+}-sensitivity of the system or from a decrease in the intraterminal Ca^{2+} concentration (Molgo and Thesleff 1984), since all other measurable parameters, including presynaptic Ca^{2+} currents, are unaffected.

BoNT(A) and (B) are targetted to motor nerve terminals via membrane acceptors

To investigate the molecular basis of their action, homogeneous samples of BoNT(A) (Williams, Tse, Dolly, Hambleton, and Melling 1983) and BoNT(B) (Evans, Williams, Shone, Hambleton, Melling, and Dolly 1986) were iodinated to high specific radioactivities with ^{125}I (500–1700 Ci mmol^{-1}) without loss of neurotoxicity under conditions optimized for the chloramine-T method. On electrophoretic analysis of each type of radioiodinated toxin (^{125}I-BoNT), both polypeptide chains were found to be labelled. Phrenic nerve–diaphragm muscle preparations were paralysed either by intraperitoneal injection of mice with ^{125}I-BoNT or after *in vitro* incubation with the toxins. After washing, sections were cut and processed for electron-microscope autoradiography. The discrete patterns of silver grains observed in the resulting autoradiograms after *in vitro* (Fig. 13.1) or *in vivo* intoxication (Black, J. D. and Dolly 1986a) showed selective labelling of nerve terminals with ^{125}I-BoNT(A) (Fig. 13.1(a)) and (B) (Fig. 13.1(c)). From the absence of grains elsewhere (such as in muscle, blood vessels or connective tissue) it was clear that each of these toxins is targetted with remarkable specificity to the unmyelinated regions of nerve terminals. This involves saturable interaction with acceptors on the neuronal membrane because inclusion of an excess of non-radioactive BoNT during the incubation with ^{125}I-BoNT totally prevented the labelling (e.g. Fig. 13.1(b)). At labelled nerve terminals grains were notably seen on the presynaptic membrane and within the cytoplasm. Quantitative analysis (Black, J. D. and Dolly 1986b) of the grain distribution showed that, under standardized conditions, *c.*40 per cent and 25 per cent internalization of radioactivity occurred with ^{125}I-BoNT(A) and (B), respectively (Table 13.1). This difference may arise from the known differences in the extent of 'nicking' in these two toxin preparations and/or distribution of

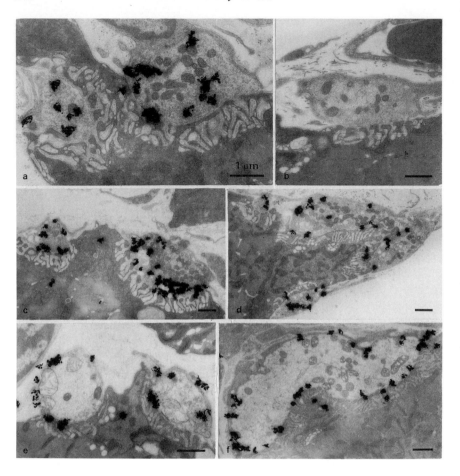

Fig. 13.1 Electron-microscope autoradiographic demonstration of saturable binding and subsequent internalization of radioactivity at motor nerve terminals labelled with ^{125}I-BoNT(A) and (B). Mouse phrenic nerve-diaphragm preparations were paralysed by incubation for 90 min at 22°C in Krebs-Ringer with ^{125}I-BoNT(A) (a, b, e) or (B) (c, d, f). After washing, fixation, and embedding, sections were cut and processed for electron-microscope autoradiography as detailed previously (Dolly *et al.* 1984a and Black and Dolly 1986a). Autoradiograms, after exposure for 3 weeks, were developed and photographed. Samples shown were treated with:

   (a) 15 nM ^{125}I-BoNT(A);
   (b) as (a) but including a 100-fold excess of unlabelled BoNT(A);
   (c) 10 nM ^{125}I-BoNT(B);
   (d) as (c) but pre-incubated (22°C for 1 h) with an excess of unlabelled BoNT(A);
   (e) 1 nM ^{125}I-BoNT(A) after pre-treatment (22°C for 30 min) with 15 nM Na azide;
   (f) 20 nM ^{125}I-BoNT(B) after treatment with 15 nM Na azide as in (e).

Table 13.1 Effects of various conditions on the binding and internalization of ^{125}I-BoNT(A) at murine motor nerve terminals.

Labelling conditions[a]	Relative number of grains per μm of plasma membrane[b] (%)	Distribution of grains with respect to the plasma membrane[c] (% of total)	
		On	Within
^{125}I-BoNT(A)			
In vivo (~1 ng)	—	63	37
In vitro (22°C unless specified)			
Control (10 nM)	100	65	35
+ BoNT large subunit (0.5 μM)	0	—	—
+ Na azide (15 mM)	100	100	0
Control (11 nM)	100	60	40
4°C	30	100	0
Control (10 nM)	100	61	39
+ Nerve stimulation	100	41	59
Control (20 nM)	—	59	41
+ Chloroquine (50 μM)	—	50	50
+ Methylamine (50 μM)	—	73	27
+ Ammonium chloride (6 mM)	—	74	26
10 nM ^{125}I-BoNT(B)	—	75	25
20 nM ^{125}I-BoNT(B) + Na azide (15 mM)	—	100	—
15 nM ^{125}I-BoNT(A)	100	—	—
+ 1.5μM BoNT(B)[d]	106	—	—
10nM ^{125}I-BoNT(B)	100	—	—
+ 1 μM BoNT(A)[d]	76	—	—

[a] Large numbers (20–50) of nerve endings from mouse diaphragm preparations treated with ^{125}I-BoNT *in vivo* (following intraperitoneal injection of the mouse) or *in vitro* (in Krebs-Ringer for 90 min), using the conditions specified, were processed for electron-microscope autoradiography as detailed elsewhere (Dolly *et al.* 1984a; Black and Dolly, 1986a) and photographed. When Na azide was included, the samples were pre-incubated for 30 min prior to additon of BoNT.

[b] Using electron-microscope autoradiograms, the total number of grains (0–200) observed on the nerve terminal membrane and enclosed within it were counted in a minimum of 30 endplates from each sample. The total length of terminal plasma membrane was measured by digitization; the number of grains per unit length, calculated for each treated sample, was expressed relative to the control (^{125}I-BoNT alone) value for that particular experiment.

[c] Silver grains on the nerve membrane and inside the synaptic bouton were counted in at least 30 endplates from each sample; these numbers were then expressed as a percentage of the total. Grains were considered to be 'on the membrane' if located within 60–70 nm of the plasma membrane.

[d] Preincubated for 1 h prior to addition of the labelled toxin.

label in their chains (Evans *et al.* 1986). The presence of some grains was also noticeable within myelinated axons after labelling *in vivo* or *in vitro*, suggesting that retrograde intra-axonal transport had taken place.

Distinct neuronal acceptors for BoNT(A) and (B): ultrastructural location and densities on the presynaptic membrane

In view of the noted similarities and differences between the structures and detailed pharmacological actions of BoNT(A) and (B), it is interesting that they bind to distinct acceptors in the peripheral and central nervous systems (see below). Addition of a large excess of unlabelled BoNT(A) caused a minimal reduction (*c.* 24 per cent) in the extent of labelling with ^{125}I-BoNT(B), as deduced from the relative number of grains observed per unit area of nerve terminal plasma membrane (Fig. 13.1(c,d)). An interaction was not detectable in the reverse experiment (Table 13.1). Treatment of the diaphragm preparation with azide abolished the internalization of radio-activity (Dolly, Black, Williams, and Melling 1984a) and resulted in a halo of grains around the plasma membrane of the nerve terminals (Fig. 13.1(e,f)). Such a dramatic inhibition of toxin uptake demonstrates directly that acceptor binding of BoNT(A) or (B) and their internalization are distinct but sequential steps.

In the presence of azide, construction of grain density histograms showed that the acceptors for both toxins reside on the presynaptic membrane (Black and Dolly 1986a), a result consistent with the lack of a direct postsynaptic action of BoNT. Moreover, when internalization was blocked, it became apparent that the location of neither acceptor type was restricted to the active zones, the regions from which transmitter release is thought to occur. Rather, the acceptors are located all around the unmyelinated areas of the nerve membrane, up to but not beyond the first node of Ranvier. Apparently, BoNT is a marker for the presynaptic membrane even in newborn rats, where myelination is incomplete (Black, J. D. and Dolly 1986a). In the presence of azide, conditions for saturable labelling of the acceptors in mouse diaphragm were established [15 and 20 nM of BoNT(A) and (B), respectively 90 min at 22°C]. When quantitative autoradiographic techniques (Fertuck and Salpeter 1976) were used, the densities of acceptors for BoNT(A) and (B) on the nerve terminals were calculated to be 152 ± 31 and 631 ± 132 per μm^2 of plasma membrane, respectively. In view of their ultrastructural location and because each of the two toxins tested apparently binds to separate sites, it is unlikely that these acceptors are directly concerned with transmitter release. They apparently serve to target the toxin to cholinergic nerves (see below).

Acceptor-mediated endocytosis: an essential step for the potent action of BoNT

The saturable binding of BoNT to ecto-acceptors, as demonstrated auto-radiographically on the presynaptic membrane, seems to be a necessary part of the intoxication process for several reasons. Thus, the acceptors reside only at cholinergic (see below) nerve terminals, where the neurotoxin acts selectively and BoNT binding is detectable under conditions of incubation time, temperature and concentration under which neuromuscular paralysis was shown to occur. In addition, extensive pharmacological investigation of the neuromuscular junction has provided indirect evidence that binding is the first of several steps in the action of BoNT in producing neuromuscular paralysis (Simpson 1980). Most importantly, the acceptors identified by means of ^{125}I-BoNT appear to be responsible for the binding recognized by electrophysiological means because the separated larger chain of the toxin antagonized the binding of the native BoNT(A) to its acceptors (L. L. Simpson and B. R. Das Gupta, unpublished). Although the heavier poly-peptide of BoNT(A) is relatively non-toxic after isolation and renaturation (Williams *et al.* 1983), it was capable of preventing ^{125}I-BoNT(A) acceptor interaction at the nerve terminals (Table 13.1). In addition to reaffirming the saturability of the binding step, the latter observation established con-clusively that the internalization is acceptor-mediated.

To investigate further the nature of the internalization process, the effects of various conditions on the distribution of silver grains in relation to the plasma membrane were quantified (Table 13.1), after labelling pieces of mouse diaphragm with ^{125}I-BoNT(A). As noted above, the uptake of radio-activity was energy-dependent. Addition to the incubation medium of inhibitors of energy production such as azide (Fig. 13.1(e,f)) or din-itrophenol (Black, J. D. and Dolly 1986b) abolished internalization with-out affecting acceptor occupancy (Table 13.1). The uptake step is also temperature-sensitive because lowering the temperature from 22°C to 4°C during incubation of the tissue with ^{125}I-BoNT(A), brought about apprecia-ble labelling but grains were not detectable intra-terminally (Table 13.1). A significant increase (*c.* 50 per cent) in the extent of internalization was induced by nerve stimulation, a condition known to accelerate endocytosis (Ceccarelli, Hurlbut, and Mauro 1973). Similarly, lysosomotropic agents altered the distribution of radioactivity (Table 13.1) in ways consistent with the uptake being endocytotic (Black, J. D. and Dolly 1986b). For example, the proportion of grains on or close to the plasma membrane was increased by short-chain amines (methylamine or ammonium chloride), at con-centrations shown in other studies (Maxfield, Willingham, Davies, and Pastan 1979) to retard endocytotic uptake and/or facilitate recycling. On the other hand, treatment of the diaphragm with chloroquine gave a small increase in the fraction of intra-terminal radioactivity (Table 13.1), in accordance with its ability to raise the pH of acidic intracellular compartments (Middlebrook and Dorland 1981) and to perturb the transport and lysosomal processing of proteins. Collectively, the available experimental data implicate *acceptor-mediated endocytosis*. This deduction is further supported by the demonstrated presence, in nerve terminals labelled with ^{125}I-BoNT, of all the component parts of the endocytosis pathway including coated pits, coated vesicles, endosomes and lysosomes, and the frequent association of silver grains with endocytotic compartments (Black, J. D. and Dolly 1986b).

An important question is whether this demonstrated endocytotic uptake of BoNT (or fragment thereof) into nerves is a prerequisite for inhibition of transmitter release. Again, pharmacological measurements of the kinetics of BoNT-induced neuromuscular paralysis, and of the influence of temperature or anti-BoNT antibodies, had implicated such an internalization step after the initial binding phase (Simpson 1980, 1981). The remarkably good correlation between the results of these electrophysiological experiments and the autoradiographic findings greatly strengthen the evidence that acceptor-mediated endocytosis is an essential step of botulinization. For instance, nerve stimulation which hastens BoNT-induced blockade of neuromuscular transmission increases the degree of internalization whilst the lysosomotropic agents found to delay the neuroparalytic action of BoNT alter the uptake phase in directions compatible (Black, J. D. and Dolly 1986b) with the neurophysiological observations. Thus, it can be concluded that inactivation of an intra-neuronal component directly or indirectly concerned with transmitter release results from exposure to BoNT. However, the nature of this target remains unknown, as does the postulated enzymic amplification system (Simpson 1981) that may underly its unique potency.

Basis of the BoNT-sensitivity of peripheral cholinergic nerves

Final proof for the importance of this multi-step scheme of botulinization was sought by demonstrating its operation in nerves vulnerable to BoNT. When sections of ileum were labelled with ^{125}I-BoNT(A) and examined autoradiographically, grains were associated with cholinergic terminals (Fig. 13.2), recognizable by the presence of agranular vesicles 45–50 nm in diameter (Burnstock 1982). Internalization of radioactivity observed in these nerves accords with the ability of BoNT to inhibit acetyl choline release from muscarinic nerves in guinea pig ileum (MacKenzie *et al.* 1982). In contrast, nerves in the ileum preparation (Fig. 13.2) that are much less sensitive or insensitive to BoNT, e.g. peptidergic and purinergic nerves, identified by their characteristic vesicles, or adrenergic varicosities in mouse *vas deferens* (Dolly *et al.* 1984a) could not be labelled specifically with ^{125}I-BoNT(A). Based on the results at present available from the peripheral

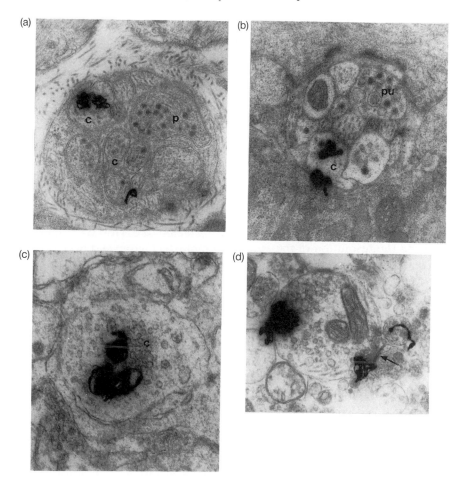

Fig. 13.2 Electron-microscope autoradiograms of ileum and synaptosome preparations after labelling with ^{125}I-BoNT(A). Pieces of mouse ileum (a–c) or rat cerebrocortical synaptosomes (d) were incubated with ^{125}I-BoNT(A), 20 nM (90 min, at 22°C) or 10 nM (40 min, at 37°C) respectively, as described in Fig. 13.1. C, P and Pu represent putative cholinergic, peptidergic and purinergic endings, respectively.

tissues examined, BoNT(A) acceptors seem to be characteristic of nerves innervating both nicotinic and muscarinic junctions. Interestingly, the inability to detect these acceptors on the cholinergic terminals of eel electroplax is consistent with their apparent insensitivity to BoNT. This observation highlights some species differences between presynaptic membranes (Black 1985).

In the rat forebrain a widespread distribution of BoNT(A) acceptors, detected by light- and electron-microscope autoradiography (Black 1985), can be correlated with the occurrence of cholinergic terminals. However, owing to uncertainty about the identity of transmitters in other brain areas, the usefulness of BoNT as a central cholinergic marker has yet to be ascertained. It is also notable that BoNT(A) does not display detectable central toxicity when injected intraventricularly into rat brain (Williams *et al.* 1983). Nevertheless, as in the periphery, distinct populations of high and low affinity acceptors for ^{125}I-BoNT(A) (Williams *et al.* 1983) and (B) (Evans *et al.* 1986) have been characterized biochemically on cerebrocortical synaptosomal membranes. At least in the case of BoNT(A), the larger subunit is responsible for the binding, as is also found for motor nerves (see above). Ultrastructural studies on rat brain slices and cerebral cortex synaptosomes (Fig. 13.2 (d)) labelled with ^{125}I-BoNT(A) demonstrated binding to acceptors, apparently located on the plasma membrane. However, notwithstanding the resolution of the autoradiography technique and peculiarities of the uptake systems in this tissue, internalization of radioactivity seemed much less than that seen with motor nerves. Thus it can be hypothesized that effective botulinization requires acceptors for targetting the toxin and, in addition, an ability to mediate the endocytotic uptake required for intraneuronal action of the active component. Exposure to high toxin concentrations for extended periods could lead to inefficient uptake by nonspecific routes. This could account for the reported inhibition of transmitter release other than acetyl choline from peripheral nerves or synaptosomes. These findings highlight the possible existence of BoNT-sensitive component(s) common to several, if not all, synapse types.

In summary, BoNT and its larger peptide chain are facilitating characterization of membrane acceptors which appear to be unique to cholinergic nerve terminals and thus undoubtedly serve an important but, as yet, unidentified role. These probes also offer a means for the study of an endocytotic process that is likely to be of functional significance. In particular, non-toxic fragments that interact with the acceptors and can become internalized could prove to be valuable agents for targetting drugs to cholinergic nerves, while neurotoxic fragments are making possible studies on the mechanism of transmitter release.

Molecular basis for the facilitatory action of dendrotoxin in the nervous system

Dendrotoxin — a convulsant protein with neurochemical applications

Dendrotoxin (DTX) purified from the venom of the Eastern green mamba (*Dendroaspis angusticeps*) and its congeners found in other *Dendroaspis* species are small proteins (*c.*60 amino acids) homologous to Kunitz-type trypsin inhibitors (Joubert and Taaljaard 1980; Harvey and Karlsson 1982). They are also structurally related to the smaller B-chain of β-bungarotoxin (β-BuTX) (Kondo, Toda, Narita, and Lee 1982), a presynaptically active protein from the venom of *Bungarus multicinctus* that exhibits phospholipase A_2 activity. Relative to all the phospholipase A_2 containing neurotoxins that affect transmitter release (cf. Tauc 1984), DTX offers many attractions as a neurochemical tool:

(a) it is a single-chain, stable polypeptide devoid of known enzymic activity (Harvey and Gage 1981);

(b) it is a potent convulsant, with a minimal lethal dose in rat brain of 2.5 ng g^{-1} body weight, that facilitates transmitter release at peripheral synapses (Harvey and Karlsson 1980, 1982; Harvey, Anderson, and Karlsson 1984) and central synapses (Dolly, Halliwell, Black, Williams, Pelchen-Matthews, Breeze, Mehraban, Othman, and Black 1984b);

(c) it is an antagonist of the inhibitory action of β-BuTX at chick neuromuscular junction (Harvey and Karlsson 1982) and a powerful inhibitor of its binding to brain synaptosomal acceptors (Othman 1983);

(d) it is one of a series of sequenced homologues that exhibit different levels of facilitatory activity (Harvey and Karlsson 1982) and central toxicity (Black, Breeze, Othman, and Dolly 1986); and

(e) it is unaffected by radioiodination to high specific radioactivity (Dolly *et al.* 1984b; Black *et al.* 1986).

Electrophysiological analysis of the central action of DTX

This was studied electrophysiologically in hippocampal slices of rat and guinea pig (Skrede and Westgaard 1971). Details of the experimental procedures used for extra- and intracellular recording of the responses of this slice preparation to DTX have been detailed (Halliwell and Adams 1982; Halliwell and Dolly 1982); voltage- and current-clamp measurements were made, with a single microelectrode, normally in the presence of tetrodotoxin.

Effects of DTX on synaptic transmission in the hippocampal slice

The normal response to stimulation of fibre afferents in stratum radiatum of the CA_1 region of the hippocampal slice includes a short-latency, triphasic compound action potential volley (CAP). This is followed by a slower negative wave (Fig. 13.3A), sometimes interrupted by positive-going notches (Fig. 13.3B), when the activity is recorded at the level of the synaptic input to the dendrites of the pyramidal cells. The negative wave reflects the summed synaptic currents in the CA_1 neurons and the superimposed notches correspond to synchronous neuronal firing (population spikes) initiated by the synaptic input (Andersen, Bliss, and Skrede 1971). When responses from CA_1 neurons are recorded intracellularly, stimulation

J. O. *Dolly* et al.

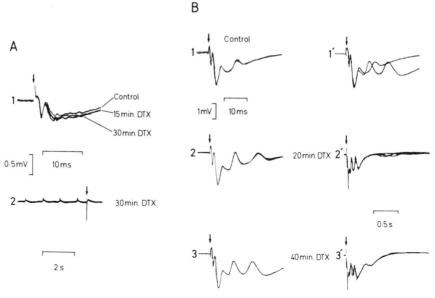

Fig. 13.3 Enhancement of synaptic transmission by DTX in the hippocampus. A₁
shows superimposed field potentials recorded in *stratum radiatum* of a rat hippocampus slice to a submaximal 50 μA, 50 μs electrical stimulus (arrowed) to the same
dendritic levels about 1 mm away. The times of recording are before (control) and 15
and 30 min (indicated) after exposure of the slice to 250 nM DTX. A₂ is a slower
single sweep showing the presence of spontaneous synaptic activity that occurs
independently of the stimulus delivery. B₁₋₃ depict supramaximal (150 μA, 50 μs)
stimulus-evoked field potentials in another rat hippocampal slice recorded as in A
before (1), 20 min after (2) and 40 min after (3) DTX (250 nM) administration. B₁'
shows the control and 40 min record superimposed for comparison and B₂'₋₃' show
the 20 min and 40 min record at slower sweeps, respectively. Note the prolongation
of the synaptic response and enhanced population spiking (see text) following
exposure to DTX.

evokes a sequence of excitatory and inhibitory postsynaptic potentials,
temporarily correlated with the extracellular wave forms. Dolly *et al.*
(1984b) have described the complex behaviour that DTX induces in the
hippocampal slice preparation. In about 50 per cent of tests fluctuations in
the efficacy of synaptic transmission were observed and at other times only
facilitation occurred (see Fig. 13.3). The CAP was not affected by exposure
to DTX but the negative synaptic wave was usually enhanced in amplitude
(Fig. 13.3A), and duration (Fig. 13.3B), with a corresponding increase in
the amplitude and number of population spikes (Fig. 13.3B). Frequently,
prolongation of the synaptic waves resulted from the development of
regenerative synaptic activity lasting for up to 1 s, where previously synaptic

responses of 20 ms duration were seen (Fig. 13.3B). Totally spontaneous extracellular waves of either polarity were also observed in stratum radiatum (Fig. 13.3A$_2$). These findings are consistent with the generation of spontaneous activity in populations of hippocampal neurones, which reactivate by way of intrinsic fibre pathways maintained in the slice.

Intracellular observations of DTX action

Concomitant behaviour, indicative of population responses, was observed by means of intracellular recordings from microelectrodes filled with potassium acetate. After 15–30 min in 250 nM DTX, cells displayed spontaneous, long-lasting hyperpolarizations (up to 500 ms) that did not depend on action potentials in the impaled neurone. Polarizing the cell with negative current reduced the hyperpolarization and revealed a clear depolarizing component preceding the hyperpolarizing phase of the response. When the cell membrane potential was close to threshold, the rhythmic spontaneous activity elicited cell firing, which indicated the presence of an excitatory influence. The hyperpolarizations were identified as inhibitory post synaptic potentials (ipsps) by their reversal potential ($c. -80$ mV) and their sensitivity to picrotoxin and bicuculline, properties shared by the stimulus-evoked ipsp. Also present, with identical characteristics, were higher frequency hyperpolarizing events that increased the level of membrane noise. Moreover, DTX induced an increase in depolarizing membrane noise when KCl-filled electrodes were used (Fig. 13.4). This, also, was sensitive to

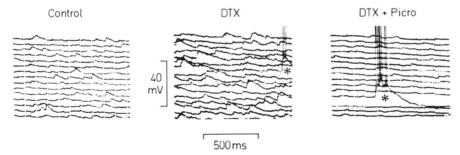

Fig. 13.4 DTX potentiates spontaneous synaptic events in hippocampal pyramidal cells. The figure shows a display of membrane potentials (average resting value in each panel -67 mV) recorded from a guinea pig CA$_1$ neurone impaled with a microelectrode containing 3 M KCl. The left-hand panel shows control spontaneous activity; the middle panel depicts the activity after 30 min in 290 nM DTX; the right-hand panel shows spontaneous potentials 15 min after 10 μM pictrotoxin (picro) has been added to the DTX-containing bathing medium. Note the increased synaptic activity induced by DTX which is mostly blocked by picrotoxin and also the burst responses (*) which are potentiated by picrotoxin. The action potentials are clipped because they are off-scale at the oscilloscope amplifier gain employed.

picrotoxin (Fig. 13.4) or bicuculline. The sensitivity of these spontaneous potentials to GABA antagonists reinforces the idea that they represent chloride-dependent ipsps inverted in polarity because of chloride-loading from the KCl-filled recording electrode (Alger and Nicoll 1980). Spontaneous burst responses were also generated in the presence of DTX (Dolly et al. 1984b). They occurred with the same frequency as the spontaneous extracellularly recorded waves and the sequence of excitatory and inhibitory post synaptic potentials observed with potassium acetate electrodes. These DTX-induced bursts were potentiated by GABA antagonists. Taken together, our findings show that synaptic transmission and cell excitability in hippocampal slices are enhanced by exposure to DTX. Such changes do not result from depression of inhibitory transmission by the toxin. Rather, the level of inhibitory activity is potentiated by the action of DTX, as indicated by the enhanced spontaneous, picrotoxin-sensitive potentials. This is presumed to originate from increased excitatory input to inhibitory neurons or potentiated output of an inhibitory transmitter, most probably GABA.

To determine whether DTX directly affects the membrane of pyramidal cells, synaptic transmission was suppressed by the addition of tetrodotoxin (TTX), to block Na^+ conductances and inhibit impulse transfer between neurons, or cadmium to block Ca^{2+}-channels. Both treatments prevented the spontaneous activity and bursting behaviour seen intracellularly when applied *before* DTX exposure and terminated the toxin-induced changes when applied *after* DTX (Dolly et al. 1984b). However, in the presence of TTX, the toxin at low doses (10–50 nM) enhanced the ability of hippocampal neurons to fire Ca^{2+} spikes (Halliwell, Othman, Pelchen-Matthews, and Dolly 1986) without other obvious changes of membrane properties (Fig. 13.5(a)), such as resting potential or input resistance. Ca^{2+}-spikes were increased in number and triggered at lower intracellular current strengths after exposure to DTX for 30–60 min. Larger doses of the toxin, up to 300 nM, sometimes produced an apparent increase in input resistance and a depolarization of up to 10–20 mV; such effects could be partially reversed with cadmium.

A selective inhibition of the A-current by DTX

Voltage-clamp of hippocampal pyramidal neurones was performed in TTX medium; Ca^{2+}-currents were recorded with electrodes containing 3 M CsC1 instead of K^+-containing solutions, to block outward currents (Tillotson 1979; Johnston, Hablitz, and Wilson 1980; Halliwell 1983). DTX did not potentiate either the sustained (Brown and Griffith 1983b) or the transient (Halliwell 1983) Ca^{2+} currents present in these neurones (Halliwell et al. 1986). Consequently, the threshold changes in Ca^{2+} spike activity induced by DTX are due to a membrane action of the toxin other than a direct effect on the Ca^{2+}-channels. Other ionic conductances present in hippocampal

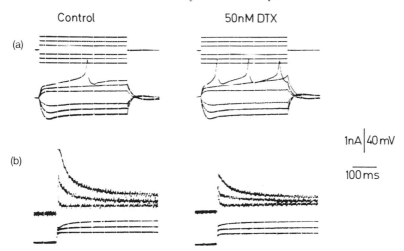

Fig. 13.5 Enhancement of Ca-spiking and suppression of I_A by DTX in hippocampal neurones. (a) potential responses recorded in a guinea pig hippocampal CA_1 neurone (lower traces) in response to depolarizing and hyperpolarizing current injection (upper traces) for 375 ms. The slice was bathed throughout in medium containing 0.5 μM TTX. The left-hand side shows records made before, and the right hand side shows records after exposing the slice to 50 nM DTX for 1 h. Resting potential in each panel was −75 mV. (b) Currents (upper traces) driven by depolarizing steps (lower traces) from −75 mV before (left) and 1 h after 50 nM DTX (right) and recorded in the same cell as in (a) under voltage clamp. I_A is the transient outward current that is activated from this negative potential by stepping to more positive potentials, at which the conductance fully inactivates (left-hand panel). Note the substantial suppression of this current by DTX.

neurones not materially affected by DTX include: Ca^{2+}-activated K^+ conductances (Brown and Griffith 1983a; Adams and Lancaster 1985), non-inactivating voltage-dependent K^+ conductance (I_M) or inward rectifier (I_Q) (Halliwell and Adams 1982). After exposure to 50 nM DTX for 1 h, the only detectable effect on an identified membrane current was a selective depression of the early transient outward current, I_A (Fig. 13.5(b)). This is an inactivating K^+ current, first described in hippocampal neurons by Gustaffson, Galvan, Grafe, and Wigstrom (1982), which is also reversibly blocked by 4-aminopyridine. Originally, it was thought that the effect of DTX on I_A was irreversible at 300 nM (Dolly *et al.* 1984b) but further experiments over longer periods and with lower doses have shown partial recovery of I_A after extensive washing (Halliwell *et al.* 1986). The slowness of the DTX-induced blockade of I_A (see above), the protracted reversibility and the apparent disparity in the minimum effective dose and the acceptor K_D have been ascribed to the high content of binding sites in the hippocampal slice (Halliwell *et al.* 1986). This leads to a reduction in the effective toxin concentration at the recording locus, which is often 200–300 μm deep. To confirm that DTX acted directly on the membrane of the impaled cell and not by direct facilitation of TTX-resistant transmitter release, further experiments established that the I_A was measurable in cadmium-containing medium and still sensitive to the toxin, even when Ca^{2+} influx into synaptic terminals was blocked in this manner (Halliwell *et al.* 1986).

Blockade of I_A by DTX probably accounts for the similarity of its action in the hippocampus to that of 4-aminopyridine (Buckle and Haas 1982). Both agents suppress I_A, which normally exerts a braking effect on cell firing (see for example Segal, Rogawski, and Barker 1984); hence, the increased cell excitability induced by DTX can be attributed to this mechanism and accounts for the effects of the toxin observed at the single cell level. Enhanced cell excitability would contribute to the convulsant effects induced by DTX. The presence of I_A or a similar conductance in terminal axonal regions that is sensitive to DTX could explain the enhanced synaptic transmission described above, an effect similar to that observed at the neuromuscular junction (Harvey and Karlsson 1982). Recently, it has been shown that at very low concentrations (1–10 nM) DTX selectively attenuates a K^+-conductance in mammalian peripheral sensory neurones and frog node of Ranvier that resembles I_A more than the delayed rectifier (Stansfeld, Marsh, Halliwell, and Brown 1986; Weller, Bernhardt, Siemen, Dreyer, Vogel, and Habermann 1985). These peripheral nerve preparations may be an appropriate model for the inaccessible terminal region and, thus, may offer an insight into the action of DTX on axons and terminals in the central nervous system. It appears that the central action of DTX is more specific than that of 4-aminopyridine. Unlike the latter (Galvan, Franz, and Vogel-Wiens 1984; Haas, Wieser, and Yasargil 1983), the toxin does not prolong the CAP volley recorded extracellularly (Fig. 13.3). On the basis of these findings it is suggested that DTX is a useful and novel biochemical probe for investigating voltage-sensitive K^+ channels responsible for I_A and certain variants of this important K^+ conductance.

Specific acceptors for DTX in neuronal membranes

Acceptors for DTX have been identified in rat brain synaptic membranes with a radioiodinated derivative (^{125}I-DTX) (Dolly *et al.* 1984b; Black *et al.* 1986). These acceptors, which are enriched in the plasma membrane fraction, are kinetically homogeneous with respect to toxin binding ($K_D = 0.3$ nM; $B_{max} = 1$–1.5 pmol mg^{-1} protein) and were recognised as proteins because of their sensitivity to proteolytic agents (Black *et al.* 1986). As observed in electrophysiological studies on chick motor nerve terminals (Harvey and Karlsson 1982), binding to these acceptors was specific for DTX and its neurotoxic homologues (see below). For example, binding was unaffected by apamin or by phospholipase A_2-containing neurotoxins in

Ca^{2+}-free medium to minimize their enzyme activity. In view of the efficacy of DTX in inhibiting the high-affinity binding of β-BuTX to rat brain synaptosomes ($K_I = 0.5$ nM), it was surprising that the potency of β-BuTX to displace ^{125}I-DTX was low ($K_I > 1$ μM as opposed to a K_D of 0.5 nM for ^{3}H-β-BuTX). However, it proved possible to elucidate the nature of the interaction between these two toxins by studying their acceptors in chick synaptic membranes.

Two classes of DTX acceptors in chick brain

Figure 13.6(a) shows the binding of ^{125}I-DTX to synaptic membranes prepared from 1-day-old chick brain. The saturable binding isotherm appears to be extended, suggesting the presence of multiple sites. A Scatchard plot of this binding (Fig. 13.6(b)) was curved upwards and could be interpreted as providing evidence for two sites, one of higher affinity (K_D ~0.5 nM; B_{max} ~90 fmol mg^{-1} protein) and another of lower affinity but higher content. The latter appeared to have a K_D of ~15 nM and a B_{max} of ~400 fmol mg^{-1} protein, although it should be noted that the parameters for these low affinity sites were poorly defined by the toxin concentrations used. This two-site model was confirmed by kinetic studies detailed elsewhere (Black, A. R. and Dolly 1986). Also consistent with the presence of multiple sites were the extended inhibition curves for DTX and its neuroactive homologues. The ratio of the concentrations of the homologues that produced 90 per cent and 10 per cent inhibition of saturable ^{125}I-DTX binding was between 155 and 165, whereas the theoretical value for interaction at a single set of sites is 81. Since these ratios were essentially identical for the three toxins tested, their relative affinities at the two sites appear to be the same (Black, A. R. and Dolly 1986). It is interesting that the rank order of affinities of these homologues for the acceptors in chick synaptic membranes is very similar to that observed with rat brain (Table 13.2), which indicates that the acceptors in these two species are related. It is also of interest that the saturable binding of ^{125}I-DTX to chick membranes could be inhibited by equimolar amounts of β-BuTX, but in contrast to that seen with active DTX homologues, this inhibition was only partial (Fig. 13.7(a)).

The antagonism is due to interaction at the set of DTX acceptors of higher affinity because the proportion of binding inhibitable by β-BuTX decreased with increasing ^{125}I-DTX concentrations. When binding (B) was taken as that prevented by 1 μM β-BuTX, a plot of B against β-BuTX concentration (Dixon plot) for the three ^{125}I-DTX concentrations used produced straight lines which intersected in the fourth quadrant (Fig. 13.7(b)). These equilibrium measurements and other kinetic analyses (Black, A. R. and Dolly 1986) show that β-BuTX competitively inhibits ^{125}I-DTX binding to a single set of acceptors. The Dixon plot gave a K_I value of 0.8 nM for β-BuTX and a B_{max} of 90 fmol mg^{-1} protein for the acceptors β-BuTX shares with DTX.

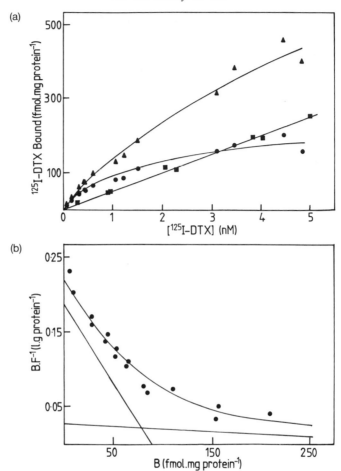

Fig. 13.6 Saturable binding of ^{125}I-DTX to chick synaptic membranes.

(a) Chick synaptic membranes (200–400 μg) were incubated in the presence of various concentrations of ^{125}I-DTX in 250 μl of assay buffer containing 2 mM CaCl$_2$. After 30 min at 23°C, bound (B) and free (F) ^{125}I-DTX were separated by rapid centrifugation through oil and quantified by γ-counting. Non-specific binding (■) was determined similarly in the presence of 400 nM DTX and was subtracted from the total binding (▲) to give the specific binding (●).

(b) The specific binding data from (a) presented on a Scatchard plot: the lines shown are derived from graphical analysis based on the presence of two independent sites.

The K_I, together with the IC$_{50}$ value for the partial inhibition, gives a K_D of 0.5 ± 0.1 nM for ^{125}I-DTX. These results show that β-BuTX binds to the higher-affinity set of DTX acceptors identified by Scatchard analysis. Moreover, the affinity and extent of β-BuTX binding agree closely with those of acceptors identified in chick membranes with ^{125}I-β-BuTX [K_D ~0.5 nM;

Table 13.2 Central neurotoxicities and membrane acceptor affinities for DTX and congeners.

	Minimum lethal dose (ng g^{-1} body wt)[a]	Rat brain acceptor K_I (nM)	Chick brain acceptors IC$_{50}$ (nM)[b]
Toxin I	0.5	0.05	0.4
DTX	2.5	0.4	3.8
Dv-14	2.5	0.4	—
Toxin B	>150	>2000	>1000

[a] Determined by intraventricular injection into rat brain.
[b] Concentrations required to inhibit 50 per cent of the specific binding of 2 nM ^{125}I-DTX to synaptic membranes.

B_{max} ~50 fmol mg^{-1} protein] (Rehm and Betz 1982). Since the latter binding can be inhibited by DTX (K_I ~0.5 nM, calculated from data in Rehm and Betz 1984), it is apparently attributable to the high-affinity acceptors described here. The potent inhibition of β-BuTX binding in rat brain by DTX suggests that a similar situation exists in rat brain as in chick brain. Failure to detect inhibition of ^{125}I-DTX binding by low β-BuTX concentrations presumably arises from the large discrepancy between the content of the two acceptor types in rat brain (B_{max} for ^{3}H-β-BuTX = 100–150 fmol mg $^{-1}$ protein; Othman *et al.* 1982), and their nearly identical affinities for the toxin (K_I for DTX = 0.4 nM and 0.5 nM when measured with ^{125}I-DTX and ^{3}H-β-BuTX, respectively) (Black *et al.* 1986; Othman 1983). However, the existence of these two sites has recently been demonstrated in solubilized extracts of rat brain membranes (Mehraban, Black, Breeze, Green, and Dolly 1985) where a proportion of ^{125}I-DTX binding could be inhibited by equimolar amounts of DTX (Black, A. R. and Dolly unpublished). In summary, there are two subtypes of DTX acceptors which can be distinguished by β-BuTX.

Structural studies on DTX acceptors

Polypeptide components of DTX acceptors have been identified by affinity labelling studies. After cross-linking of ^{125}I-DTX to membranes with *bis*-imido esters, the membrane extracts were subjected to electrophoresis and autoradiography. Electrophoresis of chick brain samples on linear SDS-polyacrylamide gels demonstrated two polypeptides with apparent m.w. of 75 000 and 69 000 (Black, A. R. and Dolly 1986). Although cross-linking to both of these polypeptides was totally inhibited by prelabelling in the presence of DTX, excess β-BuTX could only *partially* inhibit their labelling. Thus, both polypeptides must be constituents of the two acceptor classes

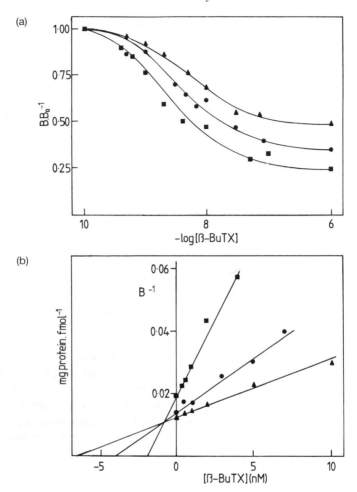

Fig. 13.7 Inhibition of the saturable binding of ^{125}I-DTX to chick synaptic membranes by β-BuTX.

(a) Chick synaptic membranes (200–400 μg protein in 250 μl) were incubated for 30 min with either 0.5 nM (■), 2 nM (●) or 3.5 nM (▲) ^{125}I-DTX in assay buffer containing $CaCl_2$ and various concentrations of β-BuTX. The specific binding shown (averages of duplicates; error is 7 per cent <), the difference between the binding seen in the presence and absence of a 100-fold excess of DTX; these were quantified as described in Fig. 13.6. Binding in the presence of β-BuTX (B) is expressed relative to the total values observed ($B_0 = 69$, 110, and 155 fmol mg^{-1} protein for 0.5, 2.0, and 3.5 nM ^{125}I-DTX, respectively).

(b) Dixon plot of the partial inhibition seen in (a), where the total binding was taken to be that inhibitable by 1 μM β-BuTX (51, 71, and 82 fmol mg^{-1} protein with 0.5, 2.0, and 3.5 nM ^{125}I-DTX, respectively).

which have some structural resemblances. The polypeptide (m.w. = 95 000) identified with ^{125}I-BuTX (Rehm and Betz 1983) would appear to be a further component of the high-affinity DTX acceptor. Cross-linking of the acceptors in rat brain also revealed two polypeptides. However, these could only be partially resolved on gradient gels (Black 1986) and appeared as a single band on linear gels with an apparent m.w. of 65 000 (Mehraban, Breeze, and Dolly 1984). This again suggests that, although some species differences are evident, the acceptors in the two species have structural similarities.

Solubilization of DTX acceptors, in an active form, from rat brain with Triton X-100 (Mehraban *et al.* 1985) has led to an estimate of their molecular weight by a combination of sucrose density-gradient centrifugation and gel filtration. This gave a m.w. value of 390 000–450 000 for the DTX acceptor (Black A. R. and Dolly, unpublished), showing that it is a large oligomeric protein. Its size is somewhat greater than that of 250 000 obtained in the membrane by radiation inactivation (Black 1986). Purification of the solubilized acceptors is in progress and should lead to a further elucidation of their structures.

Physiological relevance of the identified DTX acceptors

Binding of ^{125}I-DTX is localized in discrete areas of rat brain as shown by light-microscope autoradiography (Dolly *et al.* 1984b; Halliwell *et al.* 1986) and this is consistent with the physiological relevance of acceptors for ^{125}I-DTX. Labelling was most prominent in synapse-rich areas, while significant levels were also found in cell body layers (e.g. in hippocampus) and white matter areas (Halliwell *et al.* 1986). Moreover, a similar study in chick brain showed a localized distribution of the acceptors. Binding of ^{125}I-DTX was widespread in forebrain, optic lobe, and brainstem, while the most striking labelling pattern was observed in cerebellum, where the synapse-rich molecular layer showed intense DTX binding. Recently, DTX acceptors have been localized by means of electron-microscope autoradiography of slices of chick cerebellum labelled with ^{125}I-DTX. Preliminary analysis of the silver grains observed indicates the presence of acceptors on the cell soma membrane (Fig. 13.8(a)). This is consistent with the demonstrated action of DTX on the I_A there (see above), and on synapses (Fig. 13.8(b)) where the toxin is known to facilitate neurotransmitter release (Docherty, Dolly, Halliwell, and Othman 1983; Dolly *et al.* 1984b; see above). However, the greater part of DTX-binding was seen on the unmyelinated axons of granule cells (Fig. 13.8(c)). Some was also visible on the myelinated fibres deep in the cerebellum and this is consistent with the recently observed action of DTX on a K^+-current at the node of Ranvier (Weller *et al.* 1985).

Further evidence that the acceptors identified using ^{125}I-DTX are responsible for the physiological actions of the toxin came from structure–activity

(a)
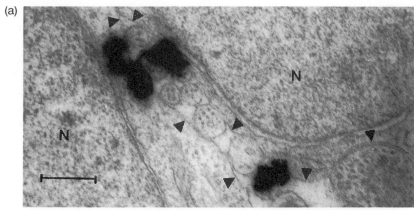

(b)
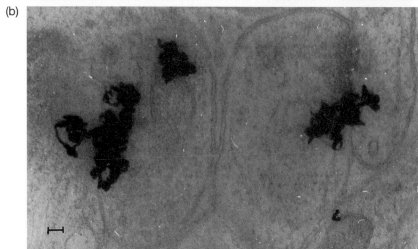

(c)
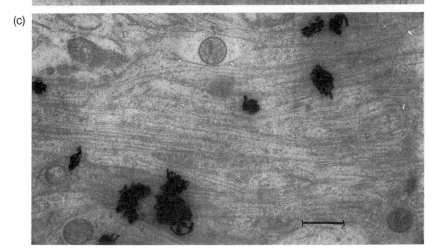

studies. These showed that the central toxicities of DTX homologues in rat brain (Black *et al.* 1986) correlate with their abilities to inhibit ^{125}I-DTX binding in both rat and chick brain (Black, A. R. and Dolly 1986) (Table 13.2). It is consistent with this that toxin I was found to be more potent than DTX in blocking I_A in hippocampal slices (Halliwell *et al.* 1986). Moreover, this correlation might be applicable to both classes of DTX acceptor in chick brain, since the ratio of the affinities of each DTX congener at the two sites is very similar (see above). Although in rat brain ^{125}I-DTX binding occurs predominantly at the acceptor class which binds only the facilitatory mamba toxins with high affinity, toxin I is more effective than DTX in antagonizing ^{3}H-β-BuTX binding to its acceptor (i.e. shared sites) in synaptosomes (Othman 1983). Hence, based on the affinities of these two toxins, the structure–activity relationship may also extend to both acceptor classes in rat brain.

Additional support for the physiological relevance of the two acceptor subtypes is provided by pharmacological studies. For example, the mutual interaction of β-BuTX and DTX at the avian neuromuscular junction (Harvey and Karlsson 1982) demonstrates the functional importance of the common acceptor. On the other hand, the ability of DTX to potentiate nerve-evoked twitch of guinea pig ileum (Black and Dolly, unpublished) may be due to sites exclusive for DTX homologues, since β-BuTX apparently has no effect on this tissue (Chang and Lee 1963). Clearly, the purification and reconstitution of these acceptors, tasks at present in progress, are necessary to decipher their precise roles. Nevertheless present evidence indicates that they are associated directly or indirectly with certain voltage-sensitive K$^+$ channels.

Acknowledgements — Research support was kindly provided by MRC and Wellcome Trust. We thank A. Breeze, D. Evans, and D. Green (Imperial College), and C. Shone, P. Hambleton, and J. Melling (CAMR, Porton Down) for help with some experiments described herein.

◀**Fig. 13.8** Localization of ^{125}I-DTX acceptors by electron-microscope autoradiography. Hand-cut 400 μm slices from one-day-old chick cerebellum were incubated in 30 nM ^{125}I-DTX in Krebs-Ringer for 1 h, washed extensively, fixed, and processed for electron-microscope autoradiography. After exposures of 4–8 weeks, silver grains were found over cell soma membrane (a) (cell membranes are indicated by ▲, N = nucleus), synpases (b), or on the unmyelinated parallel fibre axons of granule cells (c). Scale bars: (a, c) 500 nm; (b) 100 nm.

References

Adams, P. R. and Lancaster, B. (1985). Components of Ca^{2+}-activated K^+-current in rat hippocampal neurones *in vitro*. *J. Physiol.* (*Lond.*) **362**, 23p.

Alger, B. E. and Nicoll, R. A. (1980). Spontaneous inhibitory postsynaptic potentials in hippocampus: mechanisms for tonic inhibition. *Brain Res.* **200**, 195–200.

Andersen, P., Bliss, T. V. P., and Skrede, K. K. (1971). Unit analysis of hippocampal population spikes. *Exp. Brain Res.* **13**, 208–21.

Black, A. R. (1986). Functional neuronal acceptors for dendrotoxin. Ph.D. Thesis, University of London.

——, Breeze, A. L., Othman, I. B., and Dolly, J. O. (1986). Involvement of neuronal acceptors for dendrotoxin in its convulsive action in rat brain. *Biochem. J.* **237**, 397–404.

—— and Dolly, J. O. (1986). Two acceptor sub-types for dendrotoxin in chick synaptic membranes distinguishable by β-bungarotoxin. *Eur. J. Biochem.* **156**, 609–17.

Black, J. D. (1985). Ultrastructural autoradiographic analysis of the interaction of botulinum neurotoxins with nerve terminals. Ph.D. Thesis, University of London.

—— and Dolly, J. O. (1986a). Interaction of ^{125}I-labelled botulinum neurotoxins with nerve terminals: I. Ultrastructural autoradiographic localization and quantitation of distinct membrane acceptors for types A and B on motor nerves. *J. cell Biol.* **103**, 521–34.

—— and —— (1986b). Interaction of ^{125}I-labelled botulinum neurotoxin with nerve terminals: II. Autoradiographic evidence for its uptake into motor nerves by acceptor-mediated endocytosis. *J. cell Biol.* **103**, 535–44.

Bon, C., Saliou, B., Thieffry, M., and Manaranche, R. (1985). Partial purification of α-glycerotoxin, a presynaptic neurotoxin from the venom glands of the polychaete annelid *Glycera convuluta*. *Neurochem. Int.* **7**, 63–75.

Brown, D. A. and Griffith, W. H. (1983a). Calcium-activated outward current in voltage-clamped hippocampal neurones of the guinea pig. *J. Physiol.* (*Lond.*) **337**, 287–301.

—— and —— (1983b). Persistent slow inward calcium current in voltage-clamped hippocampal neurones of the guinea pig. *J. Physiol.* (*Lond.*) **337**, 303–20.

Buckle, P. J. and Hass, H. L. (1982). Enhancement of synaptic transmission by 4-aminopyridine in hippocampal slices of the rat. *J. Physiol.* (*Lond.*) **326**, 109–22.

Burnstock, G. (1982). Cytochemical studies in the enteric nervous system. In *Cytochemical methods in neuroanatomy* pp. 129–49. Alan R. Liss, New York.

Catterall, W. A. (1984). The molecular basis of neuronal excitability. *Science* **223**, 653–61.

Ceccarelli, B., Hurlbut, W. P., and Mauro, A. (1973). Turnover of transmitter and synaptic vesicles at the frog neuromuscular junction. *J. cell Biol.* **57**, 499–524.

Chang, C. C. and Lee, C. Y. (1963). Isolation of neurotoxins from the venom of *Bungarus multicinctus* and their modes of neuromuscular blocking action. *Arch. int. Pharmacodynam.* **144**, 241–57.

Docherty, R. J., Dolly, J. O., Halliwell, J. V., and Othman, I. B. (1983). Excitatory effects of dendrotoxin on the hippocampus *in vitro*. *J. Physiol.* (*Lond.*) **336**, 58–9p.

Dolly, J. O. and Barnard, E. A. (1984). Nicotinic acetylcholine receptors: an overview. *Biochem. Pharmacol.* **33**, 841–58.

——, Black, J. D., Williams, R. S., and Melling, J. (1984a). Acceptors for botulinum neurotoxin reside on motor nerve terminals and mediate its internalization. *Nature (Lond.)* **307**, 457–60.

——, Halliwell, J. V., Black, J. D., Williams, R. S., Pelchen-Matthews, A., Breeze, A. L., Mehraban, F., Othman, I. B., and Black, A. R. (1984b). Botulinum neurotoxin and dendrotoxin as probes for studies on transmitter release. *J. Physiol. (Paris)* **79**, 280–303.

——, Lande, S., and Wray, D. (1985). A population of miniature end-plate potentials unaffected by botulinum neurotoxin at mouse motor nerve terminals. *J. Physiol. (Lond.)* 365, 80p.

Dreyer, F. and Schmitt, A. (1981). Different effects of botulinum A toxin and tetanus toxin on the transmitter releasing process at the mammalian neuromuscular junction. *Neurosci. Lett.* **26**, 307–11.

Evans, D. M., Williams, R. S., Shone, C. C., Hambleton, P., Melling, J., and Dolly, J. O. (1986). Botulinum neurotoxin type B. Its purification and interaction with rat brain synaptosomal membranes. *Eur. J. Biochem.* **154**, 409–16.

Fertuck, H. C. and Salpeter, M. M. (1976). Quantitation of junctional and extrajunctional acetylcholine receptors by electron-microscope autoradiography after ^{125}I-α-bungarotoxin binding at mouse neuromuscular junctions. *J. cell Biol.* **69**, 144–58.

Galvan, M., Franz, P., and Vogel-Wiens, C. (1984). Actions of potassium channel blockers on guinea-pig lateral olfactory tract axons. *Naunyn Schmiedeberg's Arch. Pharmacol.* **325**, 8–11.

Gustaffson, B., Galvan, M., Grafe, P., and Wigstrom, H. (1982). A transient outward current in a mammalian central neurone blocked by 4-aminopyridine. *Nature* **299**, 252–4.

Haas, M. L., Wieser, H. G., and Yasargil, M. G. (1983). 4-aminopyridine and fibre potentials in rat and human hippocampal slices. *Experientia (Basle)* **39**, 114–15.

Halliwell, J. V. (1983). Calcium-loading reveals two distinct Ca^{2+}-currents in voltage-clamped guinea-pig hippocampal neurones *in vitro*. *J. Physiol. (Lond.)* **341**, 10–11p.

—— and Adams, P. R. (1982). Voltage-clamp analysis of muscarinic excitation in hippocampal neurons. *Brain Res.* **250**, 71–92.

—— and Dolly, J. O. (1982). Preferential action of β-bungarotoxin at nerve terminal regions in the hippocampus. *Neurosci. Lett.* **30**, 321–7.

——, Othman, I. B., Pelchen-Matthews, A., and Dolly, J. O. (1986). Central action of dendrotoxin: selective reduction of a transient K conductance in hippocampus and binding to localized acceptors. *Proc. nat. Acad. Sci. USA* **83**, 493–7.

Harris, A. J. and Miledi, R. (1971). The effect of type D botulinum toxin on frog neuromuscular junctions. *J. Physiol. (Lond.)* **217**, 497–515.

Harvey, A. L., Anderson, A. J., and Karlsson, E. (1984). Facilitation of transmitter release by neurotoxins from snake venoms. *J. Physiol. (Paris)* **79**, 222–7.

—— and Gage, P. W. (1981). Increase of evoked release of acetylcholine at neuromuscular junctions by a fraction from the venom of the Eastern green mamba snake (*Dendroaspis angusticeps*). *Toxicon* **19**, 373–81.

—— and Karlsson, E. (1980). Dendrotoxin from the venom of the green mamba, *Dendroaspis angusticeps*. *Naunyn-Schmiedeberg's Arch. Pharmacol.* **312**, 1–6.

—— and —— (1982). Protease inhibitor homologues from mamba venoms. Facilitation of acetylcholine release and interactions with prejunctional blocking toxins. *Br. J. Pharmacol.* **77**, 153–61.

Johnston, D., Hablitz, J. J., and Wilson, W. A. (1980). Voltage-clamp discloses slow inward current in hippocampal burst-firing neurones. *Nature (Lond.)* **286**, 391–3.

Joubert, F. J. and Taaljaard, N. (1980). Snake venoms. The amino acid sequences of two proteinase inhibitor homologues from *Dendroaspis angusticeps* venom. *Hoppe-Seyler's Z. physiol. Chem.* **361**, 661–74.

Kondo, K., Toda, H., Narita, K. and Lee, C. -Y (1982). Amino-acid sequence of β_2-bungarotoxin from *Bungarus multicinctus* venom. The amino-acid substitutions in the B chains. *J. Biochem.* **91**, 1519–30.

MacKenzie, I., Burnstock, G., and Dolly, J. O. (1982). The effects of purified botulinum neurotoxin type A on cholinergic, adrenergic and non-adrenergic, atropine-resistant autonomic neuromuscular transmission. *Neuroscience* **7**, 997–1006.

Maxfield, F. R., Willingham, M. C., Davies, P. J. A., and Pastan, I. (1979). Amines inhibit the clustering of α_2 macroglobulin and EGF on the fibroblast cell surface. *Nature (Lond.)* **277**, 661–3.

Mehraban, F., Breeze, A. L., and Dolly, J. O. (1984). Identification by cross-linking of a neuronal acceptor protein for dendrotoxin, a convulsant polypeptide. *FEBS Letts.* **174**, 116–22.

——, Black, A. R., Breeze, A. L., Green, D. G., and Dolly, J. O. (1985). A functional membraneous acceptor for dendrotoxin in rat brain: solubilization of the binding component. *Biochem. Soc. Trans.* **13**, 507–08.

Middlebrook, J. L. and Dorland, R. B. (1981). In *Receptor-mediated binding and internalization of toxins and hormones* (ed. J. L. Middlebrook and L. D. Kohn), pp. 15–30. Academic Press, London.

Miller, R. J. (1984). Toxin probes for voltage-sensitive calcium channels. *Trends Neurosci.* **7**, 309.

Molgo, J. and Thesleff, S. (1984). Studies on the mode of the action of botulinum toxin type A at the frog neuromuscular junction. *Brain Res.* **297**, 309–16.

Othman, I. B. (1983). Interactions of β-bungarotoxin and dendrotoxin with nerve terminals. Ph.D. Thesis, University of London.

——, Spokes, J. W., and Dolly, J. O. (1982). Preparation of neurotoxic ^{3}H-β-bungarotoxin: demonstration of saturable binding to brain synapses and its inhibition by toxin I. *Eur. J. Biochem* **128**, 267–76.

Rehm, H. and Betz, H. (1982). Binding of β-bungarotoxin to synaptic membrane fractions of chick brain. *J. biol. Chem.* **257**, 10 015–22.

—— and —— (1983). Identification by cross-linking of a β-bungarotoxin binding polypeptide in chick brain membranes. *EMBO J.* **2**, 1119–22.

—— and —— (1984). Solubilization and characterization of the β-bungarotoxin-binding protein of chick brain membranes. *J. biol. Chem.* **259**, 6865–9.

Scheer, H. and Meldolesi, J. (1985). Purification of the putative α-latrotoxin receptor from bovine synaptosomal membranes in an active binding form. *EMBO J.* **4**, 323–7.

Schmid-Antomarchi, H., Hugues, M., Norman, R., Ellory, C., Borsotto, M., and Lazdunski, M. (1984). Molecular properties of the apamin-binding component of the Ca^{2+}-dependent K^+ channel. *Eur. J. Biochem.* **142**, 1–6.

Segal, M., Rogawski, M. A., and Barker, J. L. (1984). A transient potassium conductance regulates the excitability of cultured hippocampal and spinal neurones. *J. Neurosci.* **4**, 604–9.

Sellin, L. C., Kauffman, J. A., and Das Gupta, B. R. (1983a). Comparison of the effects of botulinum neurotoxin types A and E at the rat neuromuscular junction. *Med. Biol.* **61**, 120–5.

——, Thesleff, S., and Das Gupta, B. R. (1983b) Different effects of types A and B botulinum toxin on transmitter release at the rat neuromuscular junction. *Acta physiol. scand.* **119**, 127–33.

Simpson, L. L. (1980). Kinetic studies on the interaction between botulinum toxin type A and the cholinergic neuromuscular junction. *J. Pharmacol. exp. Ther.* **212**, 16–21.

—— (1981). The origin, structure, and pharmacological activity of botulinum toxin. *Pharmacol. Rev.* **33**, 155–88.

Skrede, K. K. and Westgaard, R. H. (1971). The transverse hippocampal slice: a well-defined cortical structure maintained *in vitro*. *Brain Res.* **35**, 589–93.

Stansfeld, C., Marsh, S. J., Halliwell, J. V., and Brown, D. A. (1986). 4-Aminopyridine and dendrotoxin induce repetitive firing in rat visceral sensory neurones by blocking a slowly inactivating outward current. *Neurosci. Lett.* **64**, 299–304.

Sugiyama, H. (1980). *Clostridium botulinum* neurotoxin. *Microbiol. Rev.* **44**, 419–48.

Tauc, L. (1984). Neurotoxins. 8th GIF lectures in neurobiology. *J. Physiol.* (*Paris*) **79**, part 4.

Thesleff, S. (1982). Spontaneous quantal transmitter release in experimental neuromuscular disorders of the rat. *Muscle and Nerve* **5**, S 12–16.

—— (1984). Transmitter release in botulinum-poisoned muscles. *J. Physiol.* (*Paris*) **79**, 192–5.

Tillotson, D. (1979). Inactivation of Ca conductance dependent on entry of Ca ions in molluscan neurones. *Proc. nat. Acad. Sci. USA* **76**, 1497–500.

Tse, C. K., Dolly, J. O., Hambleton, P., Wray, D., and Melling, J. (1982). Preparation and characterisation of homogenous neurotoxin type A from *Clostridium botulinum*. *Eur. J. Biochem.* **122**, 493–500.

——, Wray, D., Melling, J., and Dolly, J. O. (1986). Actions of β-bungarotoxin on spontaneous release of transmitter at botulinised muscle endplates. *Toxicon* **24**, 123–30.

Weller, U., Bernhardt, U., Siemen, D., Dreyer, F., Vogel, W., and Habermann, E. (1985). Electrophysiological and neurobiochemical evidence for the blockade of a potassium channel by dendrotoxin. *Naunyn-Schmiedeberg's Arch. Pharmacol.* **330**, 77–83.

Williams, R. S., Tse, C. K., Dolly, J. O., Hambleton, P., and Melling, J. (1983). Radioiodination of botulinum neurotoxin type A with retention of biological activity and its binding to brain synaptosomes. *Eur. J. Biochem.* **131**, 437–45.

14

The structure and physiology of toxin binding sites on voltage-gated sodium channels

G. R. Strichartz

Introduction

The role of sodium channels in action potentials

Action potentials are the regenerative membrane depolarizations employed by many neural and endocrine tissues for the transmission of information and the control of secretion. In the axons of most neurons and in mammalian skeletal and cardiac muscles are found ionic sodium channels, which are essential components for the generation and propagation of action potentials (Hille 1984). During an action potential the cell's plasma membrane depolarizes relatively rapidly, yet transiently, from its resting value (-50 to -100 mV) to a potential more positive than 0 mV. This depolarization occurs because of an influx of a small number of positive sodium ions down their electrochemical gradient through discrete sites in the membrane called sodium channels (Na channels). Sodium channels are thus catalysts of a reaction, the passage of ions through an otherwise insulating high-resistance membrane. As catalysts they are much like other enzymes; they discriminate among various substrates (ions), are inhibited by certain agents, activated by others, may have regulatory components (if not separable subunits) and, uniquely, are remarkably sensitive to changes in the membrane potential. Recently these membrane-intrinsic glycoproteins have been isolated and purified from a number of excitable tissues (Agnew, Levinson, Brabson, and Raftery 1978; Barchi, Cohen, and Murphy 1980; Hartshorne and Catterall 1981). Reconstitution of their full functions in systems of artificial membranes is approaching, and will provide the pure molecular substrate for the study of neuronal excitability.

Physiological properties of the Na channel

Ionic Na channels possess three physiological attributes:

(a) they conduct ions;

(b) they select among the various cations present (effectively excluding anions but having untested permeability to non-electrolytes); and

(c) they undergo conformational transitions between plural 'states', at least one of which is the ion-conducting, or 'open' state, in response to the membrane potential.

The third activity, the 'gating' of Na channels by voltage, is the prime property for their function as mediators of regenerative electrical signals. Although the quantitative values of channel permeability and voltage dependence may vary from tissue to tissue and among different organisms, a general behaviour can be summarized for almost all cells with Na^+-dependent action potentials.

Sodium channels exist in three physiologically defined states. *Resting* channels are closed but may open in response to membrane depolarization; *inactivated* channels are closed and will not open, directly; *open* channels are in an ion-conducting state. A simplified representation of the kinetic relationships between these states is shown in Fig. 14.1. Ample evidence suggests that plural conformations occur in each of the three classes (Sigworth 1980), and there are slower and faster transitions, occurring sequentially and in parallel among several different states, but the simplified scheme shown here serves the purposes of the present description.

During a constant membrane depolarization, rapidly established from the resting potential by application of voltage-clamp instrumentation, the sodium permeability (P_{Na}) changes with the time course shown in Fig. 14.2. The rapid initial rise in P_{Na} is called 'activation' and reflects the occupancy of *open* (O) states by a fraction of *resting* (R) channels. The subsequent decrease in P_{Na}, called 'inactivation', represents the transition of *open* channels to the closed *inactivated* conformations (Hodgkin and Huxley 1952). To the extent that conformations that are intermediate between R and O (and not specifically shown in Fig. 14.1) can convert to an inactivated form, inactivation is a process paralleling activation. To the extent that only

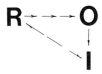

Fig. 14.1 A modest kinetic scheme to describe the gating of sodium channels during a membrane depolarization. Channels in the resting state (R) are converted, by multistep reactions, to open states (O) or inactivated states (I). Open channels will eventually inactivate, but inactivated channels cannot open directly in response to a depolarization.

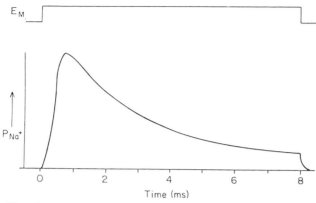

Fig. 14.2 The time-course of the sodium permeability change during a constant depolarization produced by voltage-clamp. The rapid rise, termed 'activation', is followed by a slower decline, termed 'inactivation'. Such a time-course follows from kinetic scheme of Fig. 14.1.

open channels can become inactivated, it is a sequential process. In reality, both parallel and sequential processes are probable (Stimers, Bezanilla, and Taylor 1985), and the actual kinetic pathway in this rate competition will depend on extrinsic conditions, e.g. Ca^{2+}, H^+, temperature, and the membrane potential, as well as intrinsic properties of the channel molecules themselves.

With regard to the last point, the probability that resting channels will be converted to open rather than inactivated states, and the time that the channels will remain open before inactivating, are major factors governing impulse patterns. The ability of action potentials to occur, to propagate through regions where sodium channels are only sparsely distributed or where individual axons branch to form multiple 'daughter' processes, and to recur repetitively at high frequency are all shaped by the kinetics of individual Na channels. Although the reactions drawn in Fig. 14.1 have relaxation times of 0.1 to 100 ms, additional, slower reactions are implied by physiological measurements (Peganov, Khodorov, and Shishkova 1973). Inasmuch as Na channels are phosphorylatable substrates of protein kinase (Costa, Casnellie, and Catterall 1982), and are regulated by changes in intracellular Ca^{2+}, cAMP (Sherman, Chrivia, and Catterall 1985), and membrane activity (Bar-Sagi and Prives 1985), they are also likely to be altered chemically and biosynthetically modulated. Biochemical reactions may provide the means for regulating membrane excitability over time spans of seconds, minutes, and hours (Seelig and Kendig 1982). The concerns of this chapter range from alterations in millisecond reactions to day-long differentiation processes.

Toxins that modify Na channel functions

A variety of natural organic and proteinaceous molecules modify all mea-surable functions of sodium channels. Many of these have been used to study the channel's physiology, to determine channel number and spatial distribution, and to isolate and purify the channel. A brief survey of these toxins follows.

Alkaloid and steroidal activators

Lipophilic molecules from plants and animals alter the gating behaviour of Na channels. The steroid batrachotoxin (BTX), from the skin of frogs of genus *Phyllobates*, and the alkaloid veratridine (VTD), from plants of genus *Liliaceae* (*inter alia*), are two well-studied examples (Strichartz, Hahin, and Cahalan 1982). An obvious action of these compounds is to induce sodium channels to open at negative membrane potentials where this process nor-mally occurs very infrequently (Khodorov 1978); this pharmacological activation directly produces membrane depolarization and I refer to these drugs as 'activators'. In truth, the full description of 'activator' effects on Na channels must include changes in all functions, gating (inactivation is slowed), ion selectivity (K^+ becomes relatively more permeant with refer-ence to Na^+), and limiting permeability (the conductance of a single open channel is decreased; Quandt and Narahashi 1982). The binding of the toxins to the different states of channels stabilizes those channel states and thus induces and alters channel gating. Batrachotoxin is both a more potent and a more effective activator than the other drugs, producing a greater steady-state P_{Na} at a lower drug concentration (Catterall and Ray 1976). It has been characterized as a 'full agonist' of open Na channels, whereas VTD appears to be a 'partial agonist'. At least part of this difference arises from the relative affinities of the two toxins for open versus inactivated Na channels. BTX addition produces a monotonically increasing depolariza-tion, VTD addition a partially transient one with peak values approaching those from BTX. One explanation for this difference may be that BTX-bound Na channels inactivate little and slowly (Dubois, Schneider, and Khodorov 1983), but VTD-bound channels inactivate substantially (Rando, Wang and Strichartz 1986).

Such specific statements are representative of a powerful general approach to channel modification called the 'modulated receptor hypo-thesis' (Hille 1977). Reciprocal actions between toxins (or any ligand) and the channel as a receptor explain the observed drug effects: toxins bind with different affinities to different channel states, thereby changing the free energy of those states and the kinetic and equilibrium relations among them. Reciprocally, channel states are populated differentially by the membrane potential, and thus is the effective drug affinity modulated by voltage. A repeat reading of the previous passage on activators will have added meaning in terms of this modulated receptor model.

Polypeptide inhibitors of inactivation

Small basic proteins are able to inhibit inactivation of Na channels specifically, with no effect on any other channel functions. The description of the inhibition differs among different organisms; inactivation may be slowed, but eventually still produce a zero P_{Na} value (Okamoto, Takahashi, and Yamashita 1977), or inactivation may be totally inhibited in some channels while remaining normal in others (Gillespie and Meves 1980), the balance depending on the toxin concentration. In yet other membranes both partial inactivation and slowing of the existing reaction are observed (Wang and Strichartz 1985a). Do these differences result from different receptor sites for a toxin on the same channel, or from the presence of two distinct types of Na channel molecule?

The toxins that specifically affect inactivation are called 'α-toxins'. (This is a convenient, brief name but a more descriptive form of nomenclature, for consistent international use, would be welcome.) Alpha-toxins have been purified from scorpion venoms (Miranda, Kupeyan, Rochat, Rochat, and Lissitzky 1970) and from sea anemone nematocysts (Schweitz, Vincent, Barhanin, Frelin, Linden, Hugues, and Lazdunski 1981). The scorpion α-toxins have a range of affinities, usually as high as $K_D = 10^{-9}$ M, and rates of reversibility (Wang and Strichartz 1983). The most potent one isolated from the venom of *Leiurus quinquestriatus* has been used for biochemical and physiological studies (Catterall 1976, 1980). Although it provides no depolarization by itself, it strongly potentiates this aspect of the channel activators (Tang, Strichartz, and Orkand 1979). Interestingly, other treatments that slow and inhibit channel inactivation do not potentiate activator depolarizations (Rando, Wang, and Strichartz 1986). This provides further evidence for the plural, complex pathways of Na channel inactivation processes (cf. Sigworth 1981).

The α-toxin from *Leiurus q.* binds to Na channels in a voltage-dependent manner (Catterall, Ray, and Morrow 1976). The affinity falls as the steady membrane potential becomes less negative. In biochemical experiments, including those measuring toxin binding directly, the voltage dependence of the K_D is superimposed directly on that for the activation of Na channels (peak P_{Na} as a function of membrane depolarization) (Catterall 1977, 1979). However, in electrophysiological experiments a much faster reversal of toxin binding occurs and at membrane potentials of +50 to +100 mV, far beyond those that saturate the activation process (Fig. 14.3) (Wang and Strichartz 1984; cf. Dodge and Frankenhaeuser 1959). In fact, no modulations of gating of Na channels have been reported within these membrane potential values; changes of activation and of inactivation probabilities

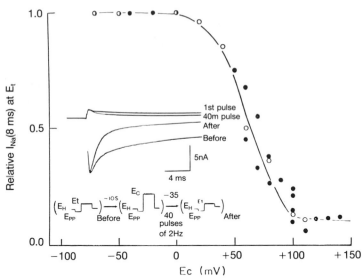

Fig. 14.3 Voltage-dependence of the action of an α-toxin, from *Leiurus* scorpion venom, on inactivation of Na currents in frog myelinated nerve. The inset shows the actual currents before, during, and after 'conditioning' by a train of large depolarizations (to E_c +100 mV). (The conditioning pulse pattern is illustrated by the square waveforms in parentheses at the lower left.) The inset current traces show Na currents with inactivation slowed by *Leiurus* toxin before and after the conditioning. The toxin acts to slow current inactivation, thereby increasing the current amplitude at later times after the peak (e.g. at 8 ms; 'before'). Conditioning procedures reverse the toxin's action, thus decreasing the current at later times ('after'). The large graph shows the final reversal of the toxin's effect after a train of conditioning pulses as a function of the conditioning potential. Note that even at the most positive conditioning potentials some effect of the toxin persists (Wang and Strichartz 1984).

occur at potentials below 0 mV. The response of the α-toxin receptor may be a case where changes in channel conformations undetected by standard electrophysiology are revealed by pharmacological probes.

Polypeptide modulators of activation

Another class of polypeptide scorpion toxins exerts its primary effects on the activation processes of sodium channels (Cahalan 1975). In the presence of these β-toxins, sodium channels, when depolarized from the resting potential, activate more slowly than they do without β-toxin. Larger depolarizing steps are required to open the same fraction of channels as were activated in the absence of toxin, and the inactivation time course is also slowed (Wang and Strichartz 1982, 1985b). These effects on channel gating are markedly dependent on the immediately previous history of the membrane potential; a large and long depolarization preceding the test depolarization changes the entire pattern of toxin-modified gating. Following such a 'conditioning' depolarization, the activation process is accelerated, now reaching rates faster than in the toxin-free control. All fractional occupancies of the open state then occur at depolarizations that are more negative than those required in toxin-free controls. In other words, the function describing the probability of activation as a function of the test potential is shifted positively along the voltage axis by the toxin alone, but shifted negatively when the toxin and a conditioning pulse are applied (Fig. 14.4). Curiously, conditioning depolarizations slow inactivation even further in the presence of β-toxins, even though activation is accelerated. Such results make it very unlikely that inactivation follows activation as a single, undimensional, sequential reaction.

Alpha- and beta-toxins have been found in the same scorpion venom, *C. sculpturatus* (Ewing) (Meves, Rubly, and Watt 1982; Wang and Strichartz 1983). The α-toxin of this venom is less potent than that of *L. quinquestriatus* and it reverses relatively rapidly upon washing. Addition of purified α- and β-toxins together to a nerve leads to spontaneously initiated impulses, often in high frequency trains, and slow waves of membrane depolarization (Wang and Strichartz 1982, 1983). Electrophysiological experiments show that α-, and β-toxins can act on the same Na channel simultaneously (Wang and Strichartz 1982) and biochemical studies show that equilibrium binding of each separate toxin is independent of the other (Jover, Couraud, and Rochat 1980). The physiological effects, however, are modestly synergistic; each aspect of gating behaviour that is modified by one toxin is exaggerated when the other toxin is also present.

This cooperative interaction is reflected in the kinetics of β-toxin action on single nerve fibres. Present alone, at 10^{-8} M, the *Centruroides* β-toxin only produces its first detectable effects after 5 min of incubation, the maximum effect being reached at 15–20 min (Fig. 5). But in nerve fibres pre-exposed to *Leiurus q.* α-toxin, the response to β-toxins occurs with latencies of less than 1 min and the maximum effect is reached after 5 min incubation. We believe that the α-toxin increases the probability of occurrence of a substate of the Na channel that reacts rapidly with β-toxin, but is not of greater equilibrium affinity than other states of the channel normally found at rest.

Other toxins that modify channel gating

Several large polycyclic ethers have been isolated from the dinoflagellates *Ptychodiscus* (previously *Gymnodinium*) and *Gambierdiscus*. These compounds, called *brevetoxins* and *ciguatoxins* respectively, have similar chemical properties; I believe that their essential mode of action will prove to be identical. They depolarize some excitable cells, e.g. nerves and muscles from live animals (Wu, Huang, Vogel, Luke, Atchison, and Narahashi

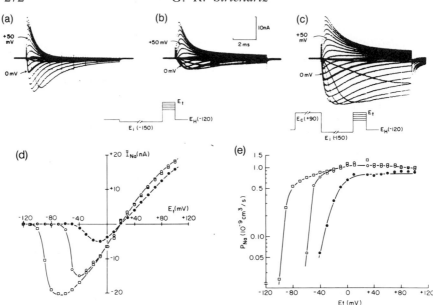

Fig. 14.4 Families of Na currents in the absence and presence of β-scorpion toxin. (a) Na currents in control frog node were measured before toxin treatment. Each voltage step was incremented by 10 mV from a holding potential of −120 mV. The numbers near the current traces indicate the corresponding membrane potentials. The pulse protocol is shown at the bottom. (b) Na currents, after exposure to 100 nM *Centruroides s.* β-scorpion toxin for 40 min, were recorded in the same node. Notice that outward Na currents are less reduced than inward Na currents and that the rising phases are slowed. The current declining phases are also slowed, with a small amount of current left at the end of the pulse. (c) Na currents in the same node were measured after a strong depolarizing conditioning pulse. The pulse program is shown under the current traces. Notice that the currents now appear in the more negative potential range and that the current peak amplitudes nearly equal the control levels. Also the current rising phases are faster and declining phases slower than those without conditioning pulses shown in (b). (d) The peak Na current–voltage relationship and (e) the peak Na permeability–voltage relationship. Data in (d) were taken from (a–c) and further calculated and plotted in (e) according to the Goldman–Hodgkin–Katz equation. Open and filled circles indicate the results before and after toxin treatment, respectively, and the open squares represent the data with a conditioning pulse. E_H = holding potential; E_c = conditoning pulse for 100 ms; E_i = interpulse for 50 ms; E_t = test pulse for 8 ms. (After Wang and Strichartz 1983, 1985b.)

1985), but do not produce a sustained P_{Na} in cultured cells (Catterall and Gainer 1985). In frog nerve they have a modest potentiating effect on the depolarizing action of veratridine (Crill and Strichartz, unpublished observation), but this effect is far more significant in the cultured cells. These

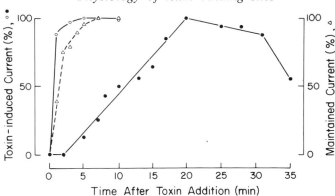

Fig. 14.5 Time course of the appearance of β-toxin modified ('induced') current and of the maintained, non-inactivating (α-toxin) current after the addition of different scorpion toxins. After addition of β-toxin (200 nM) at time $t = 0$, the peak induced current was measured (upon repolarization to −95 mV from a 20 ms depolarization to +5 mV), and is plotted here as a percentage of the maximal induced current. Induced current in a node treated with β-toxin (●) and in a node that had been exposed to *Leiurus* α-toxin (200 nM) for 15 minutes before the *Centruroides* β-toxin (○). Induced currents in both situations declined in time after reaching a maximal value. △ = Normalized amplitude of the maintained α-toxin current after addition of *Leiurus* α-toxin at 400 nM; the rate of appearance of the maintained current produced by 200 nM α-toxin was similar, demonstrating that the rate-limiting reaction that inhibits sodium channel inactivation is not diffusion of the toxin molecules to their receptor sites. (From Wang and Strichartz 1983.)

differences may arise from the detailed differences in channel gating pathways between the two types of cells, rather than from any intrinsic difference in receptor sites for these polyether toxins. The synergism seen with the brevetoxins and veratridine, considered in addition to interactions with other drugs, requires that the brevetoxins (and ciguatoxins) bind to sites separate from those for the activators or the two types of polypeptide toxins.

Tetrodotoxin and saxitoxin

Two small cationic organic molecules, tetrodotroxin (TTX), and saxitoxin (STX), inhibit most sodium channels reversibly but with high affinity (10^{-9}– 10^{-8} M; Kao 1966). The inhibition is a constant factor at all membrane potentials and times, and appears as a reduction in the number of ion-conducting channels (Hille 1968). The remaining functional channels gate normally and have the same single-channel conductance value. The small electrical signals from the membrane, which reflect the conformational changes of Na channels during activation, are not affected by saturating concentrations of TTX (Armstrong and Bezanilla 1974). Inhibited channels thus appear to undergo all the usual electrically coupled conformational changes, but not to yield an ion-conducting pathway. Often the channel's pore is said to be 'blocked' or 'occluded', but there is no test of this concept.

The molecular mechanism of the action of TTX and STX has been investigated for 20 years. The two toxins bind to a common receptor and mutually exclude each other (Henderson, Ritchie, and Strichartz 1973; Wagner and Ulbricht 1975), but the chemistry of binding differs between toxins. Binding and blocking of both are inhibited at low (5.5) and high (8.5) pH (Hille 1968; Kao, James-Kracke, and Kao, 1983; Strichartz 1984), and by elevated polyvalent cations in the bathing solution (Henderson, Ritchie, and Strichartz 1974). But the binding of STX is more sensitive than that of TTX to elevated cations (Hille, Ritchie, and Strichartz 1975) and less sensitive to increases in temperature (Hansen Bay and Strichartz 1980). Replacement of water by D_2O doubles the equilibrium blocking affinity of STX for neuronal Na channels (by halving the rate of dissociation), but is without effect on TTX action (Hahin and Strichartz 1981). Excitable tissues from certain animals that are less sensitive to the effects of one of these toxins sometimes show near normal sensitivity to the other toxin (Kao and Fuhrman 1967; Twarog, Hidaka, and Yamaguchi 1972; Harris and Thesleff 1971). The different bond energies and enthalpies demonstrated experimentally show that the molecular interaction between the Na channel and the two toxins cannot be identical.

Studies with a series of naturally occurring saxitoxin homologues and with several synthetic STX analogues have contributed to a current view of the inhibitory mechanism (Kao and Walker 1982; Strichartz, Hall, and Shimizu 1984). Molecules having –OH substituents at the R1 position tend to be more potent than their hydrogenated parents (Table 14.1). Those having $-OSO_3^-$ additions at the C11 position are 1.4 to 0.25 times as potent as their unsulphated counterparts, whereas $-SO_3^-$ additions to the N21 carbamyl group reduce the potency to 10 to 2 per cent of that of STX (Strichartz 1984; Moczydlowski, Hall, Garber, Strichartz, and Miller 1984). Reduction of the gem-diol at C12 to an alcohol has stereospecific effects; the α-OH compound has about one-fifth of the potency of STX, the β-OH derivative only one-hundredth (Kao and Walker 1982; Strichartz 1984). Altogether these observations, along with others, have led me to a hypothesis for STX binding that is shown diagrammatically in Fig. 14.6. The toxin molecule, which exists as the gem-diol more than 99 per cent of the time in solution (Shimizu, Hsu, and Genenah 1981), tends towards the dehydrated ketone form as a result of initial formation of an ionic bond between an anionic receptor group and the toxin's 7,8,9 guanidinium group. The keto group rapidly reacts with adjacent amino or hydroxy groups on the receptor to form a hemiketal or a Schiff base. This two-stage reaction is reversible, because the covalent bond is relatively weak and easily hydrolyzed. Synthetic analogues of STX that have only a $-CH_2$ group at C12 are 10^5–10^6

Table 14.1 Structures of the twelve naturally occurring homologues of saxitoxin and their equilibrium dissociation constants (K_1).

Toxin	$\bar{K}_{1-9}$ (10 M)	$\bar{q}=\overline{K_1/K_D}$ a*STX[†]	N
°STX	0.96 ± 0.07	≡ 1	5
B1	48.0 ± 9.7	39.5 ± 6.9	6
GTX2	3.6 ± 0.31	2.92 ± 0.20	17
C1	781 ± 141	720 ± 124	13
GTX3	0.80 ± 0.09	0.54 ± 0.04	6
C2	12.4 ± 1.3	10.8 ± 1.4	5
NEO·STX	0.29 ± 0.02	0.23 ± 0.01	12
B2	49.0 ± 6.3	45.1 ± 5.8	14
GTX1	2.76 ± 0.31	2.46 ± 0.23	15
C3	330 ± 41.4	343[a*] ± —	6
GTX4	1.04 ± 0.042	1.20 ± 0.058	10
C4	12.9 ± 0.75	15.0 ± 0.92	9

*K_{STX} not measured simultaneously, but average value used.

	R1	R2	R3	R4	
1	H	H	H	H	STX
2	H	H	H	SO₃⁻	B1
3	H	H	OSO₃⁻	H	GTX 2
4	H	H	OSO₃⁻	SO₃⁻	C1
5	H	OSO₃⁻	H	H	GTX 3
6	H	OSO₃⁻	H	SO₃⁻	C2
7	OH	H	H	H	NEO
8	OH	H	H	SO₃⁻	B2
9	OH	H	OSO₃⁻	H	GTX 1
10	OH	H	OSO₃⁻	SO₃⁻	C3
11	OH	OSO₃⁻	H	H	GTX 4
12	OH	OSO₃⁻	H	SO₃⁻	C4

The dissociation constants were determined by the competitive displacement, by several inhibitory toxin concentrations, of ³H-STX from high-affinity sodium channel receptors of rabbit brain. The means of the ratios of each dissociation constant to that of radiolabelled STX (*STX) (measured for each separate experiment) are listed in column 3 ($\bar{q}$) followed by the standard error of that mean; N lists the number of separate competition curves used to compute $\bar{q}$ (after Strichartz *et al.* 1984).

G. R. Strichartz

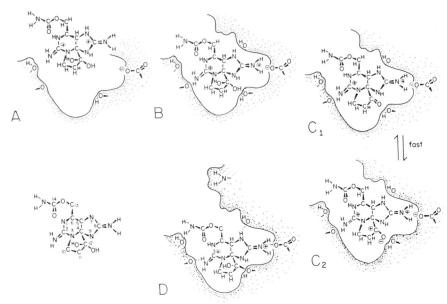

Fig. 14.6 Two-stage binding reaction of STX with receptor. The charged guanidinium at C8 binds at an acidic group on the receptor in the initial step (A → B). This binding induces the dehydration of the gem-diol with concomitant formation of the ketone, which exists as a resonance hybrid of carbonyl (C_1) and carbo-cation (C_2) species. The ketone carbon at C12 is then susceptible to attack, for example, by an alcohol on the receptor with the eventual formation of a hemilactal (D). The amine group on the membrane above the binding site represents the fixed basic charge that modifies the pH dependence of STX potency (from Strichartz 1984).

times less potent than identical compounds having hydrated ketones at C12, proving that this group contributes about half the free energy of equilibrium binding (Strichartz, Rando, Hall, Gitschier, Hall, Magnani, and Hansen Bay 1986).

Beyond this description of a toxin binding site, is there a mechanism for channel inhibition? I believe that the receptor for STX molecules is a flexible region of the outer opening of the ion pathway, and involves two zones of the channel that normally catalyze the primary dehydration of permeant metal cations (Figure 14.7, E–H). When the first ionic bond is initially made between toxin and receptor, the channel responds by changing conformation. It 'puckers up' to the toxin, forming a second ionic bond with the 1,2,3 guanidinium group and, perhaps, another hydrogen bond with the atoms of the carbamyl 'tail'. Synthetic STX analogues having –CH_2OH groups on the C6 position are about equipotent with STX, but those having only –CH_3 or –H_2 are less potent by two orders of magnitude. This implies an important role for this hitherto undistinguished region of the molecule.

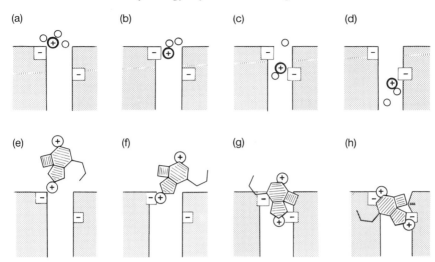

Fig. 14.7 Hypothetical mechanism for the inhibition of sodium channels by saxitoxin. Two anionic sites near the channel's outer opening process the rate-limiting dehydration steps involved in the influx of a Na ion (a–d). The initial binding and dehydration of Na^+ at the outer site (a–b) leads to a conformational shift of the inner site (c) as the ion passes through the pore, finally dissociating from this narrowest region into the channel's cytoplasmic 'lumen' (d). The binding of STX involves analogous steps (e–h). Following initial ionic binding (f), a covalent bond (dashed lines) is formed with the receptor (g) and, perhaps, a second ionic bond with the other anionic site (h). Conformational stabilization of the carbamyl 'tail' may also result from toxin binding (h). The essence of this mechanism is that just as the receptor induces configurational changes in the toxin molecule (Fig. 14.6), so does the toxin molecule induce a conformational change in the receptor.

Thus the binding reaction for STX is composed of a series of interactions between toxin moieties and receptor regions whose configurations have been induced by the preceding steps in the binding process. As a further elaboration of this hypothesis, I believe that the toxin exploits the normal configurational changes in the channel that occur during ion permeation (Fig. 14.7, A–D). Initial ionic binding of a hydrated sodium ion is followed rapidly by polarization of its water of hydration by a receptor group, the same one that forms a covalent bond with STX's C12 ketone. Just as the toxin becomes dehydrated in response to ionic bonding, so the channel changes its configuration in response to the bound Na^+ ion. A second anionic group, 'deeper' in the pore, moves near to the partially dehydrated Na^+ ion, binds it, and then shifts it towards the cytoplasmic end of the channel. The first dehydration site returns towards its original position, achieving it when the ion leaves the second site. Bonds between Na^+ ions and the channel are about as strong as those between Na^+ ions and water.

The channel's configurational changes are modest and of short extent, so the permeation sequence occurs at high velocity and the occupancy time for ions in the channel is relatively brief. The primary hydration site is located superficially at the channel surface and is not essential for ion permeation; when this site is modified chemically the channel conducts Na^+ ions inwards at a slower rate (Sigworth and Spalding 1980) but discriminates among metal cations in the same order (Spalding 1980). It is, however, an obligatory site for toxin binding and its chemical modification renders channels insensitive to STX and TTX at 10^3 times the normal blocking concentrations (Baker and Rubinson 1975; Spalding 1980).

Summarizing the molecular hypothesis for guanidinium toxin action, binding of toxin molecules to the channel is a multi-step process involving induced configurational changes in both toxin and receptor. The receptor is a sequence of sites at the channel's outer opening, normally involved in the primary dehydration of Na^+ ions as they enter the channel mouth. Toxin molecules form ionic and covalent and, perhaps, hydrogen bonds with multiple sites on the receptor and therefore remain bound for tens of seconds; Na^+ ions form weaker bonds with fewer, more restricted regions at any one time and occupy their sites for less than microseconds.

Interactions between different toxins on the Na channel

The potentiation of activator actions by *Leiurus* α-toxin was described previously in this chapter (section B.3). Such potentiation is only seen with the toxin and does not occur in channels where inactivation is slowed by oxidants or transition metals (Rando *et al.* 1986). Thus, potentiation is due to a unique interaction of toxins on the channel, and not to changes in inactivation kinetics *per se*.

Interactions between α-toxins and β-toxins provide another example of synergistic interactions on the Na channel. Beta-toxins act much more rapidly in nerves previously exposed to α-toxins than in unexposed nerves. Since the equilibrium binding of each of these toxins is unaffected by the presence of the other (Jover *et al.* 1980), the accelerated rate of β-toxin action is not symptomatic of an affinity change related to conformational modulation, but rather appears to involve changes in the population of β-toxin reactive states.

The actions of TTX and STX are also modulated by toxins, at least by BTX. In single channels reconstituted into lipid bilayers and activated by BTX, the inhibition by individual STX or TTX molecules can be observed directly as the times that a channel is in the blocked or unblocked state. (With such BTX-modulated channels the duration of an open-state is much longer than the time required for toxin molecules to bind or dissociate from the channel.) Blockade of the channels by the guanidinium toxins depends on the membrane potential (Krueger, Worley, and French 1983), being weaker as the potential becomes less negative. The equilibrium binding affinity is reduced because of voltage-dependent changes in the rate constants for binding and dissociation, of equal but opposite voltage-dependence. This modulation of toxin affinity does not seem to be a direct electrostatic effect of membrane potential on the charged toxin, for toxin molecules ranging in net valence from +2 to 0 exhibit identical voltage dependences (Moczydlowski *et al.* 1984). One explanation is that the membrane voltage regulates the channel distribution between states of high and low affinity for the guanidinium toxins (Moczydlowski *et al.* 1984). When these experiments are conducted in single axons rather than in reconstituted channels, analogous results are observed for macroscopic currents in the presence of BTX, with one noteworthy exception; the blocking action of STX is not voltage-dependent in the negative potential range where channels are not open (Rando and Strichartz 1986). In the potential range where channels are open the same fractional change in channel blocking with changing potential is observed as in the reconstituted, BTX-activated channels. Although one might think that this voltage-dependence is a property of open channels *per se*, and not previously observed in any experiments because unmodified channels are normally open for times ($1-5 \times 10^{-3}$ s) short compared to the relaxation time for toxin binding (10 s; Hille 1975), in fact this is not the case. When the channel open time is prolonged by treatment with the oxidant chloramine-T (Wang 1984), no voltage-dependent blockade by STX is observed (Rando and Strichartz 1985). Thus, the modulation of action of the guanidinium toxins by membrane potential is so far a unique feature of BTX-modified Na channels.

Summary

A broad variety of natural molecules modify the actions of voltage-gated sodium channels of excitable membranes. Some of these are small organic cations, carrying guanidinium moieties (e.g. tetrodotoxin and saxitoxin), which block ion permeation at the outer opening of the channel, without seeming to alter channel gating. Others are small, basic polypeptides that alter the activation and inactivation gating of channels, with no effect on ion permeation through open channels. These, like STX and TTX, also act exclusively from the external solution. And a third type of toxin is represented by the lipophilic activator drugs, batrachotoxin and veratradine, which probably bind at more hydrophobic regions of the channel within the membrane interior. These drugs appear to modify the gating, permeation and selectivity properties, in short, all the measurable functions of the Na channel. Polycyclic ethers like brevetoxin and ciguatoxin also modify channel gating properties, but appear to act at sites separate from those of the traditional activators.

All the toxins that modify channel gating have actions that may be modulated by the membrane potential. Such modulation is probably mediated through potential-dependent changes in channel conformation and hence, toxin binding affinity (the modulated receptor mechanism). The membrane potential may also exert a direct, electrostatic influence on the binding of certain charged toxins.

Toxin molecules also influence each other's action on and binding to the Na channel. Synergistic relations have been observed between activators and α-toxins, and brevetoxins and activators. The onset of β-toxin action is accelerated by α-toxins, and the blocking potency of TTX and STX becomes voltage-sensitive in the presence of BTX. Even though the Na channel is a large protein (m.w. ~ 300 000 daltons) with separate binding sites for five different classes of toxins, these sites interact to influence each other's chemistry. Such interactions probably also occur in the absence of exogenous toxin ligands, and the channel functions of gating and ion selectivity may correspond to the concerted molecular arrangements of a single, narrow ion pore region of the entire channel.

Acknowledgements — This article summarizes research in many laboratories, but the author wishes to recognize collaborations with Professor Yuzuru Shimizu, University of Rhode Island, Drs Sherwood Hall, FDA, and Edward Moczydlowski, Univerisity of Cincinnati, and particularly with Drs Ging Kuo Wang and Thomas Rando of Harvard Medical School. Synthetic saxitoxin analogues were synthesized and generously provided by Professor Yoshito Kishi, Department of Chemistry, Harvard University. Financial support has come from USPHS NIH grants GM 15904, NS 18467 (NS 12828) and from a grant from the US National Multiple Sclerosis Society.

References

Agnew, W. S., Levinson, S. R., Brabson, J. S., and Raftery, M. A. (1978). Purification of the tetrodotoxin binding component associated with the voltage-sensitive sodium channel from *Electrophorus electricus* electroplax membranes. *Proc. nat. Acad. Sci. USA* **75**, 2606–10.

Armstrong, C. M. and Bezanilla, F. (1974). Charge movement associated with the opening and closing of the activation gates of the Na channels. *J. gen. Physiol.* **63**, 533–52.

Baker, P. F. and Rubinson, K. A. (1975). Chemical modification of crab nerves can make them insensitive to the local anesthetics tetrodotoxin and saxitoxin. *Nature* **257**, 412–14.

Barchi, R. L., Cohen, S. A., and Murphy, L. E. (1980) Purification from rat sarcolemma of the saxitoxin binding component of the excitable membrane sodium channel. *Proc. nat. Acad. Sci. USA* **77**, 1306–10.

Bar-Sagi, D. and Prives, J. (1985). Negative modulation of sodium channels in cultured chick muscle cells by the channel activator batrachotoxin. *J. biol. Chem.* **260**, 4740–4.

Cahalan, M. D. (1975) Modification of sodium channel gating in frog myelinated nerve fibres by *Centruroides sculpturatus* scorpion venom. *J. Physiol.* **244**, 511–34.

Catterall, W. A. (1976). Purification of a toxic protein scorpion venom which activates the action potential N^+ ionophore. *J. biol. Chem.* **251**, 5528–36.

—— (1977). Membrane potential-dependent binding of scorpion toxin to the action potential Na^+ ionophore. *J. biol. Chem.* **252**, 8860–8.

—— (1979). Binding of a scorpion toxin to receptor sites associated with sodium channels in frog muscle. Correlation of voltage-dependent binding with activation. *J. gen. Physiol.* **74**, 375–92.

—— (1980). Neurotoxins that act on voltage-sensitive sodium channels in excitable membranes. *A. Rev. Pharmacol. Toxicol.* **20**, 15–43.

—— and Gainer, M. (1985). Interaction of brevetoxin A with a new receptor site on the sodium channel. *Toxicon* **23**, 497–504.

—— and Ray, R. (1976). Interactions of neurotoxins with the action potential Na^+ ionophore. *J. supramol. Struct.* **5**, 397–407.

——, ——, and Morrow, C. S. (1976). Membrane potential dependent binding of scorpion toxin to action potential Na^+ ionophore. *Proc. nat. Acad. Sci. USA* **73**, 2682–6.

Costa, M. R. C., Casnellie, J. E., and Catterall, W. A. (1982). Selective phosphorylation of the α-subunit of the sodium channel by cAMP-dependent protein kinase. *J. biol. Chem.* **257**, 7918–21.

Dodge, F. A. and Frankenhaeuser, B. (1959). Sodium currents in the myelinated nerve fibre of *Xenopus laevis* investigated by the voltage clamp technique. *J. Physiol.* (*Lond.*) **148**, 188–200.

Dubois, J. M., Schneider, M. F., and Khodorov, B. I. (1983). Voltage-dependence of intramembrane charge movement and conductance activation of batrachotoxin-modified sodium channels in frog node of Ranvier. *J. gen. Physiol.* **81**, 829–44.

Gillespie, J. I. and Meves, H. (1980) The effect of scorpion venoms on the sodium currents of the squid giant axon. *J. Physiol.* **308**, 479–99.

Hahin, R. and Strichartz G. R. (1981) Effects of deuterium oxide on the rate and dissociation constants for saxitoxin and tetrodotoxin action. *J. gen. Physiol.* **78**, 113–39.

Hansen Bay, C. M. and Strichartz, G. R. (1980). Saxitoxin binding to sodium channels of rat skeletal muscles. *J. Physiol.* **300**, 89–103.

Harris, J. B. and Thesleff, S. (1971). Studies on tetrodotoxin resistant action potentials in denervated skeletal muscle. *Acta physiol. scand.* **83**, 382–8.

Hartshorne, R. P. and Catterall, W. A. (1981). Purification of the saxitoxin receptor of the sodium channel from rat brain. *Proc nat. Acad. Sci. USA* **78**, 4620–4.

Henderson, R., Ritchie, J. M., and Strichartz, G. R. (1973). The binding of labelled saxitoxin to the sodium channels in nerve membranes. *J. Physiol.* (*Lond.*) **235**, 783–804.

——, —— and —— (1974). Evidence that tetrodotoxin and saxitoxin act at a metal cation binding site in the sodium channels of nerve membrane. *Proc nat. Acad. Sci. USA* **71**, 3936–40.

Hille, B. (1968). Pharmacological modification of the sodium channels of frog nerve. *J. gen. Physiol.* **51**, 199–219.

—— (1975). The receptor for tetrodotoxin and saxitoxin: a structural hypothesis. *Biophys. J.* **15**, 615–19.

—— (1977). Local anesthetics: hydrophilic and hydrophobic pathways for the drug–receptor reaction. *J. gen. Physiol.* **69**, 497–515.

—— (1984). *Ionic channels of excitable membranes.* Sinauer Associates, Sunderland, Massachussetts.

——, Ritchie, J. M., and Strichartz, G. R. (1975) The effect of membrane surface charge on the action of tetrodotoxin and saxitoxin on frog myelinated nerve. *J. Physiol.* **250**, 34P–35P.

Hodgkin, A. L. and Huxley, A. F. (1952) A quantitative description of membrane current and its application to conduction and excitation in nerve. *J. Physiol.* **117**, 500–44.

Jover, E., Couraud, F., and Rochat, H. (1980). Two types of scorpion neurotoxins characterized by their binding to two separate receptor sites on rat brain synaptosomes. *Biochem. Biophys. Res. Commun.* **95**, 1607–14.

Kao, C. Y. (1966). Tetrodotoxin, saxitoxin and their significance in the study of excitation phenomena. *Pharm. Rev.* **18**, 997–1049.

—— and Fuhrman, F. A. (1967). Differentiation of the actions of tetrodotoxin and saxitoxin. *Toxicon* **5**, 25–34.

—— and Walker, S. E. (1982). Active groups and saxitoxin and tetrodotoxin as deduced from actions of saxitoxin analogues on frog muscle and squid axon. *J. Physiol.* **323**, 619–37.

Kao, P. N., James-Kracke, M. R., and Kao, C. Y. (1983). The active guanidinium group of saxitoxin and neosaxitoxin identified by the effects of pH on their activities on squid axon. *Pflüg. Arch. ges. Physiol. Menschen Tiere* **398**, 199–203.

Khodorov, B. I. (1978). Chemicals as tools to study nerve fiber sodium channels: effects of batrachotoxin and some local anesthetics. In *Membrane transport processes* (ed. D. C. Tosteson, Y. A. Ovchinnikov, and R. Latorre), pp. 153–74. Ravens Press, New York.

Krueger, B. K., Worley, J. F., and French, R. J. (1983). Single sodium channels from rat brain incorporated into planar lipid bilayer membranes. *Nature* **303**, 172–5.

Meves, H., Rubly, N., and Watt, D. D. (1982). Effect of toxins isolated from the venom of the scorpion *Centruroides sculpturatus* on the Na currents of the node of Ranvier. *Pflüg. Arch. ges. Physiol. Menschen Tiere* **393**, 56–62.

Miranda, F., Kupeyan, C., Rochat, H., Rochat, C., and Lissitzky, S. (1970). Purification of animal neurotoxins. *Eur. J. Biochem.* **16**, 514–23.

Moczydlowski, E., Hall, S., Garber, S. S., Strichartz, G. R. and Miller, C. (1984). Voltage-dependent blockade of muscle Na^+ channels by guanidinium toxins. Effect of toxin charge. *J. gen. Physiol.* **84**, 687–704.

Okamoto, H., Takahashi, K., and Yamashita, N. (1977). One-to-one binding of a purified scorpion toxin to the Na channels. *Nature* **266**, 465–8.

Peganov, E. M., Khodorov, B. I., and Shishkova, L. (1973). Slow sodium inactivation in the Ranvier node membrane: role of extracellular potassium. *Bull. exp. Biol. Med.* **76**, 1014–17.

Quandt, F. N. and Narahashi, T. (1982). Modification of single Na⁺ channels by batrachotoxin. *Proc. nat. Acad. Sci. USA* **79**, 6732–6.

Rando, T. A. and Strichartz, G. R. (1985). Voltage-dependence of saxitoxin block of Na⁺ channels appears to be a property unique to batrachatoxin-modified channels. *J. gen. Physiol.* **86**, 14a.

—— and —— (1986). Saxitoxin blocks batrachatoxin-modified Na⁺ channels in the node of Ranvier in a voltage dependent manner. *Biophys. J.* **49**, 785–94.

——, Wang, G. K., and Strichartz, G. R. (1986). The interaction of alkaloid neurotoxins batrachatoxin and veratridine with gating processes of neuronal Na⁺ channels. *Molec. Pharmacol.* **29**, 467–77.

Schweitz, H., Vincent, J. -P., Barhanin, J., Frelin, C., Linden, G., Hugues, M., and Lazdunski, M. (1981). Purification and pharmacological properties of eight sea anemone toxins from *Anemone sulcata*, *Anthopleura xanthogrammica*, *Stoichatus giganteus* and *Actinodendron plumosum*. *Biochemistry* **20**, 5245–52.

Seelig, T. L. and Kendig, J. J. (1982). Cyclic nucleotide modulation of Na⁺ and K⁺ currents in the isolated node of Ranvier. *Brain Res.* **245**, 144–7.

Sherman, S. J., Chrivia, J., and Catteral, W. A. (1985). Cyclic adenosine 3′, 5′-monophosphate and cytosolic calcium exert opposing effects on biosynthesis of tetrodotoxin-sensitive sodium channels in rat muscle cells. *J. Neurosci.* **5**, 1570–6.

Shimizu, Y., Hsu, C.-P., and Genenah, A. (1981). Structure of saxitoxin in solutions and stereochemistry of dihydrosaxitoxins. *J. Am. chem. Soc.* **103**, 605–9.

Sigworth, F. J. (1980). The variance of sodium current fluctuations at the node of Ranvier. *J. Physiol* **307**, 97–129.

Sigworth, F. J. (1981). Covariance of nonstationary sodium current fluctuations at the node of Ranvier. *Biophys. J.* **34**, 111–33.

—— and Spalding, B. C. (1980). Chemical modification reduces the conductance of sodium channels in nerve. *Nature* **283**, 293–5.

Spalding, B. C. (1980). Properties of toxin-resistant sodium channels produced by chemical modification in frog skeletal muscle. *J. Physiol.* **305**, 485–500.

Stimers, J. R., Bezanilla, F., and Taylor, R. E. (1985). Sodium channel activation in the squid giant axon. Steady-state properties. *J. gen. Physiol.* **85**, 65–82.

Strichartz, G. (1984). Structural determinants of the affinity of saxitoxin for neuronal sodium channels: electrophysiological studies on frog peripheral nerve. *J. gen. Physiol.* **84**, 281–305.

——, Hahin, R., and Cahalan, M. (1982). Pharmacological models for sodium channels producing abnormal impulse activity. In *Abnormal nerves and muscles as impulse generators* (ed. W. J. Culp and J. Ochoa) pp. 98–129. Oxford University Press, New York.

——, Hall, S., and Shimizu, Y. (1984). Evidence for covalent bonding of saxitoxin to the neuronal sodium channel. *Biophys. J.* **45**, 286a.

——, Rando., T., Hall, S., Gritschier, J., Hall, L., Magnani, B. and Hansen Bay, C. (1986). On the mechanism by which saxitoxin binds to and blocks Na⁺ channels. In

Tetrodotoxin, saxitoxin and the molecular biology of the sodium channel (eds. C. Y. Kao and S. R. Levinson). *N.Y. Acad. Sci.* (In press.)

Tang, C. M., Strichartz, G. R., and Orkand, R. K. (1979). Sodium channel in axons and glial cells of the optic nerve of *Necturus maculosa. J. gen. Physiol.* **74**, 629–42.

Twarog, B., Hidaka, T., and Yamaguchi, H. (1972). Resistance to tetrodotoxin and saxitoxin in nerves of bivalve molluscs. *Toxicon* **10**, 273–8.

Wagner, H.-H. and Ulbricht, W. (1975). The rates of saxitoxin action and of saxitoxin–tetrodotoxin interaction at the node of Ranvier. *Pflüg. Arch. ges. Physiol. Menschen Tiere* **359**, 297–315.

Wang, G. K. (1984). Irreversible modification of sodium channel inactivation in toad myelinated nerve fibres by the oxidant chloramine-T. *J. Physiol. (Lond.)* **346**, 127–41.

—— and Strichartz, G. R. (1982). Simultaneous modifications of sodium channel gating by two scorpion toxins. *Biophys. J.* **40**, 175–9.

—— and —— (1983). Purification and physiological characterization of neurotoxins from venoms of the scorpions *Centruroides sculpturatus* and *Leiurus quinquestriatus. Mol. Pharmacol.* **23**, 519–33.

—— and —— (1984). Rapid voltage-dependent binding of α-scorpion toxins to Na^+ channels. *Soc. Neurosci. Ann. Mtg. Abst.* **255**, 8.

—— and —— (1985a). Kinetic analysis of the action of *Leiurus* scorpion α-toxin on ionic currents in myelinated nerve. *J. gen. Physiol.* **86**, 739–62

—— and —— (1985b). The actions of an isolated β-scorpion toxin on Na^+ channel activation. *Biophys. J.* **47**, 438a.

Wu, C. H., Huang, J. M. C., Vogel, S. M., Luke, V. S., Atchison, W. D., and Narahashi, T. (1985). The actions of *Ptychodiscus brevis* toxins on nerve and muscle membranes. *Toxicon* **23**, 481–8.

Part V

On the treatment of natural poisoning

15

Characterization of venoms and standardization of antivenoms

R. D. G. Theakston

Introduction

For many years there has been a need for the production of international standard antivenoms active against the major medically important venoms so that the efficacy of commercial products can be properly evaluated. In 1962 Christensen first produced a proposed international standard antivenom (ISA) from eight horses which had already been immunised against the venoms of *Naja nivea*, *Haemachatus haemachatus* and *Bitis arietans* and which were subsequently immunized against *N. naja* venom. This pooled polyspecific serum was purified by pepsin digestion, heat coagulation and ammonium sulphate precipitation (Pope 1939a, b; Harms 1948). Lethal toxicity tests (LD_{50}s) were first carried out on the venoms under test by both intravenous and subcutaneous routes, and serum potency assays (ED_{50}s) were subsequently carried out against five intravenous and subcutaneous LD_{50}s. The ED_{50}s of eight different antisera, including the proposed ISA were compared against eight different venoms. It was concluded that the proposed ISA behaved satisfactorily in tests with some venoms and less so with others. The production of monospecific ISAs was not at this time proposed.

In 1979 a WHO coordination meeting was held in Zurich to examine the work in progress throughout the world on the characterization of medically important venoms and the standardization of antivenom preparations. As a direct result of this meeting it was decided that bulk amounts of eight venoms of medical importance should be collected. These International Reference Venoms (IRVs) should be biologically characterized using simple tests capable of being carried out in any laboratory throughout the world; monospecific antivenoms should also be raised against each one, these to be termed International Standard Antivenoms (ISAs). Each antivenom should be tested for its ability to prevent lethality in experimental animals, and to neutralize the pathological activities of the individual IRV (WHO 1981).

One of the main aims of the WHO-based project was, therefore, to prepare International Standard reagents which would enable accurate comparisons to be made between both currently available and new commercial antivenoms. The report also emphasised the importance of (1) the collection of reliable data on morbidity and mortality due to bites and stings by venomous animals, (2) the more widespread epidemiological studies using immunodiagnostic tests such as enzyme-linked immunosorbent assay (ELISA) for evaluating the extent of the snake bite problem and the species involved, (3) the use of such tests in aiding clinical treatment of poisoning due to bites and stings by venomous animals, (4) the increasing use of clinical trials as opposed to results obtained using animal models, (5) determining the correct route of administration of antivenom following systemic poisoning and the effect of both early and late serum reactions, and (6) education of medical workers and the lay public with respect to snake bites and other venomous bites and stings.

WHO International Reference Venoms (IRVs)

Choice of venoms

Venoms of snakes of the same species from different geographical areas often have different pharmacological, pathological, and antigenic properties. For example, the venom of Saudi Arabian *Echis carinatus* does not cause significant clotting of normal plasma whereas Ghanaian, Nigerian, Iranian, Indian, Pakistani, Omani, and Kenyan species are all very active in this respect. Moreover, venoms from different individual snakes originating in the same area vary considerably (Taborska 1971); likewise as individuals age the venom characteristics change. Reid and Theakston (1978) and Theakston and Reid (1978) reported that in specimens of *Crotalus atrox* up to 2 months old, the venom had a direct thrombin-like action on fibrinogen, between two and eight months it exerted a prothrombin-like action, clotting only plasma and not fibrinogen, and when the snakes reached 9 months the venom had no detectable plasma coagulant activity. Because of this type of variation in venom properties many of the clinical reports on snake bite envenoming in man are conflicting and confusing.

In spite of this type of regional, individual, and age variation, the majority of venoms, providing they are obtained from a large number of snakes of different age groups from the same area and pooled, do possess recognizable biological activities and produce reasonably clear clinical symptoms in human victims of snake bite as well as in experimental animals. For this reason it was decided initially to collect bulk amounts of eight venoms of major medical importance throughout the world and establish these as major reference reagents.

Collection of IRVs

The first eight IRVs and their sources are shown in Table 15.1. These are currently held at the WHO Collaborative Centre for the Control of Anti-venoms (CCCA), Liverpool School of Tropical Medicine, Liverpool, UK. It was estimated that the amount of each IRV required should be enough to allow for the production of 1000 ampoules of freeze-dried material for an international reagent and some ampoules for biological characterization by collaborating laboratories. In addition some of each venom should be reserved for the production of a standard monospecific antivenom preparation. The total amounts of each IRV collected for this purpose as well as the amounts of venom per ampoule for each species are shown in Table 15.1. *Crotalus adamanteus* venom was originally selected as an IRV but insufficient amounts of this venom were available; it was therefore decided to replace this with *C. atrox* venom as the IRV for the USA.

Processing of IRVs

Following collection, the IRVs were centrifuged and subsequently lyophilized. Prior to distribution into ampoules, the venoms were dissolved in distilled water and sterilized by Millipore filtration (0.22 μm filter); 40 ml of the solution was tested for sterility following the procedures adopted by Rijksinstituut voor Volksgezondheid en Milieuhygiene, Bilthoven, Holland (personal communication, E. J. Ruitenberg). Aliquots (1.0 ml) containing the required amount of venom were dispensed into all-glass 7.5 ml ampoules, frozen in liquid nitrogen and freeze-dried. The ampoules were subsequently heat-sealed. It is intended that the lyophilized venom will be tested for stability by accelerated degradation tests and also for accuracy of fill by weighing the quantity of venom contained in 10 ampoules (WHO 1981).

Inter-laboratory scheme for characterization of venoms

Samples of the eight IRVs will be sent to the 17 collaborating laboratories based in Czechoslavakia, Switzerland, Yugoslavia, UK, France, W. Germany, USA, Japan, Brazil, Pakistan, Iran, and Costa Rica. The venoms will be tested according to the schedule outlined in pp. 289–97, and the results of the tests will be co-ordinated by the WHO CCCA in Liverpool.

Venom characterization tests

At the WHO co-ordination meeting in 1979 (WHO 1981) it was concluded that methods for the estimation of lethal, defibrinogenating, procoagulant, haemorrhagic and necrotizing activities of venoms should be standardized

Table 15.1 Proposed international reference venoms (IRVs).

Species	Source	Area collected	Number of snakes	Length (cm)	Weight of venom (g)	Amount per ampoule (mg)
N. n. kaouthia	Thailand	Samutprakaan	15	90–100	10	1
N. scutatus	Australia	Portsea (S. Victoria) Lake George (Central New South Wales)	110	1000	10	1
E. carinatus	Mali		245	50–65	10	2
E. carinatus	Iran	Zabol (S.E. Iran)	3440	30–65 (adult) 20 <1 year)	10	2
V. russelli	Thailand	Saraburi Lopburi	20	90–100	15	2
C. atrox	Mexico	North	22	100–165 (adult)	30	10
B. atrox asper	Costa Rica	Atlantic	104	50–1000 41 per cent adult, 40 per cent middle, 20 per cent young)	30	10
T. flavoviridis	Japan	Ryukyu Is.			27	10

(Theakston and Reid 1983). It was also concluded that these tests should be simple and reproducible and capable of being carried out in collaborating laboratories throughout the world as part of the interlaboratory scheme for biological characterization of IRVs.

Tests for the estimation of neuromuscular paralytic activity of elapid venoms and for measuring systemic myotoxic activity are in the process of development in collaboration with Professor J. B. Harris of the University of Newcastle, UK. The former test will involve the use of mouse hemidiaphragm preparations to study the effect of whole venoms and venom fractions on the neuromuscular junction and the latter will most probably involve histopathological studies on the effect of venoms and muscles and/or the use of creatine phosphokinase (CPK-MM) estimations in experimental animals injected with different doses of venom.

A total of 53 venoms from 30 different species of snake, 20 of which are maintained at the Liverpool School of Tropical Medicine, were evaluated by the WHO CCCA during 1982/83 (Table 15.2). Six of the venoms were IRVs, tested before being dispensed into ampoules. The following tests were made (Theakston and Reid 1983).

Median lethal dose (LD_{50})   Lethal toxicity was assessed by the injection of different venom doses in 0.2 ml physiological saline (PSS) into the tail vein of male CFW-strain mice, using six 18–20 g animals at each dose level. The LD_{50} was calculated by probit analysis (Finney 1971) of deaths occurring within 24 h of venom injection.

Minimum coagulant does (MCD)   This is defined as the smallest amount of venom (in mg dry weight per litre of test solution) that clots either a solution of bovine fibrinogen (2 g l^{-1}) in 60 s at 37°C (MCD-F) and/or a standard citrated solution of human plasma (fibrinogen content 2.8 g l^{-1}) in 60 s at 37° (MCD-P). For measurement of the MCD-F, 50 μl of PSS with final venom concentrations ranging from 240 to 0.5 mg l^{-1} was added to 0.2 ml of bovine fibrinogen solution (2 g l^{-1}) at 37°C. The solutions were mixed thoroughly and the clotting time recorded. The MCD-P was estimated by adding the same venom concentrations to 0.2 ml of a standard human plasma solution under the same conditions and recording the clotting time. In each case, the MCD was calculated by plotting clotting time against venom concentration and reading off the level at the 60-s clotting time.

Minimum haemorrhagic dose (MHD)   This is defined as the smallest amount of venom (μg dry weight) which, when injected intradermally into rats, results in a haemorrhagic lesion of 10 mm diameter 24 h later. The method of Kondo, Kondo, Ikezawa, and Murata (1960) was used in rats. Aliquots of 0.1 ml of PSS containing between 120 and 5 μg of venom were

Table 15.2 Lethal, procoagulant, and necrotizing effects of 53 snake venoms[a].

Species	Source	No. of samples	LD$_{50}$[b] (µg/ mouse)	MDD (µg/ mouse)	MCD-P (mg/ litre)	MCD-F (mg/ litre)	MND (µg/ rat)	MHD (µg/ rat)
Colubrine:								
Rhabdophis subminiatus	Hong Kong	8	150.6 (136–172)	13.3	3.4	NA	NA	118.0
Viperine:								
Agkistrodon rhodostoma	Malaysia	50	107.5 (104–111)	0.9	18.4	32.6	48.0	60.0
Bitis arietans (immature)	Saudi Arabia	1	20.3 (16–24)	5.6	NA	NA	40.0	13.5
B. arietans (mature)	Nigeria	3	25.0 (20–29)	tr	NA	NA	25.5	26.5
B. gabonica	Nigeria	10	35.2 (29–40)	NA	tr	NA	39.0	20.4
Bothrops atrox asper	Costa Rica	?	43.0 (41–46)	7.8	1.4	18.0	40.0	70.0
B. nasutus	Costa Rica	?	135.1 (128–144)	NA	tr	NA	92.5	23.2
B. schlegelii	Costa Rica	?	39.0 (38–40)	12.2	13.2	153.0	60.0	28.2
Cerastes cerastes	Oman	12	10.0 (6–14)	5.8	152.0	NA	30.5	12.0
C. cerastes	Saudi Arabia	1	5.0 (3–7)	4.1	NA	NA	31.3	8.2
C. cerastes	Libyan Arab Jamahiriya	1	12.5 (8–15)	8.2	NA	NA	27.3	24.0
C. vipera	Israel	4	10.0 (6–12)	4.1	tr	NA	29.5	12.5
Crotalus adamanteus	N. America	2	50.4 (41–59)	27.8	73.0	84.0	45.0	40.0
C. adamanteus[c]	N. America	40	57.6 (54–63)	7.5	37.0	40.8	42.5	15.5
C. atrox (immature)	N. America	3	25.0 (21–28)	25.6	38.4	86.0	64.2	31.0
C. atrox (mature)	N. America	3	72.5 (69–76)	NA	NA	NA	30.5	25.5
C. atrox[d]	N. America	58	56.0 (42–65)	47.5	tr	tr	50.0	22.5
C. durissus	Costa Rica	3	28.1 (22–35)	11.6	59.0	55.0	37.5	29.0
C. viridis helleri	N. America	1	22.3 (20–25)	7.5	106.0	tr	NA	31.2
C. v. viridis (immature)	N. America	5	26.3 (24–28)	NA	NA	NA	28.0	77.5
C. v. viridis (mature)	N. America	5	25.0 (23–29)	NA	NA	NA	10.0	41.0
Echis carinatus	India	10+	19.0 (16–24)	3.0	14.0	NA	28.0	17.8
Echis carinatus	Islamic Republic of Iran	10+	12.2 (6–17)	1.6	2.0	NA	27.6	14.0
E. carinatus[d]	Islamic Republic of Iran	3440	17.9 (16–20)	2.5	2.2	NA	27.5	46.5
E. carinatus	Kenya	10	14.0 (12–15)	6.0	16.0	NA	26.0	18.2
E. carinatus	Kenya	61	12.0 (10–14)	1.2	14.0	NA	25.0	19.0
E. carinatus	Nigeria	13	8.1 (7–9)	5.3	3.0	NA	32.3	9.8
E. carinatus	Nigeria	4	17.3 (14–21)	2.9	4.0	NA	30.0	11.0

Table 15.2 (*continued*)

Species	Source	No. of samples	LD$_{50}$[b] (µg/ mouse)	MDD (µg/ mouse)	MCD-P (mg/ litre)	MCD-F (mg/ litre)	MND (µg/ rat)	MHD (µg/ rat)
E. carinatus	Oman	6	15.7 (14–18)	11.0	14.0	NA	12.0	4.6
E. carinatus	Pakistan	?	38.0 (30–46)	1.8	7.6	NA	50.0	23.0
E. carinatus	Saudi Arabia	5	75.3 (69–82)	9.0	NA	NA	22.0	18.6
E. coloratus	Saudi Arabia	3	24.9 (21–30)	3.0	13.0	NA	43.0	16.4
Lachesis muta	Costa Rica	?	110.0 (61–139)	4.0	17.5	17.0	37.0	16.5
Trimeresurus albolabris	Thailand	14	12.5 (9–15)	15.0	58.0	77.0	85.0	70.0
T. flavoviridis	Ryukyu Islands	?	75.1 (65–80)	163.0	NA	NA	50.0	40.8
T. flavoviridis[d]	Ryukyu Islands	?	183.0 (175–191)	95.0	NA	NA	35.0	160.0
T. macrops	Thailand	5	175.0 (140–192)	40.0	146.0	NA	146.5	23.5
T. popeorum/stejnegeri	Thailand	5	30.0 (21–39)	22.5	58.0	98.0	38.5	26.5
T. purpureomaculatus	Thailand	2	25.0 (14–36)	22.5	59.0	98.0	71.0	18.0
T. stejnegeri	?	?	90.0 (67–121)	0.8	29.0	35.0	55.0	62.0
T. wagleri	Thailand	2	12.5 (8–15)	NA	NA	NA	NA	NA
T. wagleri	Malaysia	?	15.0 (9–12)	NA	NA	NA	NA	NA
Vipera palaestinae	Israel	4	15.0 (13–18)	NA	NA	NA	60.0	15.8
V. russelli	India	10+	5.2 (4–6)	8.7[c]	NA	NA	4.0	21.5
V. russelli[d]	Thailand	20	2.7 (2–3)	4.4	NA	NA	38.0	39.0
V. russelli	Burma	?	4.0 (3–5)	95.0	tr	NA	23.0	3.0
Elapine:								
Micrurus nigrocinctus	Costa Rica	?	9.8 (8–13)	NA	tr	NA	60.0	NA
Naja naja naja	Malaysia	30	15.2 (14–17)	NA	NA	NA	50.0	NA
N. n. kaouthia[d]	Thailand	15	3.5 (3–4)	NA	NA	NA	30.0	NA
N. nigricollis	Nigeria	1	25.4 (20–29)	NA	NA	NA	14.5	NA
Notechis scutatus	Australia	?	4.5 (4–6)	tr	95.0	tr	30.0	NA
N. scutatus[d]	Australia	110 approx	0.8 (0.7–0.8)	NA	16.5	NA	35.5	42.3
Oxyuranus scutellatus	Australia	?	3.1 (2–4)	tr	13.8	NA	NA[f]	NA[f]

[a] NA = No activity; tr = trace activity, i.e., 1.2–2.0 LD$_{50}$ (MDD), 240 mg/litre (MCD), and 120 µg (MND, MHD).
[b] 95% confidence limits are given in parentheses.
[c] Previous international standard venom, now replaced by *C. atrox*.
[d] International reference venom.
[e] Result obtained by extrapolation (FPT test).
[f] No activity with 5-µg dose; rat died with 10 µg.

injected into the shaved dorsal skin of 250 g male Sprague Dawley rats under light ether anaesthesia. After 24 h the animals were killed, the dorsal skin removed, and the diameter of the lesion measured on the inner surface of the skin, in two directions at right angles, using callipers and background illumination. Care was taken not to stretch the skin. The mean diameter of the haemorrhagic lesion was calculated for each venom dose and the MHD estimated by plotting mean lesion diameter against venom dose and reading off the dose corresponding to the 10 mm diameter.

Minimum necrotizing dose (MND)   This is defined as the smallest amount of venom (μg dry weight) which, when injected intradermally into rats, results in a necrotic lesion of 5 mm diameter 3 days later. The method used was the same as that for the MHD except that the dorsal skin was removed three days after intradermal injection of venom. The MND was calculated by plotting mean lesion diameter against venom dose and reading off the dose corresponding to a diameter of 5 mm.

Minimum defibrinogenating dose (MDD)   For measurement of the MDD, a wide range of doses was selected for each venom tested and each dose was injected intravenously into four mice. One hour after injection, the mice were anaesthetized with ether and bled by cardiac puncture. The blood was pooled and divided into two equal portions, one of which was tested using the whole blood clotting method (MDD-WBC), while the other was mixed with citrate containing 50 g l^{-1} aminocaproic acid to prevent fibrinolysis, and tested using the fibrin polymerization time test (MDD-FPT).

In the whole blood clotting method, the blood was placed in a clotting tube and left at room temperature for 1–2 h. The clot quality was then recorded using the '1–5' grading system (Reid 1967). The MDD-WBC was defined as the minimum dose of venom that produced non-clotting blood within 60 minutes of intravenous injection.

To determine the fibrin polymerization time (FPT), blood was taken from 10 normal mice, mixed with citrate containing 50 g l^{-1} aminocaproic acid, and pooled. The plasma was diluted with PSS to give final plasma concentrations ranging from 100 per cent to 10 per cent. An aliquot of 0.4 ml of each plasma dilution was added to 0.9 ml of PSS, followed by 0.1 ml of thrombin (600 IU ml^{-1}). The time taken for a web of fibrin to form on a gently agitated glass rod was then plotted against log plasma concentration to give a standard curve (Vermylen, Vreker, and Verstraete 1963). The actual amount of fibrinogen present in the sample was determined by carrying out a similar assay using known amounts of bovine fibrinogen. Aliquots of 0.4 ml of each unknown citrated test portion were treated as described above. Using the computed standard curve, the fibrinogen content of the test sample was determined 1 h after injection of venom. The

MDD-FPT was defined as the dose of venom resulting in a decrease in the fibrinogen level to 10 per cent of that for the standard plasma fibrinogen solution.

The results of these tests carried out on the 53 venoms are shown in Table 6.2. A close correlation was observed between the results of the two tests for defibrinogenating activity ($r = 0.99$, $p<0.001$). The advantages of the whole blood clotting method are that it is simpler, does not necessitate expert supervision, and is much more economical in terms of materials — the method has also been used extensively on snake bite patients (Reid *et al.* 1963a). For the majority of situations this is, therefore, the method of preference. The main advantage of the FPT method is that it gives a direct estimation of fibrinogen levels — non-coagulability may, in certain situations, be due to lack of procoagulant factors other than fibrinogen and antithrombin may interfere (Blomback, personal communication 1980). Of 45 viperine venoms 35 (78 per cent) had defibrinogenating activity, the most active being the IRV, *Vipera russelli* (Thailand). None of the elapine venoms possessed more than a trace of this activity (Table 15.2).

Although defibrinogenation following snake bite is remarkably benign and is not in itself a primary cause of spontaneous bleeding (Reid *et al.* 1963a; Reid, Thean, Chan, and Baharom 1963b), the results suggest that if the MDD is near to or greater than the LD_{50}, then defibrinogenation in humans following a bite has serious clinical implications (Theakston and Reid 1983); this observation would apply to the venoms of *V. russelli*, *E. carinatus* (Nigeria and Oman), immature *C. atrox* (Reid and Theakston 1978), *Cerastes cerastes*, *Trimeresurus flavoviridis*, and *C. adamanteus*. The venoms of *Oxyuranus scutellatus*, mature *B. arietans*, and *Notechis scutatus* possess a trace of defibrinogenating activity, and if this effect was observed in snake bite victims bitten by these species, the prognosis would be extremely grave. Conversely when the MDD is much less than the LD_{50}, defibrinogenation is unlikely to have serious clinical implications (e.g. *Calloselasma rhodostoma* venom). It should also be noted that the defibrinogenating capacity of some venoms may change as the snakes age, as for example in the case of *C. atrox* (Reid and Theakston 1978; Theakston and Reid 1978) and *B. arietans*.

Seven venoms from five species had defibrinogenating activity but no detectable *in vitro* clotting activity as assessed by the MCD test. It seems likely that, in some cases, other factors may be involved in defibrinogenation or that the MDD test is more sensitive than that used for the MCD. The MCD test showed that 12 venoms had a direct thrombin-like action on fibrinogen and therefore also clotted plasma. Twelve viperine venoms including the IRV *E. carinatus* (Iran), two elapid venoms including *N. scutatus* (IRV) and the venom of the colubrid, *Rhabdophis subminiatus*, exerted a thromboplastic-like action only; two venoms had a milder thromboplastic-like action on plasma and trace activity on fibrinogen. Trace procoagulant activity was detected in the venoms of five viperine and three elapine species (including the IRVs, *T. flavoviridis*, and *N. kaouthia*). At the limits of the test, the venom of Saudi Arabian *E. carinatus* was remarkable in that no significant clotting action on plasma was recorded unlike the venoms of *E. carinatus* from six other geographical areas (in fact, plasma was clotted by the Saudi Arabian venom, but only with venom concentrations of three times the maximum amount normally used in the test; MCD-P 870 mg l^{-1}). It should be noted, however, that the Saudi Arabian venom did cause defibrinogenation *in vivo*. Similarly, of 12 specimens of *C. cerastes* from Oman only one had strongly procoagulant venom. Likewise Taborska (1971) reported that of venoms from 21 individual specimens of *E. carinatus* collected from Karachi, Pakistan, eight showed no detectable clotting activity on human oxalated plasma. This again implies a considerable amount of both inter- and intra-regional variation in venom clotting activity. The age of the snake may also contribute to this (Reid and Theakston 1978; Theakston and Reid 1978).

The only elapid venom showing haemorrhagic activity was the IRV from *N. scutatus*, whereas almost all the viperine venoms tested has some activity in this respect (Table 15.2). These observations are supported by the observation of Reid (1968) that haemorrhage caused by the action of powerful proteases on the vascular endothelium is the outstanding feature of viperine poisoning. It is not a general characteristic of elapid envenoming. Although haemorrhage following viperine poisoning is frequently accompanied by a clotting defect and may indeed aggravate it, these activities are not necessarily related, and often the factors responsible for haemorrhage can be separated from those responsible for the coagulation defect (Esnouf and Tunnah 1967). A coagulation defect in itself does not lead to haemorrhage. The most haemorrhagic venom studied was that of Burmese *V. russelli*; venom from immature *B. arietans* was twice as haemorrhagic as that from mature snakes, although it should be noted that these snakes originated in different geographical areas (Nigeria and Saudi Arabia).

Forty-eight out of 53 (91 per cent) of the venoms tested caused local necrosis following intradermal injection, and the MND test proved reasonably reliable for assessing this activity. The assay should have application for estimating the rather doubtful neutralizing ability of most commercial antivenoms against the local necrotizing action of many medically important venoms. Local necrotizing activity is not necessarily related to local haemorrhagic activity.

For estimation of the minimum neuromuscular paralytic dose (MNPD) it is hoped to develop an *in vitro* assay using the mouse hemidiaphragm; the muscle will be mounted so that it can be stimulated either directly (by appropriate electrodes applied to the muscle) or indirectly (by stimulating the phrenic nerve). Such preparations can be stimulated both before and after addition of the venom suspected to initiate neuromuscular blockade. If both direct and indirect responses are reduced, this will indicate that the venom is causing direct suppression of the contractibility of the muscle; if only the indirect nerve response is inhibited, this will imply that the venom is inhibiting neuromuscular transmission either by blockade of transmitter receptor or by suppression of transmitter release, or both. This assay system is being developed in collaboration with Professor J. B. Harris, of the University of Newcastle, UK. Likewise it is also intended to develop a simple procedure for assaying the minimum systemic myotoxic dose (MSMD) of venoms using either histological techniques and/or CPK-MM isoenzyme estimations.

The development of reliable tests is necessary if antivenoms are to be graded easily and consistently in different laboratories in terms of their venom neutralizing abilities. This applies especially to the IRVs that have been selected because of their medical importance worldwide. As with all animal-based studies, however, great caution is urged when extrapolating the results of venom characterization tests to envenoming in humans.

WHO International Standard Antivenoms (ISAs)

Production of ISAs

The WHO standard monospecific antivenoms are being manufactured by different laboratories against each of the IRVs, using the methods described by the WHO (1981). Table 15.3 shows the laboratories concerned in the scheme for ISA production. Each ISA will comprise an almost pure F(ab)$_2$ plasma fraction, the volume of fill being 5 ml of a 100 g l^{-1} protein solution in a 20-ml vial. The 5 ml volume will be isotonic and will contain 20 g l^{-1} glycine at pH 6.4–6.8. The final preparation will be freeze-dried.

Following preparation each ISA will be assayed for protein nitrogen,

Table 15.3 International Standard Antivenoms (ISAs).

Antivenom	Laboratory
Naja naja kaouthia	Commonwealth Serum Laboratories, Australia
Notechis scutatus	Commonwealth Serum Laboratories, Australia
Echis carinatus (Mali)	Pasteur Institute, France
Echis carinatus (Iran)	Razi Institute, Iran
Vipera russelli	Razi Institute, Iran
Crotalus atrox	Gerencia General de Biologicos y Reactivos, Mexico
Bothrops atrox asper	Instituto National de Higine, Mexico
Trimeresurus flavoviridis	National Institute of Health, Japan

moisture content, and sterility. Purity will also be determined by immunoelectrophoresis, polyacrylamide gel electrophoresis, and analytical centrifugation.

At least 5500 vials of each ISA will be maintained at the Copenhagen Serum Institute as international standard preparations, and it is estimated that these stocks should last for at least 10 years. This means that a pooled stock of 27.5 l of each ISA will be required; at the Zurich meeting it was suggested that producers should aim for 30 l so that 5500 vials remain after antivenom standardization.

Proposed inter-laboratory scheme for the standardization of antivenom

It is hoped that all the laboratories involved in the venom characterization tests will also carry out the neutralization tests on the ISAs. The results of these assays will be co-ordinated by the WHO CCCA. The tests will first be used to assay the neutralizing potency of the ISAs, so that these are completely standardized. These antivenoms will therefore act as true standards, with which both newly developed and currently available antivenoms can be compared. It is hoped that this will eventually result in the development and production of more potent antivenoms for use in developing countries and thus improve the understanding and management of snake bite throughout the world.

Antivenom standardization tests

Each ISA will be tested for its ability to neutralize the pharmacological properties of the respective IRV using the tests already developed for the characterization of IRVs. It is important that for each test the same weight and type of animal and route of injection is used in *in vivo* tests as was used previously in the venom characterization tests. Likewise, mixtures of venom and antivenom should be incubated for 1 h at 37°C before being inoculated into animals or before being used in *in vitro* tests.

Median effective dose (ED_{50}) Five intravenous mouse ED_{50}s are to be mixed with different doses of antivenom, incubated at 37°C for 1 h and injected in 0.2 ml PSS into the tail vein of 18–20 g male white mice. Six animals are to be used at each venom dose. The ED_{50} will be calculated by a probit analysis (Finney 1971) of deaths occurring within 24 h of the injection of the venom/antivenom mixture.

Neutralization of coagulant activity (ANA-MCD-P/F) IRV at the MCD-F and MCD-P concentrations will be mixed with different amounts of antivenom (ISA), incubated together at 37°C for 1 h, and subsequently used in the MCD tests to determine the neutralizing activity of the ISA on procoagulant activity. The antivenom neutralizing activity (ANA-MCD-P/F) is defined as the amount of standard antivenom in μl that reduces the MCD to zero (i.e. complete neutralization of procoagulant activity).

Neutralization of haemorrhagic activity (ANA-MHD)   IRV at the MHD is to be mixed with different amounts of antivenom (ISA). These are then incubated together at 37°C for 1 h and subsequently used in the MHD test to determine the neutralizing activity of the ISA on haemorrhagic activity. The antivenom neutralizing activity (ANA-MHD) is defined as the amount of standard antivenom in μl that reduces the MHD to zero (i.e. no haemorrhagic lesion, no haemorrhagic effect) in rats injected intradermally with the venom/antivenom mixture and examined for the presence of a haemorrhagic lesion 24 h later.

Neutralization of necrotizing activity (ANA-MND)   The method is the same as that used for estimation of neutralizing potency against venom haemorrhagic activity, except that the rats are examined for the presence/ absence of the necrotic lesion 3 days after injection of the venom/antivenom mixture. The antivenom neutralizing activity (ANA-MND) is defined as the amount of standard antivenom (in μl per rat) that reduces the MND to zero.

Neutralization of defibrinogenating activity (ANA-MDD)   Venom at the MDD is to be mixed with different amounts of ISA; the mixture is then incubated at 37°C for 1 h before intravenous injection into four mice at each dose. The antivenom neutralizing activity (ANA-MDD) is defined as the minimum amount of standard antivenom (in μl per mouse) that results in fully non-clotting blood (ANA-MDD-WBC) or 100 per cent fibrinogen levels (ANA-MDD-FPT) within 60 min of intravenous injection of the mixture.

Future developments

It is understood that antivenom producers have to make some estimation of neutralizing potency with respect to their products; usually this is presented as the number of lethal doses or the dry weight of a particular venom neutralized by a known volume of antivenom. Christensen (1968) rightly stated that such measures of potency are pointless unless the different laboratories use identical methods in relation to the test animal, route of injection, and the composition of the venom/antivenom mixtures. He also stressed that the same venom sample must be used in the assays. It is well established that considerable biological variation exists in venoms from the same species in different biological areas, as well as between individuals from the same area (Taborska 1971). Venoms also change in biological characteristics as snakes age (Reid and Theakston 1978; Theakston and

Reid 1978). In 1968 Christensen proposed that such problems may be avoided by expressing potencies of commercial products against a standard antivenom preparation. Even when it is possible to determine the potency of an antivenom against an individual pharmacological component of the venom concerned, a standard serum would still be useful; but it could then be expected that potency estimates would be to an extent independent of such factors as test level, test animal and route of injection.

Christensen considered that eventually the use of animals could largely be replaced by *in vitro* methods for estimation of antivenom neutralizing activity. This is not simply of importance because of the difficulty of extrapolating between non-human species and humans; it is highly desirable to avoid the suffering and death of animals. If *in vitro* methods measure life-saving capability with a precision similar to that of *in vivo* methods, a major reason for the continued use of animals would be eliminated. That such a system is possible was demonstrated by Theakston and Reid (1979), who investigated ELISA as a screen of antivenom potency. These workers used one batch of antivenom from each of three commercial sources (SAIMR, Behringwerke, Haffkine) and two antisera raised in rabbits in research laboratories. The five sera were used as reference antivenoms, and the ED_{50}s for neutralizing four venoms of medical importance in Africa (*E. carinatus*, *B. arietans*, *N. nigricollis*, *N. naje*), were estimated in mice. Reference curves were prepared relating ED_{50}s to optical densities with ELISA. The ED_{50}s of 38 different batches of test antivenom were estimated by ELISA, and 'ELISA ED_{50}s' were then compared with *in vivo* mouse ED_{50}s. Excellent correlation was obtained ($r = 0.96$; $p<0.001$) and the method proved to be rapid, cheap, simple, economic in amounts of venom used, and most importantly, greatly reduced the need for live animals. If validated in an extended range of venoms and antivenoms, ELISA screening of antivenom potency could be a useful standard procedure. ELISA measures antibody (or antigen), and it is realized that antigen–antibody reactions of venoms and their degree of toxicity are two distinct and sometimes unrelated phenomena (Schottler 1951). Antigens may be non-toxic and toxins may be non-antigenic. Nevertheless, these preliminary studies suggest sufficient correlation between *in vivo* mouse ED_{50}s and ELISA optical density readings to warrant further exploration of this system.

Further possibilities as far as the improvement of the quality of antivenoms are concerned involve the development of new methods of immunization, including the possible use of specially treated membrane-stabilized liposomes for stimulating a rapid and sustained high-titre protective antibody response in experimental animals following a single immunizing injection. Research on this subject is being carried out at the present (New, Theakston, Zumbuehl, Iddon, and Friend 1984, 1985), and it is hoped to extend the study into larger animals. It may eventually be of use in immunization of humans in areas where snake bite is a high risk factor. A further possibility is that it may well be possible to freeze-dry such preparations. The possibility of oral immunization using these procedures is also being investigated (New *et al.* 1984). Antivenoms developed using this or similar methods should result in cheaper, more avid antivenoms, which would be greatly welcomed in developing countries where snake bite is a serious problem.

The development of avid monoclonal antibodies active against pathological venom fractions may be a further possibility. The mode of action of antivenom, i.e. how antibodies neutralize venom toxins, is not known and is probably variable from one toxin to another. To improve antivenom serotherapy, it is critically important to determine whether antibodies interact at the toxic or enzymatic site of the molecule or at an unrelated antigenic site, and which isotype of immunoglobulin is most effective in its neutralizing activity. Recent work by Boulain, Ménez, Couder, Faure, Liacopoulos, Fromageot (1982) and Boulain and Ménez (1982) in France suggest that in the case of the α-neurotoxin of *N. nigricollis* venom, a monoclonal antibody with an epitope localized at a distance from the ACH-binding site can effectively interact with venom-ACH binding, either by inhibition of binding or by dislocation of the association when binding has already occurred (see Ménez *et al.* pp. 332–45 of this volume). This latter mode of action is consistent with the kinetics of antivenom activity after neurotoxin poisoning in humans, in that serum remains beneficial for several days after snake bite. The major implication of the results obtained in this model system (the venom of *N. nigricollis* is one of the few elapid venoms that apparently lacks neurotoxic activity in humans) is that a well-chosen polypeptide fraction of a toxin, could, when linked to a suitable carrier/adjuvant, be used for immunization to prepare antivenom without the usual toxic side effects. Such a molecule could possibly be used for preventive immunization of individuals at high risk.

The immunization procedures used for the commercial production of antivenom (mostly in horses) generally use whole venom (WHO 1981). Consequently the antivenom produced is often not very effective in its venom-neutralizing activity and large amounts have to be used in therapeutic treatment of seriously poisoned snake-bite victims. This increases the risks of both immediate (life-threatening) and delayed serum reactions (Sutherland and Lovering 1979). For example, in *E. carinatus* envenoming in W. Africa 20 ml of SAIMR monospecific anti-*Echis* administered by slow intravenous infusion are usually required, and 40 ml of Behringwerke polyvalent (*Bitis-Echis-Naja*) (Warrell, Davidson, Greenwood, Ormerod, Pope, Watkins, and Prentice 1977); in poisoning by elapids such as the Thai cobra (*N. kaouthia*), up to 450 ml may have to be used to reverse the symptoms of severe systemic poisoning, and a total 1150 ml has been reported necessary for the treatment of poisoning due to the king cobra, *Ophiophagus hannah* (Ganthavorn 1971). Moreover, in view of the high toxicity of the antigen to the animal, it is often necessary to immunize with atoxic venom (i.e. venom which has been chemically detoxified causing a reduction in antigenicity, or adsorbed to some inert carrier such as bentonite (Christensen 1966). The use of avid monoclonal antibodies either alone, as a mixture, or as an additive to currently available commercial preparations, may result in the use of smaller volumes of antivenom being required for treatment of patients.

References

Boulain, J.-C. and Ménez, A. (1982). Neurotoxin-specific immunoglobulins accelerate dissociation of the neurotoxin-acetylcholine receptor complex. *Science* **217**, 732–3.

——, ——, Couderc, J., Faure, G., Liacopoulos, P., and Fromageot, P. (1982). Neutralizing monoclonal antibody specific for *Naja nigricollis* Toxin α: preparation, characterization and localization of the antigenic binding site. *Biochemistry* **21**, 2910–15.

Christensen, P. A. (1962). Antivenom standardization. Progress report, WHO Expert Committee on Biological Standardization. Geneva, 10–15 December.

—— (1966). The preparation and purification of antivenoms. *Mem. Inst. Butantan. Simp. Int.* **33**, 245–50.

—— (1968). The venoms of Central and South African snakes. In *Venomous animals and their venoms. Vol. 1 Venomous vertebrates* (ed. W. Bucherl, E. E. Buckley, and V. Deulofeu), pp. 437–461. Academic Press, New York.

Esnouf, M. P. and Tunnah, G. W. (1967). The isolation and properties of the thrombin-like activity from *Ancistrodon rhodostoma* venom. *Br. J. Haematol.* **13**, 581–90.

Finney, D. J. (1971). *Probit analysis* (3rd edn). Cambridge University Press, Cambridge.

Ganthavorn, S. (1971). A case of king cobra bite. *Toxicon* **9**, 293–4.

Harms, A. J. (1948). The purification of antitoxic plasmas by enzyme treatment and heat denaturation. *Biochem. J.* **42**, 390–7.

Kondo, H., Kondo, S., Ikezawa, H., and Murata, R. (1960). Studies on the quantitative method for determination of haemorrhagic activity of Habu snake venom. *Jap. J. Med. Sci. Biol.* **13**, 43–51.

New, R. R. C., Theakston, R. D. G., Zumbuehl, O., Iddon, D., and Friend, J. (1984). Immunization against snake venoms. *New Eng. J. Med.* **311**, 56–7.

——, ——, ——, ——, and —— (1985). Liposomal immunization against snake venoms. *Toxicon* **23**, 215–19.

Pope, C. G. (1939a). The action of proteolytic enzymes on the antitoxins and proteins of immune sera. I. True digestion of the proteins. *Br. J. exp. Pathol.* **20**, 132–49.

—— (1939b). The action of proteolytic enzymes on the antitoxins and proteins of immune sera. II. Heat denaturation after partial enzyme action. *Br. J. exp. Pathol.* **20**, 201–12.

Reid, H. A. (1967). Defibrination by *Agkistrodon rhodostoma* venom. In *Animal toxins. First International Symposium on Animal Toxins*, Atlantic City, New Jersey, 9–11 April 1966 (ed. F. E. Russell, and P. R. Saunders). Pergamon Press, Oxford.

—— (1968). Pathology and treatment of land snake bite in India and Southeast Asia. In: *Venomous animals and their venoms. Vol. 1, Venomous vertebrates* (ed. W. Bucherl, E. E. Buckley, and V. Deulofeu), pp. 611–42. Academic Press, New York.

—— and Theakston, R. D. G. (1978). Changes in coagulation effects by venoms of *Crotalus atrox* as snakes age. *Am. J. trop. Med. Hyg.* **27**, 1053–7.

——, Chan, K. E., and Thean, P. C. (1963a). Prolonged coagulation defect (defibrination syndrome) in Malayan viper bite. *Lancet* **1**, 621–6.

——, Thean, P. C., Chan, K. E., and Baharom, A. R. (1963b). Clinical effects of bites by Malayan viper (*Ancistrodon rhodostoma*). *Lancet* **1**, 617–21.

Schottler, W. H. A. (1951). Antigen-antibody relations in the present antivenin production of Brazil. *Am. J. trop. Med. Hyg.* **31**, 500–9.

Sutherland, S. K. and Lovering, K. E. (1979). Antivenoms: use and adverse reactions over a 12-month period in Australia and Papua New Guinea. *Med. J. Austr.* **2**, 671–4.

Taborska, E. (1971). Intraspecies variability of the venom of *Echis carinatus*. *Physiol. bohemoslov.* **20**, 307–18.

Theakston, R. D. G. and Reid, H. A. (1978). Changes in biological properties of venom from *Crotalus atrox* with ageing. *Period. biol.* **80**, 123–33.

—— and Reid, J. A. (1979). Enzyme-linked immunosorbent assay (ELISA) in assessing antivenom potency. *Toxicon* **17**, 511–15.

—— and Reid, H. A. (1983). Development of simple standard assay procedures for the characterization of snake venoms. *Bull. WHO* **61**, 949–56.

Vermylen, C., Vrcker, R. A. D., and Verstracte, M. (1963). A rapid enzymatic method for assay of fibrinogen. Fibrin Polymerisation Time (FPT Test). *Clin. chim. acta*, **8**, 418–24.

Warrell, D. A., Davidson, N. McD., Greenwood, B. M., Ormerod, L. D., Pope, H. M., Watkins, B. J., and Prentice, C. R. M. (1977). Poisoning by bites by the saw-scaled or carpet viper (*Echis carinatus*) in Nigeria. *Q. J. Med.* **46**, 33–62.

WHO (1981). *Progress in the characterization of venoms and standardization of antivenoms.* Offset Publication No. 58. World Health Organization, Geneva.

16

Live oral cholera vaccines: a new toxin produced by candidate strains

Suhas C. Sanyal

Introduction

Justification for live oral cholera vaccine

For the past 100 years, since the first trial by Ferran (1885), attempts to immunize against cholera have relied upon parental vaccines. These have included a killed *Vibrio cholerae* vaccine (Oseasohn, Benenson, and Fahimuddin 1965), a purified lipopolysaccharide vaccine (Benenson, Mosley, Fahimuddin, and Oseason 1968), an adjuvanted toxoid vaccine (Curlin, Levine, Aziz, Rahman, and Verwey 1976) and two aluminium-adjuvanted killed *V. cholerae* vaccines (Joó and Csizér 1978; Saroso, Bahrawi, Witjaksono, Budiarso, Brotowasisto, Benćić, Dewitt, and Gomez 1978; Pal 1977). Although each evoked high titres of serum antibody, none was protective for more than a few months (Feeley and Gangarosa 1980).

Two lines of evidence suggest that the goal of immunization should be stimulation of an immune response in intestinal lymphoid tissue and that this may be best done by giving antigen orally (Sack 1980; Pierce 1981). First, it is known that *V. cholerae* is non-invasive (Gangarosa, Biesel, Benyajati, Spring, and Piyaratn 1960) — it causes diarrhoea by colonizing the small intestine (Freter and Jones 1976; Schrank and Verwey 1976) and secreting cholera toxin, which acts directly upon intestinal epithelium to stimulate water and electrolyte secretion (Sack 1980). Any immunological defence against this process would have to work at the mucosal surface or within the bowel lumen.

Second, lymphoid tissues closely associated with mucosal surfaces appear to play a major role in mucosal surface defence (Gearheart and Cebra 1979). A major product of this system is s1gA antibody, which is stimulated by absorbed antigens and actively secreted onto the mucosal surface (Pierce and Koster 1981). Present evidence indicates that immunity to cholera is mediated largely or entirely by sIgA antibodies (Cray, Tokunaga, and Pierce 1983).

Support for the possible effectiveness of oral immunization against cholera also comes from evidence that enteric exposure to *V. cholerae* causes substantial immunity to cholera. In endemic areas, multiple accidental ingestions of the organism cause an age-related acquisition of immunity (Mosley 1969). Studies in volunteers show that persons convalescent from a single episode of induced cholera are highly protected against rechallenge for at least 1–3 years (Cash, Music, Libonati, Craig, Pierce, and Hornick 1974; Levine, Black, Clements, Nalin, Cisneros, and Finkelstein 1981).

Protective antigens of Vibrio cholerae

The antigens of *V. cholerae* that evoke protective immune responses are only partly understood. Best studied amongst them are lipopolysaccharide (Holmgren and Svennerholm 1977; Chitnis, Sharma, and Kamat 1982), which includes serogroup and serotype antigens, and cholera toxin (Lange and Holmgren 1978; Pierce 1978). Both antigens have been shown to be capable of evoking protective antibodies. Other antigens that may also stimulate protective immune responses but are incompletely studied include cell-associated haemagglutinins (Chaicumpa and Attasishtha 1977; Foo and Chaicumpa 1981), flagellar sheath protein, and other flagellar antigens (Eubanks, Guentzel and Berry 1977; Hranitzky, Mulholland, Larson, Eubanks, and Hart 1980; Attridge and Rowley 1983), other membrane proteins (Kabir 1980, 1983; Kelley and Parker 1981), cholera lectin (Finkelstein, Boesman-Finkelstein, and Holt 1983), and various extracellular enzymes such as proteases (Schneider and Parker 1978), neuraminidase (Burnet and Stone 1947; Freter 1955), and mucinase (Jensen 1953).

Available strains for live oral cholera vaccine

Isolation of nontoxigenic *Vibrio cholerae* 01 strains from diverse environmental sources, such as sewage, oysters, and brackish water, has been reported from Bangladesh, Brazil, Guam, UK, India, Japan, USA, USSR, and Australia (WHO Scientific Working Group 1980). Such strains were also isolated from human intestinal and extra-intestinal infections. Many of them failed to demonstrate any homology with *Escherichia coli* heat-labile toxin (LT) and cholera toxin (CT) genes (Kaper and Levine 1981; Kaper, Mosley, and Falkow 1981). These strains, therefore, had not been recognized as a cause of acute diarrhoea, even though, for almost a decade, numerous cases of acute diarrhoea had been attributed to unexplainable contamination of the very types of marine environments where the mutant *V. cholerae* 01 varieties were known to exist. Especially in the United States, Western Europe, and Australia, which have been free of cholera epidemics for decades, minor cholera outbreaks were thought to have been caused by bacteria that had somehow been imported to the area. No one believed the bacteria to be indigenous. This was the case with minor outbreaks in Louisiana and Texas that began in 1973, continued each year, and culminated in a total of 21 cases in 1981 alone (WHO 1982). The first scientific report to the contrary appeared in 1980 (Blake, Allegra, Snyder, Barrett, McFarland, Caraway, Feeley, Craig, Lee, Puhr, and Feldman 1980), concerning a mini-outbreak in Louisiana in 1978. There, the disease was traced to cooked crabs from local marshes. Investigators concluded that the bacteria responsible had been indigenous to the area for at least 8 years. Nevertheless, most scientists did not connect this finding with the toxin-gene deficient mutant cholera strains found in the marine environments.

The genetic evidence for the absence of CT or LT genes in the mutant *V. cholerae* strains has encouraged researchers to use them (or laboratory tailored CT gene-deletion mutant strains of *V. cholerae* 01 possessing other functions, such as the ability to colonize the small intestine) as potential candidates for a live oral cholera vaccine (Kaper and Levine 1981; Levine, Black, Clements, Cisneros, Saah, Nalin, Gill, Craig, Young, and Ristaino 1982; Mekalanos, Mosley, Murphy, and Falkow 1982).

Live oral cholera vaccines

Critera for an ideal vaccine strain

In principle, a live oral vaccine must be (a) non-pathogenic for humans, (b) genetically stable, (c) able to proliferate in the upper small bowel, (d) able to induce local antibodies to both anti-colonizing and anti-subunit B activity, and (e) capable of stimulating long-term protection (Levine, Black, Clements, Cisneros, Nalin, and Young 1981).

While no naturally occurring or laboratory derived *V. cholerae* strain has yet been identified that fulfils all these criteria, certain candidate vaccine strains show much promise that they exhibit many of the above-mentioned qualities. These candidate vaccine strains have been isolated as (a) naturally occurring avirulent strains, (b) plasmid or phage-induced attenuated strains, (c) chemically mutagenized strains, and (d) genetically engineered strains.

Naturally occurring avirulent strains

Mukerjee (1963, 1965) isolated several strains of *V. cholerae* biotype *eltor* from the Middle East and Calcutta. These proved to be apathogenic in adult rabbit ileal loops (De and Chatterjee 1953) and infant rabbits (Dutta and Habbu 1955), and this characteristic was stable even after several serial passages through these animal models. Intraduodenal immunization of rabbits with the non-pathogenic strains conferred antitoxic immunity (Bhattacharya, Narayanaswami, and Mukerjee 1968; Sanyal, Narayanaswami, and Mukerjee 1969a,b; Bhattacharya and Mukerjee 1970). The vaccine strains colonized and multiplied in the ligated intestinal loops of adult rabbits and in the intestine of infant rabbits without producing pathogenic reactions; immunization with a single dose of live vaccine could protect the animals against subsequent challenge with virulent *V. cholerae* strains of both classical and *eltor* biotypes. Immunization was further found to inhibit the growth of homologous strains in the ligated ileal loop and to reduce markedly the growth rate of pathogenic classical and *eltor* biotype *V. cholerae* strains (Bhattacharya and Mukerjee 1968b; Sanyal *et al.* 1969b). Administration of live vaccine was followed by a significant rise in antibody titre in serum as well as in intestinal secretions (Bhattacharya and Mukerjee 1968a; Sanyal *et al.* 1969b). After vaccination with *V. cholerae* strain EW-6, cell-bound antibodies could be demonstrated in intestinal epithelial cells of adult rabbits by immunofluorescent technique (Sanyal, Narayanaswami, and Mukerjee 1969c). In view of the promising results of animal experiments, a systematic volunteer trial of strain EW-6 was carried out in 25 adult humans. It showed a statistically significant increase in serum vibriocidal titres on oral administration of the vaccine strain EW-6 in doses of 10^9 or 10^{10} colony-forming units (c.f.u.) after neutralization of stomach acidity (Sanyal and Mukerjee 1969). Co-proantibodies, including IgA, were also present in the stool samples (Sanyal, Narayanaswami, and Mukerjee 1971). Serum antibody and co-proantibody titres persisted throughout the observation periods of 3 and 6 months, respectively. None of the volunteers suffered any inconvenience during the trial. Despite two successive passages through human intestine there was no change in pathogenicity of the strain. However, in only four of the 25 volunteers could viable vibrios be isolated from the stool.

Although this vaccine showed promising results, it did not go to field trial, probably because the idea of using live vaccine was not popular in the 1960s and because, at that time, the toxoid appeared to be a good immunizing agent.

Two strains (nos. 1196–78 and 1074–78) of *V. cholerae* biotype *eltor*, serotype Ogawa, were isolated from sewage water in Santos, Brazil (WHO 1979). The strains were found to be non-enterotoxigenic (Levine 1980) in the Y1 adrenal cell assay (Sack and Sack 1975), GM1 ganglioside enzyme-linked immunosorbent assay (Sack, Huda, Neogi, Daniel, and Spira 1980), pigeon erythrocyte lysate assay (Gill and King 1975) and the rabbit skin permeability factor (PF) assay (Craig, Yamamoto, Takeda, and Miwatani 1981). Both the strains were found to lack tox genes (Kaper *et al.* 1981). When fed to 20 human volunteers in doses of 10^6 or 10^8 c.f.u. with $NaHCO_3$ these strains did not induce clinical illness (Levine *et al.* 1982). Eight of the

13 volunteers who ingested strain 1196–78 had a few vibrios each in co-pro-cultures and an increase in vibriocidal antibody, but none had a rise in serum antitoxin. Four volunteers who excreted strain 1196–78 and six controls were challenged one month later with 10^6 c.f.u. of *V. cholerae* eltor E7946, a strain isolated during a cholera epidemic in Bahrain. Attack rates and severity of cholera were similar in both groups.

It appears, therefore that the lack of antitoxin response and a minimal degree of intestinal colonization by 1196–78 were responsible for the failure to prevent clinical infection due to pathogenic *V. cholerae*.

Attenuation following conjugation

Srivastava, Sinha, and Srivastava (1979) isolated two avirulent strains *V. cholerae* (no CDI and CD3) after bacterial mating between a virulent donor and an attenuated slow growing recipient strain of low adherence. The strains proved to be nontoxigenic in experimental models. Rabbits immunized orally with three doses at 21 days apart, when challenged at regular intervals up to 90 days with virulent Ogawa and Inaba strains of classical and *eltor* biotypes showed 60–89 per cent protection (Srivastava 1981). The strains were not tested in humans.

Plasmid-induced attenuation

Some strains of *V. cholerae* are known to harbour P and V plasmids (Bhaskaran 1960; Bhaskaran and Sinha 1971). When P and V plasmids were introduced into the pathogenic *V. cholerae* strains KB9 and 569B through conjugation, pathogenicity was suppressed (Sinha and Srivastava 1978). The strains proved to be non-toxigenic in animal experiments and anti-genically similar to their parent strains (Sinha and Srivastava 1979). This plasmid-induced suppression was found to be a general phenomenon in *V. cholerae*, but the mechanism is not known (Sinha and Srivastava 1983). The degree of suppression varied from strain to strain or among different P + V + clones of the same strain. Possible explanations for this include: (a) the plasmids code for repressors which repress operons for toxin bio-synthesis, alternately: (b) the plasmids like Mu and vibriophage VcAI might integrate at chromosomal site(s) causing mutation in structural gene(s) for toxin production (Johnson, Liu, and Romig 1981).

Phage-induced attenuation

Johnson, Liu, and Romig (1981) observed that vibriophage VcA1 induces mutation in the *V. cholerae* chromosome. Following this initial observation, phenotypically non-toxigenic mutants of *V. cholerae* were isolated after infection with either of the two mutagenic vibriophages VcA1 and VcA2ctsl (Mekalanos *et al.* 1982). DNA isolated from these mutants was analysed for toxin gene sequences by the Southern blotting method with ^{32}P-labelled probes derived from the cloned A and B subunit genes for the heat labile enterotoxin of *E. coli*. Several of the mutant isolates were shown by this method to have lost all sequences hybridizing to the LT probes, indicating that these clones contain deletion mutations that removed the structural gene(s) coding for cholera toxin. The mutants were prototrophic and grew normally *in vitro*, demonstrating that the toxin is not essential for the growth and viability of *V. cholerae*. Moreover, the toxin gene deletion mutants multiplied well *in vivo* in ligated rabbit intestine. Because of these growth properties and the stability of deletion mutations, these strains are promising candidates for testing as live oral vaccine for protection against cholera.

Chemically attenuated mutant strains

Bhaskaran and Sinha (1967) isolated a dwarf colony mutant of a pathogenic *V. cholerae* strain by means of *N*-methyl-*N*-nitro-*N*-nitrosoguanidine. The mutant was apathogenic in adult rabbit ileal loop (De and Chatterjee 1953). The mutant character appeared to be stable and the avirulence of the strain probably resulted from its inability to multiply in the gut of experimental animals. The strain has not been tested in humans.

Finkelstein, Vasil, and Holmes (1974) isolated a mutant of *V. cholerae* strain 569B designated M 13 following mutagenesis with nitrosoguanidine. The strain produced no detectable enterotoxin in the Oakley–Fulthrope test (Oakley and Fulthrope 1953) or in the rabbit skin test, and was avirulent for infant rabbits (Dutta and Habbu 1955) although it colonized their intestines. Massive oral doses of this strain conferred only 60 per cent protection in volunteers (Woodward, Gilman, Hornick, Libonati, and Cash 1976). This relatively poor protection as compared to that conferred by fully virulent strains could be due to an associated defect in one of the colonization or non-stimulation of antitoxin response.

Honda and Finkelstein (1979) isolated an avirulent strain designated Texas Star-SR after mutagenesis with nitrosoguanidine. This strain produced no detectable A (active, ADP-ribosylating) region of the cholera enterotoxin (choleragen) but produced the B region (choleragenoid) at the toxin in amounts similar to the hypertoxigenic wild type parent *V. cholerae eltor* Ogawa strain no. 3083. The mutant retained the colonizing ability, motility, prototrophy, and serologic characteristics of the parent strain. It was found to be non-toxigenic in immunological tests, tissue culture assays, and animal systems such as adult rabbit ileal loops (De and Chatterjee 1953) and infant rabbits (Dutta and Habbu 1955). The organism multiplied in the gut of infant rabbits and in the gut of chinchillas it induced significant resistance to challenge with a virulent *V. cholerae* strain. Texas Star-SR successfully colonized the gut of infant mice and did not elicit diarrhoea even after 10 successive passages through their intestines. The strain was, however, slightly temperature-sensitive (Siegel, Finkelstein, and Parker 1981).

In adult rabbit intestine the strain multiplied poorly, evoked very small mucosal antitoxin responses, and was only partially protective against experimentally induced cholera even when immunization was done with 10^{10} viable bacteria (Tokunaga, Cray, and Pierce 1984).

A volunteer trial with Texas Star-SR was conducted on 33 humans (Levine, Black, Clements, Lanata, Sears, Honda, Young and Finkelstein, 1984). Doses of 10^5–10^{10} viable organisms were fed to volunteers with $NaHCO_3$ and the strain could be recovered from stools of only 10 subjects. Mild diarrhoea was observed in 25 per cent of recipients. Vibriocidal antibody response was noted in sera of 85 per cent of recipients but antitoxin in only 21 per cent of them, IgA-type antitoxin could be detected in the jejunal fluid of only three volunteers.

Unfortunately, Texas Star-SR suffers from certain drawbacks. Nitrosoguanidine mutagenesis inflicts multiple genetic changes, not all of which are known, and the precise genetic lesion responsible for the attenuation of the strain is unknown, and in theory it could revert. Further the immunogenicity of the parent strain 3084 has not been tested in volunteers.

Genetically engineered Vibrio cholerae *strains*

The other most recent approach to the development of new oral cholera vaccines involves the use of recombinant DNA techniques to attenuate virulent *V. cholerae* 01 by removing specific virulence properties (Mekalanos, Swartz, Dearson, Harford, Groyne, and de Wilde 1983; Kaper and Levine 1981). The parent strains are those shown to be pathogenic in volunteers and capable of stimulating solid protection (WHO 1982).

Genes encoding the production of cholera holotoxin or the enzymatically active A subunit were deleted to give rise to *eltor* Inaba JBK 70, classical Ogawa NT (A⁻ B⁻), and classical Ogawa CVD101 and N1 (A⁻ B⁻) vaccine strains. These recombinant strains, unlike the chemically induced mutants, evoked immunity that more nearly resembled that caused by fully virulent strains. They colonized the intestine and induced serum vibriocidal responses equal to those seen after clinical cholera. A single dose of JBK 70 provided a high degree of protection (89 per cent) against experimental challenge with virulent *V. cholerae* 01 of the Inaba serotype. JBK 70 caused mild diarrhoea in a proportion of volunteers receiving 10^6, 10^8 or 10^{10} viable organisms with $NaHCO_3$. CVD 101 induced comparable rates of diarrhoea in vaccines who received between 10^4 and 10^8 organisms.

These strains seem to be very promising candidates for live oral vaccine against cholera but have an unacceptably high rate of adverse reactions. Both JBK 70 and CVD 101 (and presumably NI and NT) produce enterotoxic and cytotoxic substances. It remains to be seen whether deletion of one or both of the possible virulence properties will further attenuate the vaccine strains.

Although non-toxigenic live bacteria obtained either from natural sources or tailored in the laboratory by chemical mutagenesis or genetic hybridization are promising for oral immunization against cholera, almost all such strains so far isolated cause diarrhoea in a portion of volunteers. As these strains lack either the toxic A subunit or the entire CT gene, the diarrhoea cannot be due to cholera toxin. We decided, therefore, to examine some of the non-toxinogenic strains in greater detail, using various animal, tissue-culture and immunological assays. The aim was to determine whether these strains lack completely the ability to produce any toxin of clinical significance.

A new virulent cholera toxin

Models for toxigenicity testing

Different methods, depending upon availability, are used to measure the enterotoxic activity of bacteria. There is no internationally accepted and standardized technique for the purpose. Such factors as inoculum size, time of incubation, medium used for preparation of culture filtrates, cell associated toxins, sources of laboratory animals, and definition of a positive response, all of which can profoundly affect the observed results, may vary from laboratory to laboratory. Thus the exact comparison of results obtained from such experiments should not be attempted.

Genetic techniques (Mosley and Falkow 1980; Mosley, Huq, Alim, So, Samadpour-Motalebi, and Falkow 1980; Kaper and Levine 1981; Gennero, Greenaway and Broadbent 1982; Kaper, Bradford, Roberts, and Falkow 1982) now are being evolved that can recognize specific genes governing toxin production. Such a genetic technique uninfluenced by physiological, cultural, and other conditions, should be an unequivocal indicator of toxigenicity. Many workers, seeking to discover potential candidates for a live oral cholera vaccine, spent much effort either trying to identify strains of *V. cholerae* 01 that would demonstrate no genetic homology with the CT or LT gene, or trying to engineer strains that lack the appropriate gene (Kaper and Levine 1981; Levine *et al.* 1982; Mekalanos *et al.* 1982; Mekalanos *et al.* 1983). Implicit in this work was the assumption that only one important enterotoxin (CT) existed in *V. cholerae*, an enterotoxin governed by one gene. However, enterotoxins by definition produce a secretory response when introduced into the lumen of the small intestine of humans and experimental animals (Holmes, Bramucci, and Twiddy 1979). Since fluid accumulation in the ligated loops of adult rabbits (De and Chatterjee 1953) and diarrhoea in infant rabbits (Dutta and Habbu 1955) are the classical bioassays for detection of LT or CT, the genetic techniques developed must corroborate with the results obtained in these assays. If a discrepancy is found then the new toxin must be purified and its gene identified (Sanyal, Alam, Neogi, Huq, and Al-Mahmud 1983; Sanyal, Neogi, Alam, Huq, and Al-Mahmud 1984).

Enterotoxin testing of CT-gene negative strains

The sources of the 13 strains tested and the results of tests for production of an enterotoxin are shown in Table 16.1. These strains were isolated from such environmental sources as sewage, oysters, and brackish water as well as from intestinal and other human infections. None of them demonstrated any homology with CT or LT genes.

Live cells with inocula of 10^6 c.f.u. and culture filtrates of the 13 CT gene-negative strains caused accumulation of fluid in rabbit ileal loop (De and Chatterjee 1953), indicating that the organisms elaborate an enterotoxic substance. This observation was further substantiated by the fact that all the strains induced either diarrhoea or fluid accumulation in the large gut of infant rabbits (Dutta and Habbu 1953). Moreover, the culture supernates increased the capillary permeability of rabbits' skin (Craig 1970).

In the rabbit ileal-loop assay the minimal loop reacting dose of the culture filtrate of the CT-negative strain X-392 could not be neutralized by four times the dilution of anti-CT that completely inactivated the minimal loop reacting dose of the CT positive *V. cholerae* strain 569B. The antisera against CT and its A and B subunits, in dilutions of 1:64 and 1:10 respectively, also failed to neutralize the skin PF activity of the 13 test culture filtrates diluted 1:2 and 1:10. However, the skin PF activity of *V. cholerae* strain 569B was completely neutralized with four times higher dilutions of the antitoxins. None of the 20-fold concentrated culture filtrates gave any precipitin band when tested against serial twofold dilutions (up to 1:32) of anti-CT in the Ouchterlony gel-diffusion test. These observations strongly suggest that the toxin is immunologically different from the known CT.

The culture filtrates did not cause any observed alteration in the morphology of CHO and Y-1 cells that would indicate cytotoxicity (Guerrant, Brunton, Schnaitman, Rebhun, and Gilman 1974; Sack and Sack 1975). These observations suggest either that the culture filtrates did not stimulate the adenylate cyclase system (as CT or LT do; Guerrant *et al*. 1974; Donta, King, and Sloper 1973) or that binding to GM_1 ganglioside receptors does not occur. The ganglioside GM_1 enzyme-linked immunoabsorbent assays performed with the cell-free culture supernates yielded negative results, indicating their receptor site to be different from that of known CT or LT (Svennerholm and Holmgren 1978).

None of the culture filtrates gave a positive result in the suckling mice assay, indicating the absence of a heat-stable toxin (Gianella 1977). This observation was confirmed by ileal loop tests using heat-treated culture filtrates.

Table 16.1 Enterotoxicity tests with cholera toxin or heat-labile toxin gene probe-negative strains of *Vibrio cholerae* Q1

Strain designation and source of isolation	Rabbit ileal loop tests				Suckling mice assay and heated culture filtrates in loops	Infant rabbit test	PFᵃ	Y-1 and CHO	GM₁ ELISA
	Live cells		Culture filtrates						
	No. of positives/ No. of tests	Range of fluid accumulation (ml/cm of gut)	No. of positive/ No. of tests	Range of fluid accumulation (ml cm⁻¹ of gut)					
VL 6007 (water, England)	2/2	1.0–2.0	5/7	1.8–1.1	0	+	+	0	0
1196-74 (sewage, Brazil)	2/3	0.8–1.5	2/3	0.6–1.2	0	+	+	0	0
X 392 (environment, Guam)	3/3	1.0–2.6	4/4	0.8–2.7	0	+	+	0	0
1727-79 (oyster, Louisiana)	2/3	0.6–1.5	2/3	0.5–2.2	0	+	+	0	0
V-69 (water, Maryland)	2/2	0.5–1.2	2/2	0.9–1.4	0	+	+	0	0
VL 6085 (water, England)	2/2	0.6–1.2	2/2	1.0–1.5	0	+	+	0	0
1528-79 (oyster, Louisiana)	3/4	0.5–1.0	2/2	0.9–1.1	0	+	+	0	0
1074-78 (sewage, Brazil)	2/5	0.5–0.9	2/2	0.4–0.8	0	+	+	0	0
X 725 (environment, Guam)	2/5	0.6–0.8	2/2	0.4–1.0	0	+	+	0	0
1077-79 (leg ulcer, Louisiana)	2/3	1.0–2.4	2/2	1.2–1.6	0	+	+	0	0
1165-77 (gall bladder, Alabama)	2/5	0.4–0.8	2/2	0.5–0.9	0	+	+	0	0
165G7 (oyster, Louisiana)	4/4	1.3–2.4	4/4	0.9–1.7	0	+	+	0	0
2740-80	2/2	1.3–1.5	3/4	0.5–1.7	0	+	+	0	0
569B (positive control) *Escherichia coli* 265,	10/10	1.2–2.5	10/10	1.3–2.5	0	+	+	0	0
physiologic saline and Richardson's medium (negative controls)	0/10	0.0	0/10	0.0	0	0	0	0	0

ᵃBlanching or necrosis, along with blueing, was noted for most of the culture supernates.

The dialysed ammonium sulphate precipitates of the culture filtrates of strains grown in syncase medium caused fluid accumulation in rabbit gut loops. The enterotoxin was heat-labile and could be precipitated with ammonium sulphate, which suggests that it is a protein (Finkelstein, Atthasampunna, Chulasamaya, and Charunmethee 1966).

The enterotoxic activity of the strains was greatly enhanced after two serial passages through rabbit gut. The strains produced quantitatively more toxin of the same kind after passage, and still failed to show any homolgy with the CT or LT genes, indicating that they did not revert to making the 'typical' toxin. This enhancement of enterotoxicity suggests that if such an organism is fed to humans for prohylaxis and is excreted into the environment, it may be ingested by others in the community and may circulate there, leading to a further increase in virulence (Singh and Sanyal 1978).

The results of this study indicate that CT-gene negative *V. cholerae* 01 strains, isolated from diverse environmental sources and from humans with intestinal and extra-intestinal infections, do possess enterotoxic activity. The diarrhoeal illness of the patient, from whom the CT-gene negative strain 2740–80 used in this study was isolated, might have been due to this toxin, possibly ingested with contaminated seafood. The chemically induced deletion mutant of the human isolate of *V. cholerae* 01 Texas Star-SR, which lacks the gene for the CT toxic A subunit (Honda and Finkelstein 1979), caused diarrhoea in a number of volunteers who were fed an inoculum of 10^5 bacteria (Levine *et al.* 1984). The other more recent deletion mutants induced by genetic recombination, such as JBK 70 and CVD101, also caused diarrhoea in a proportion of the recipients. The possibility that these mutant strains elaborated this toxin, which was then responsible for the diarrhoeal episodes, cannot be excluded. The strain 1074–78, isolated from sewage in Brazil, was administered orally, in a dose of 10^6 bacteria to seven volunteers, after neutralization of stomach acidity (Levine *et al.* 1982). None of the volunteers excreted the organism, indicating that it did not colonize in their guts. However, in the present study, this strain caused fluid accumulation after only one passage in rabbit gut loop, suggesting enhancement of its virulence factors. The strain also multiplied by 3–4 orders of magnitude in the loops upon passage, thus indicating that it retained its colonizing capability. The result might have been similar if the strain could have been passed through a human gut, as expected of an oral vaccine strain fed to members of a community.

It is thus demonstrated that the CT-gene negative *V. cholerae* 01 strains produce a toxin that has not been previously recognized. This new toxin is a heat-labile protein, and differs from the known CT in (i) antigenicity, (ii) receptor site, (iii) mode of action, and (iv) genetic homology. Therefore, before a direct vaccine development program based on CT-gene negative *V. cholerae* 01 strains is embarked upon, the immunobiological and genetic aspects of this toxin should be defined.

References

Attridge, S. R. and Rowley, D. (1983). The role of the flagellum in adherence to *V. cholerae. J. infect. Dis.* **147**, 864–72.

Benenson, A. S., Mosley, W. H., Fahimuddin, M., and Oseasohn, R. O. (1968). Cholera vaccine field trials in East Pakistan, 2. Effectiveness in the field. *Bull. WHO.* **38**, 359–72.

Bhaskaran, K. (1960). Recombination of characters between mutant stocks of *Vibrio cholerae* strain 162. *J. gen. Microbiol.* **23**, 47–54.

—— and Sinha, V. B. (1967). Attenuation of virulence in *Vibrio cholerae. J. Hyg.* **65**, 135–48.

—— and Sinha, V. B. (1971). Transmissible plasmid factors and fertility inhibition in *Vibrio cholerae. J. gen. Microbol.* **69**, 89–97.

Bhattacharya, P. and Mukerjee, S. (1968a). Production of antibodies after live enteral cholera vaccination. *J. infect. Dis.* **118**, 271–79.

—— and —— (1968b). Further studies on the development of a live oral cholera vaccine. *J. Hyg.* **66**, 307–18.

—— and —— (1970). Quantitative differences in antitoxic and antibacterial immunogenesis after live and killed enteral cholera vaccination. *Indian J. med. Res.* **58**, 1569–77.

——, Narayanaswami, A., and Mukerjee, S. (1968). Production of antitoxic immunity by live oral cholera vaccine. *J. Bacteriol.* **95**, 255–7.

Blake, P. A., Allegra, D. T., Snyder, J. D., Barrett, T. J., McFarland, L., Caraway, C. T., Feeley, J. C., Craig, J. P., Lee, J. V., Puhr, N. D., and Feldman, R. A. (1980). Cholera — a possible endemic focus in the United States. *New Engl. J. Med.* **302**, 305–9.

Burnet, F. M. and Stone, J. D. (1947). Desquamation of intestinal epithelium *in vitro* by *V. cholerae* filtrates: characterization of mucinase and tissue disintegrating enzyme. *Aust. J. exp. Biol. med. Sci.* **25**, 219–26.

Cash, R. A., Music, S. I., Libonati, J. P., Craig, J. P., Pierce, N. F., and Hornick, R. B. (1974). Response of man to infection with *Vibrio cholerae*. II. Protection from illness afforded by previous disease and vaccine. *J. infect. Dis.* **130**, 325–33.

Chaicumpa, W. and Atthasistha, N. (1977). Study of intestinal immunity against *V. cholerae*: role of antibody to *V. cholerae* haemagglutinin in intestinal immunity. *S.E. Asian J. trop. Med. publ. Hlth.* **8**, 13–8.

Chitnis, D. S., Sharma, K. D., and Kamat, R. S. (1982). Role of somatic antigen of *Vibrio cholerae* in adhesion to intestinal mucosa. *J. med. Microbiol.* **5**, 53–61.

Craig, J. P. (1970). Some observations on the neutralization of cholera vascular permeability factor *in vivo. J. infect. Dis.* **121** (Suppl.), 100–10.

——, Yamamoto, K., Takeda, Y., and Miwatani, T. (1981). Production of cholera-like enterotoxin by a *Vibrio cholerae* non-01 strain isolated from the environment. *Infect. Immunol.* **34**, 90–97.

Cray, W. C., Tokunaga, E., and Pierce, N. F. (1983). Successful colonization and immunization of adult rabbits by oral inoculation with *Vibrio cholerae* 01. *Infect. Immunol.* **41**, 735–41.

Curlin, G., Levine, M. M., Aziz, K. M. A., Rahman, A. S. M. M., and Verwey,

W. F. (1976). Field trial of cholera toxoid. In *Proceedings of the 11th US— Japan cholera conference*. New Orleans 1975. pp. 314–29. US Department of Health, Education, and Welfare.

De, S. N. and Chatterjee, D. N. (1953). An experimental study on the mechanism of action of *Vibrio cholerae* on the intestinal mucous membranes. *J. Pathol. Bacteriol.* **66**, 559–62.

Donta, S. T., King, M., and Sloper, K. (1973). Induction of steroidogenesis in tissue culture by cholera enterotoxin. *Nature (New Biol.)* **243**, 246–7.

Dutta, N. K. and Habbu, M. K. (1955). Experimental cholera in infant rabbits: a method for chemotherapeutic investigation. *Br. J. Pharmacol. Chemother.* **10**, 153–9.

Eubanks, E. R., Guentzel, M. N., and Berry, L. J. (1977). Evaluation of surface components of *Vibrio cholerae* as protective immunogens. *Infect. Immunol.* **15**, 533–8.

Feeley, J. C. and Gangarosa, E. J. (1980). Field trials of cholera vaccine. In *Cholera and related diarrhoea. 43rd Nobel symposium* (ed. O. Ouchterlony and J. Holmgren), pp. 204–10. Karger, Basel.

Ferrán, J. (1885). Note sobre la profilasis del cholera per medio di invecciones hipodérmicas de cultivo puro del bacilo virgula. *Siglo Med.* **32**, 480–5.

Finkelstein, R. A., Atthasampunna, P., Chulasamaya, M., and Charunmethee, P. (1966). Pathogenesis of experimental cholera: biologic activities of purified procholeragen A. *J. Immunol.* **96**, 440–9.

——, Boesman-Finkelstein, M., and Holt, P. (1983). *Vibrio cholerae* haemagglutinin/lectin/protease hydrolyses fibronectin and ovomucin: F. M. Burnet revisited. *Proc. nat. Acad. Sci. USA.* **80**, 1092–5.

——, Vasil, M. L., and Holmes, R. K. (1974). Studies on toxigenesis in *Vibrio cholerae*. I. Isolation of mutants with altered toxigenicity. *J. infect. Dis.* **129**, 117–23.

Foo, E. S. A. and Chaicumpa, W. (1981). Protection against *Vibrio cholerae* infection afforded by fragments of antihaemagglutinin. *S.E. Asian J. trop. med. publ. Hlth.* **12**, 506–12.

Freter, R. (1955). The serologic character of cholera vibrio mucinase. *J. infect. Dis.* **97**, 238–45.

—— and Jones, G. W. (1976). Adhesive properties of *Vibrio cholerae*: nature of the interaction with intact mucosal surfaces. *Infect. Immunol.* **14**, 246–56.

Gangarosa, E. J., Biesel, W. R., Benyajati, C., Spring, H., and Piyaratn, P. (1960). The nature of the gastrointestinal lesion in Asiatic cholera and its relation to pathogenesis. *Am. J. trop. Med. Hyg.* **9**, 125–35.

Gearhart, P. J. and Cebra, J. J. (1979). Differentiated B lymphocytes: potential to express particular antibody variable and constant regions depends on site of lymphoid tissue and antigen load. *J. exp. Med.* **149**, 216–27.

Gennaro, M., Greenaway, P., and Broadbent, D. A. (1982). Expression of cloned cholera enterotoxin gene in *Escherichia coli* and possibilities of vaccine development. *Lancet* **i**, 1239–40.

Gianella, R. A. (1977). Specificity of suckling mouse assay (SMA) for heat stable

E. coli enterotoxin (ST) and mode of action of the toxin. *Gastroenterology* **72**, 1062.

Gill, D. M. and King, C. A. (1975). The mechanism of action of cholera toxin in pigeon erythrocyte lysates. *J. biol. Chem.* **250**, 6424–32.

Guerrant, R. L., Brunton, L. L., Schnaitman, T. C., Rebhun, L. L., and Gilman, A. G. (1974). Cyclic adenosine monophosphate and alteration of Chinese hamster ovary cell morphology: a rapid, sensitive *in vitro* assay for the enterotoxins of *Vibrio cholerae* and *Escherichia coli*. *Infect. Immunol.* **10**, 320–7.

Holmes, R. K., Bramucci, M. G., and Twiddy, E. M. (1979). Genetics of toxigenesis in *Vibrio cholerae* and *Escherichia coli*. *Contrib. Microbiol. Immunol.* **6**, 165–77.

Holmgren, J. and Svennerholm, A. M. (1977). Mechanisms of disease and immunity in cholera. *J. infect. Dis.* **136** (Suppl.), 105–12.

Honda, T. and Finkelstein, R. A. (1979). Selection and characteristics of a *Vibrio cholerae* mutant lacking the A (ADP-ribolysating) portion of the cholera enterotoxin. *Proc. nat. Acad. Sci. USA.* **76**, 2052–6.

Hranitzky, K. W., Mulholland, A., Larson, A. D., Eubanks, E. R., and Hart, L. T. (1980). Characterization of a flagellar sheath protein of *Vibrio cholerae*. *Infect. Immunol.* **27**, 597–603.

Jensen, K. E. (1953). Immunological characterization of a mucinolytic enzyme of *Vibrio cholerae*. *J. infect. Dis.* **93**, 107.

Johnson, S. R., Liu, B. C. S., and Romig, W. R. (1981). Auxotrophic mutations induced *Vibrio cholerae* mutator phage VcA1. *FEMS microbiol. Lett.* **11**, 13–16.

Joó, I. and Csizer, Z. (1978). Preparation and laboratory testing of a plain and aluminium hydroxide-adsorbed cholera vaccine used in a field trial in Indonesia. *Bull WHO* **56**, 615–18.

Kabir, S. (1980). Composition and immunochemical properties of outer membrane proteins of *Vibrio cholerae*. *J. Bacteriol.* **144**, 283–9.

—— (1983). Immunochemical properties of the major outer membrane protein of *Vibrio cholerae*. *Infect. Immunol.* **39**, 452–5.

Kaper, J. B. and Levine, M. M. (1981). Cloned cholera enterotoxin genes in the study and prevention of cholera. *Lancet* **ii**, 1162–3.

——, Mosley, S. L., and Falkow, S. (1981). Molecular characterization of environmental and nonenterotoxigenic strains of *Vibrio cholerae*. *Infect. Immunol.* **32**, 661–7.

——, Bradford, H. B., Roberts, N. C., and Falkow, S. (1982). Molecular epidemiology of *Vibrio cholerae* in the US Gulf Coast. *J. clin. Microbiol.* **16**, 129–34.

Kelley, J. T. and Parker, C. D. (1981). Identification of *Vibrio cholerae* outer membrane protein. *J. Bacteriol.* **145**, 1018–24.

Lange, S. and Holmgren, J. (1978). Protective antitoxic cholera immunity in mice: influence of route and number of immunizations and mode of action of protective antibodies. *Acta path. microbiol. scand.* **E86**, 145–52.

Levine, M. M. (1980). Immunity to cholera as evaluated in volunteers. In *Cholera and related diarrhoeas, 43rd Nobel Symposium* (ed. O. Ouchterlony and J. Holmgren), pp. 195–203. Karger, Basel.

——, Black, R. E., Clements, M. L., Cisneros, L., Nalin, D. R., and Young, C. R.

(1981). Duration of infection derived immunity to cholera. *J. infect. Dis.* **143**, 818–20.

——, ——, ——, Nalin, D. R., Cisneros, L., and Finkelstein, R. A. (1981). Volunteer studies in development of vaccines against cholera and enterotoxigenic *Escherichia coli*: A review. In *Acute enteric infections in children. New prospects for treatment and prevention* (ed. T. Holme, M. R. Merson, and R. Mollby), pp. 443–59. Elsevier/North Holland Biomedical Press, Amsterdam.

——, ——, ——, Lanata, C., Sears, S., Honda, T., Young, C. R., and Finkelstein, R. A. (1984). Evaluation in humans of attenuated *Vibrio cholerae* E1 Tor Ogawa strain Texas Star-SR as a live oral vaccine. *Infect. Immunol.* **43**, 515–22.

——, ——, ——, Cisneros, L., Saah, A., Nalin, D. R., Gill, D. M., Craig, J. P., Young, C. R., and Ristaino, P. (1982). The pathogenicity of non-enterotoxigenic *Vibrio cholerae* serogroup 01 biotype E1 Tor isolated from sewage water in Brazil. *J. infect. Dis.* **145**, 296–9.

Mekalanos, J. J., Mosley, S. L., Murphy, J. R., and Falkow, S. (1982). Isolation of enterotoxin structural gene deletion mutations in *Vibrio cholerae* induced by two mutagenic vibriophages. *Proc. nat. Acad. Sci. USA.* **79**, 151–55.

——, Swartz, D. T., Dearson, G. D. N., Harford, N., Groyne, F., and de Wilde, M. (1983). Cholera toxin genes: nucleotide sequencing, deletion, analysis, and vaccine development. *Nature (Lond.)* **306**, 551–7.

Mosley, W. H. (1969). The role of immunity in cholera. A review of epidemiological and serological studies. *Tex. Rep. Biol. Med.* **27** (Suppl.), 227–74.

Mosley, S. L. and Falkow, S. (1980). Nucleotide sequence homology between the heat-labile enterotoxin gene of *Escherichia coli* and *Vibrio cholerae* deoxyribonucleic acid. *J. Bacteriol.* **144**, 444–6.

——, Huq, I., Alim, A. R. M. A., So, M., Samadpour-Motalebi, M., and Falkow, S. (1980). Detection of enterotoxigenic *Escherichia coli* by DNA colony hybridization. *J. infect. Dis.* **142**, 892–8.

Mukerjee, S. (1963). Preliminary studies on the development of a live oral vaccine for anti-cholera immunization. *Bull WHO* **29**, 753–66.

—— (1965). Living oral cholera vaccine. In *Proceedings of the cholera research symposium*, Honolulu, pp. 167–70. Public Health Service Publication No.1328. U.S. Government Printing Office, Washington, D.C.

Oakley, C. L. and Fulthrope, A. J. (1953). Antigenic analysis by diffusion. *J. Pathol. Bacteriol.* **65**, 49–60.

Oseasohn, R. O., Benenson, A. S., and Fahimuddin, M. (1965). Field trial of cholera vaccine in East Pakistan. First year of observation. *Lancet* i, 450–3.

Pal, S. C. (1977). Annual Report of the Cholera Research Centre, Calcutta, p. 5. Indian Council of Medical Research.

Pierce, N. F. (1978). The role of antigen form and function in the primary and secondary intestinal immune responses to cholera toxin and toxoid in rats. *J. exp. Med.* **148**, 195–206.

—— (1981). The experimental basis for oral immunization against cholera. In *Proceedings of the conference on experimental cholera vaccines* (ed. S. Rahman), pp. 23–39. ICDDR, B, Dhaka.

—— and Koster, F. T. (1981). Stimulation of intestinal immunity. In *Acute enteric infections in children. New prospects for treatment and prevention* (ed. T. Holme, M. H. Merson, and R. Mollby), pp. 413–23. Elsevier/North Holland Biomedical Press, Amsterdam.

Sack, R. B. (1980). Pathogenesis and pathophysiology of diarrhoeal diseases caused by *Vibrio cholerae* and enterotoxigenic *Escherichia coli*. In *Cholera and related diarrhoeas, 43rd Nobel symposium* (ed. O. Ouchterlony and J. Holmgren), pp. 53–63. Karger, Basel.

Sack, D. A. and Sack, R. B. (1975). Test for enterotoxigenic *Escherichia coli* using Y1 adrenal cells in mini culture. *Infect. Immunol.* **11**, 334–6.

——, Huda, S., Neogi, P. K. B., Daniel, R. R., and Spira, W. M. (1980). Microtiter ganglioside enzyme-linked immunosorbent assay for *Vibrio* and *Escherichia coli* heat-labile enterotoxins and antitoxin. *J. clin. Microbiol.* **11**, 35–40.

Sanyal, S. C., and Mukerjee, S. (1969). Live oral cholera vaccine: Report of a trial on human volunteer subjects. *Bull WHO* **40**, 503–11.

——, Narayanaswami, A., and Mukerjee, S. (1969a). Antigenic analysis of *Vibrio* culture filtrate and vaccine E1 Tor vibrios. *J. Hyg.* **67**, 539–44.

——, ——, and —— (1969b). Comparative study on the protective value of different antigenic preparations from cholera vibrios. *Indian J. med. Res.* **57**, 1621–8.

——, ——, and —— (1969c). Demonstration of cell-bound antibody by fluorescent microscopy in the intestine of rabbits following live enteral cholera vaccination. *Experientia.* **25**, 860–61.

——, ——, and —— (1971). Nature of coproantibodies appearing after live oral cholera vaccination in human volunteers. ICMR Technical Report Series No. 9, pp. 52–4.

——, Alam, K., Neogi, P. K. B., Huq, M. I., and Al-Mahmud, K. A. (1983). A new cholera toxin. *Lancet* **i**, 1337.

——, Neogi, P. K. B., Alam, K., Huq, M. I., and Al-Mahmud, K. A. (1984). A new enterotoxin produced by *Vibrio cholerae 01. J. Dir. Dis. Res.* **2**, 3–12.

Saroso, J. S., Bahrawi, W., Witjaksono, H., Budiarso, R. L. P., Brotowasisto., Benćić, Z., Dewitt, W. E., and Gomez, C. Z. (1978). A controlled field trial of plain and aluminium hydroxide adsorbed cholera vaccines in Surabaya, Indonesia, during 1973–75. *Bull WHO* **56**, 619–27.

Schneider, D. R. and Parker, C. D. (1978). Isolation and characterization of protease deficient mutants of *Vibrio cholerae. J. infect. Dis.* **143**, 143–51.

Schrank, G. D. and Verwey, W. F. (1976). Distribution of cholera organisms in experimental *Vibrio cholerae* infections: proposed mechanism of pathogenesis and antibacterial immunity. *Infect. Immunol.* **13**, 195–203.

Siegel, S. P., Finkelstein, R. A., and Parker, C. D. (1981). Ability of an avirulent mutant of *Vibrio cholerae* to colonize in the infant mouse upper bowel. *Infect. Immunol.* **32**, 474–9.

Singh, S. J. and Sanyal, S. C. (1978). Enterotoxicity of the so-called NAG vibrios. *Ann. Soc. Belg. Med. trop.* **58**, 133–40.

Sinha, V. B. and Srivastava, B. S. (1978). Plasmid induced loss of virulence in *Vibrios cholerae. Nature (Lond.)* **276**, 708.

—— and —— (1979). Attenuation of virulence by P and V plasmids in *Vibrio cholerae*: strains suitable for oral immunization. *Bull WHO* **57**, 643–7.

—— and —— (1983). Plasmid associated suppression of pathogenicity of wild-type strains of *Vibrio cholerae* from cholera patients. *Indian J. med. Res* **77**, 1–4.

Srivastava, B. S. (1981). Two classes of attenuated strains of *Vibrio cholerae* which possess potential of live vaccine. In *Proceedings of the conference on experimental cholera vaccines*. (ed. S. Rahman), pp. 149–53. ICDDR, B, Dhaka.

—— Sinha, V. B., and Srivastava, R. (1979). Attenuated recombinant strains of *Vibrio cholerae* for oral immunization. *Bull WHO* **57**, 649.

Svennerholm, A.-M. and Holmgren, J. (1978). Identification of *Escherichia coli* heat-labile enterotoxins by means of a ganglioside immunosorbent assay (GM1 ELISA) procedure. *Curr. Microbiol.* **1**, 19–24.

Tokunaga, E., Cray, W. C. and Pierce, N. F. (1984). Compared colonizing and immunizing efficiency of toxigenic (A$^+$ B$^+$) *Vibrio cholerae* and A$^-$ B$^-$ mutant (Texas Star-SR) studied in adult rabbits. *Infect. Immunol.* **44**, 364–9.

Woodward, W. E., Gilman, R., Hornick, R., Libonati, J., and Cash, R. (1976). Efficacy of a live oral cholera vaccine in human volunteers. In *Proceedings of 11th US–Japan cholera Conference*, New Orleans, 1975. pp. 330–35. US Department Health, Education and Welfare.

WHO (1979). Cholera surveillance. *Wkly. epidemiol. Rec.* **54**, 257.

WHO (1982). Cholera in 1981. *Wkly. epidemiol. Rec.* **57**, 131–2.

WHO Scientific Working Group (1980). Cholera and other associated diarrhoeas. *Bull WHO* **58**, 353–74.

17

The role of enterotoxin components in future vaccines against enterotoxigenic *Escherichia coli*-induced diarrhoea and cholera

Gordon Dougan

Introduction

Enteric bacterial infections that lead to diarrhoeal diseases such as dysentery and enteric fevers are important health problems throughout the world, especially in young children in the Third World and in travellers to Third World countries. Amongst the most important enteric bacterial pathogens recognised are the enterotoxigenic *Escherichia coli* (ETEC) as a cause of diarrhoea in travellers, infant humans, and animals, and *Vibrio cholerae* 01, responsible for endemic and epidemic cholera. Both of these bacterial pathogens establish their infection in the small bowel of the host. Small bowel colonization normally involves specific adhesion to the brush-border enterocytes lining the bowel lumen. This process of adhesion allows the bacteria to resist the normal gut clearing mechanisms active at this site. Once established and almost certainly during the active process of colonization, the bacteria synthesize one or more enterotoxins that play a role in the development of the diarrhoeal symptoms normally associated with infections caused by ETEC and *V. cholerae*. These enterotoxins can be assigned to a number of classes according to their biological, biochemical, and immunological properties.

For many years attempts were made to develop immunizing agents against these infections with variable results. In many cases, especially for cholera vaccines, empirical approaches were taken with no recognizable scientific basis for that approach. An example of this is the phenolized heat-killed *V. cholerae* currently used as a parenteral vaccine. More recently, however, there have been major advances in our understanding of the pathogenesis of infections caused by these organisms. This information can allow a fresh evaluation of how new vaccines should be designed. In this short review I will discuss some of the recent work on the characterization of *V. cholerae* and ETEC enterotoxins and discuss how this information may be used to develop more effective vaccines against diseases caused by these organisms.

Pathogenesis of infection

Before an attempt can be made to evaluate how effective new vaccines based on enterotoxins may be, it is important to understand the pathogenic mechanisms by which these organisms cause diseases.

ETEC

The mechanisms by which ETEC strains infect the host are well understood as a result of careful genetic studies by a number of groups, but especially by the Ørskovs and co-workers (Ørskov and Ørskov 1966; Ørskov, Ørskov, Smith, and Sojka 1975). In addition, excellent studies in relevant animal model systems by H. Williams-Smith and co-workers allowed the identification of some of the important virulence factors possessed by ETEC strains (Williams-Smith and Linggood 1971). The important first step in the establishment of infection in the small bowel of the host by ETEC strains is attachment to the brush-border enterocytes. For many ETEC strains this attachment is mediated by proteinaceous surface-associated fimbriae, often referred to as adhesion antigens because they can be identified using immunological techniques (Gaastra and DeGraaf 1982; Dougan and Morrissey 1985). ETEC produce a number of species specific, immunologically distinct adhesion fimbrial types. For example, porcine ETEC strains produce K88 or 987P fimbriae, bovine isolates produce K99 and F41, and human isolates can produce an array of immunologically distinct adhesins. Vaccination with purified preparations of one adhesion fimbriae has proved to be effective in protecting against challenge with ETEC expressing the same but not immunologically distinct fimbrial types (Nagy, Walker, Bhogal, and McKenzie 1978; Morgan, Isaacson, Moon, Brinton, and To 1978). Thus anti-adhesive rather than anti-toxic immunity presents an option for vaccination against ETEC strains.

ETEC strains can secrete at least two classes of recognized enterotoxins. H. Williams-Smith and co-workers were able to establish a role for these enterotoxins in induction of severe diarrhoeal symptoms in young animals. (Williams-Smith and Gyles 1970; Williams-Smith and Linggood 1971). One class, known as the heat-labile enterotoxins (LT toxins) are inactivated by heating at 60°C for 30 min. LT toxins are structurally and immunologically highly related to cholera enterotoxins (Gyles 1974; Dallas and Falkow 1980). The second class are known as heat-stable enterotoxins (ST toxins) and they retain their activity even after boiling. ST toxins have been purified in an active form as small peptides and as a consequence they are poor immunogens (Dougan and Morrissey 1985). Sub-types are known to exist within the two recognized classes of *E. coli* enterotoxins, although they form a more immunologically homogenous group in comparison to adhesion fimbriae. This factor may affect their value as vaccine components. Other potential classes of *E. coli* enterotoxins have been identified but they will not be considered here.

Cholera

Cholera infections essentially follow the same pattern as ETEC infections. There is a preliminary phase of colonization of the small bowel and attachment to the mucosal surface. Exactly how *V. cholerae* cells attach to the mucosal surface is unclear. No adhesin that has a clear role in attachment has been identified. This factor alone has inhibited the development of new subunit cholera vaccines. *V. cholerae* secretes a number of extracellular products, which may play a role in disease pathogenesis, but undoubtably the most important amongst these is the cholera enterotoxin. Indeed, oral ingestion of as little as 25 μg of cholera enterotoxin by human volunteers can lead to the development of the full symptoms of cholera (Levine, Kaper, Black, and Clements 1983). There has been a debate as to whether anti-enterotoxin immunity alone is enough to prevent cholera or whether anti-adhesin immunity is also required. This will be discussed later.

Structure of the enterotoxin families

Heat-labile toxin and cholera toxin

The heat-labile toxins of ETEC were classically grouped together because of their sensitivity to heat and because they cause fluid accumulation in a ligated intestinal loop assay. The LT toxins isolated from humans or animal ETEC form a homogenous group of molecular weight about 84 000. The holotoxins contain two distinct subunits and both are related structurally and immunologically to cholera enterotoxin (Dallas and Falkow 1979). LT toxins are composed of an enzymatically active A subunit polypeptide of 27 000 dalton and five identical B subunits of 11 500 dalton. The A subunit is responsible for solute efflux from the epithelial brush-border cells and ultimately diarrhoeal symptoms (Dallas, Gill, and Falkow 1979). In cholera toxin the equivalent A polypeptide is nicked to form an A_1 component of 24 000 dalton and an A_2 component of 5 000 dalton. In both toxins the B complex can be separated from the A by biochemical means. The B subunits appear to be non-toxic and have a role in binding holotoxin to GM1-ganglioside receptors present in the membrane of susceptible cells. The B subunits are the immuno dominant parts of the holotoxins (Clements and

Finkelstein 1979). Porcine LT, human LT, and cholera toxin, although highly related, can be distinguished from each other biochemically and immunologically. For example cholera toxin is more active than LT toxin, and some monoclonal antibodies identify only one of the toxins whereas others recognize all three (Lindholm, Holmgren, Wilkstrom, Karlsson, Andersoon, and Lycke, 1983). DNA sequence analysis of the toxins show that LT toxins are almost identical as a group, and they show 70 per cent homology with cholera toxin DNA sequences. The same is true at the amino acid level (Dallas and Falkow 1980).

Heat-stable toxins

ST toxins are classified as a group because of their resistance to short periods of boiling. Most ST toxins can be detected using the suckling mouse assay. These form the ST_I group of toxins (Burgess, Bywater, Cowley, Mullan, and Newsome 1978). Some porcine isolates of ETEC produce ST_{II} toxin which can be detected biologically using a pig ligate-loop assay (Williams-Smith and Hall 1967). Since most work has been carried out on ST_I toxins, these will be considered here, as they are of more relevance to vaccine development. Gene cloning techniques helped greatly in the elucidation of the structures of ST-toxins (So and MacCarthy 1980; Moseley, Hardy, Imdadul Hug, Escheverria, and Falkow 1983; Lee, Moseley, Moon, Whipp, Gyles, and So 1983). ST_I can be purified as a peptide 18 or 19 amino acids in length. The peptide is unusual in that it contains six cysteine residues. Disulphide bonding plays a critical role in determining the tertiary structure of active ST toxin. Attempts to immunize animals with crude or purified ST toxin failed probably because of their small size. ST toxins, however, can be made immunogenic by chemically coupling them to larger protein carriers (Frantz and Robertson 1981). This technique was used to show that ST toxins isolated from different sources were antigenically related.

This factor increases their potential value as vaccine components especially as coupled ST toxin was found to be less toxic than uncoupled ST toxin.

Role of enterotoxins as vaccine components

Because enterotoxins play a major role in the pathogenesis of diseases caused by ETEC and *V. cholerae* they have received a great deal of attention as potential vaccine components. There are important considerations to bear in mind when considering vaccinating against an enteric infection. If the disease is established in a very young animal or human, active immunity cannot be considered for protection. Protection can be acquired in a passive manner by suckling milk or colostrum from an immune mother. This is the normal means for protecting neonatal farm animals such as pigs and calves against ETEC infections, as such infections are most hazardous in the first few days after birth. In these cases immunogens delivered to the mother must stimulate antibody production in the milk. For older animals it is necessary to stimulate active immunity. It has been long recognized that in order to stimulate long-lasting and solid immunity in animals against enteric infections it is best to deliver antigens via the oral rather than the parenteral route. Live attenuated bacterial strains can be developed for this purpose. Oral challenge stimulates the local gut immune system. It should be bourne in mind that this whole area is controversial with different people favouring different approaches to vaccination. This controversy can be extended to the question, is there any role at all for enterotoxins as vaccine components? Some people claim vaccination with enterotoxins is not required but only anti-adhesive immunity is needed whereas others are developing vaccines entirely based on toxin components. Central to this problem is whether anti-toxic immunity can (a) prevent totally disease symptoms and (b) prevent colonization of the small bowel. All these points should be considered when assessing the following sections.

Immunity to ETEC: role of LT and ST toxins

A number of approaches have been taken to adapt the *E. coli* LT and ST toxins for use as immunogens. Genetic manipulation has proved to be extremely useful for creating *E. coli* strains that synthesize LT toxoid rather than LT toxin. LT toxin is composed of two different polypeptides, A single A polypeptide which contains the enzymatic component of the toxin and five copies of B subunit which form the B pentamer. The genes for these two polypeptides map next to each other in the genome of ETEC (Dallas *et al.* 1979). Indeed, the LT toxin genes are normally encoded or extrachromo-somal plasmid DNA.

The two genes form a single operon, with the A polypeptide cistron being proximal to the B cistron. This is shown in Fig. 17.1. Gene cloning has been used to characterize the LT toxin operon. Simple manipulations have been used to construct recombinant plasmids that express B polypeptide in the absence of the A cistron. Normally expression of B is made dependent on a strong *E. coli* promoter such as the *trp* or *lac* promoter. Figure 17.1 shows a plasmid where B cistron expression is under control of the artificial *tac* promoter. Cells harbouring this plasmid synthesize high levels of B but not A polypeptide. Because B subunit is the immunodominant portion of the toxin and is a strong immunogen, and because B alone is non toxic, these cells synthesize a LT toxoid based on the B pentamer, which can be readily purified.

The LT toxin B subunit has now been used for several years as a component of commercially available vaccines designed to protect neonatal piglets

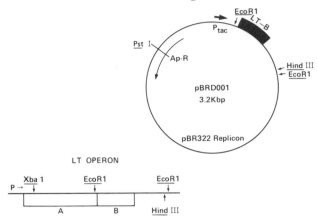

Fig. 17.1 Map of the recombinant plasmid which directs the expression of LT-B from the *tac* promoter. The plasmid is a pBR322-based replicon. Ap-R is the ampicillin resistance gene. The arrow designates the direction of transcription from the tac promoter. The closed box designates the LT-B cistron. In the bottom left of the diagram is a representation of the organization of the LT toxin operon. P shows the position of the natural LT promoter in front of the A subunit cistron.

against ETEC infections. The antigen is usually used together with other components such as the K88 and 987P adhesion antigens of these strains. Little published data is available on the efficacy of the LT-B component alone or in combination with other antigens (Dougan and Morrissey 1985; Winther and Dougan 1984). The LT-B is normally administered parenterally to the sow, who protects her suckling offspring via antibodies in her colostrum.

ST toxin presents a different problem to that of the LT toxins. ST toxin is poorly immunogenic in its native form. However, its immunogenicity is increased greatly if it is coupled chemically to a larger carrier molecule. Klipstein and co-workers have published a series of papers describing work in which they coupled ST to the LT-B subunit. Coupled ST was highly immunogenic and its toxicity was greatly reduced (Klipstein, Engert, and Houghten 1983b). These workers also employed an ST toxin that has been synthesised *de novo* from amino acids using a peptide synthesizer. This synthetic ST behaved in an identical manner to purified ST toxin in biological and biochemical assays (Klipstein, Engert, and Houghten 1983a, b). Small animals including rats and rabbits were immunized with coupled LT-ST preparations, and ST and LT neutralising antibody was detected in the serum of the vaccinated animals. These animals were also protected in ligated loop assays as fluid accumulation was prevented when an LT-toxin, ST-toxin-producing *E. coli* was inoculated into the loops (Klipstein *et al.* 1983b). Preliminary studies in cattle failed to show protection against

ST-toxin challenge, but the conditions of toxoid preparation were different, thus the results are not directly comparable. More recently these workers have developed a completely synthetic LT-ST toxoid based on synthetic ST toxin joined to the sequence representing amino acids 58–83 of the LT-B polypeptide (Houghten, Engert, Ostresh, Haffman, and Klipstein 1985). It will be interesting to see how these preparation perform when administered to humans.

Cholera toxoids

Early attempts to immunize humans against cholera with cholera entero-toxin used chemically inactivated material. Cholera toxin can by toxoided using either formaldehyde or glutaraldehyde. Work in humans using for-maldehyde-inactivated toxin was halted in part due to problems with rever-sion to toxicity. Work with glutaradehyde-prepared toxoid was better evaluated in humans but the antigen alone failed to induce significant protection against cholera in several trials, whether administered orally or parenterally (Levine *et al.* 1983). More recently purified cholera B subunit has been used as an immunogen in humans, although work is still going on to assess its value as a vaccine component.

Procholeragenoid is a high molecular weight toxoid that results when cholera enterotoxin is heated to 65°C for at least 5 min (Finkelstein, Fujita, and Lospallutlo 1971). This antigen has been used in pigs to protect them against ETEC infections with promising results in field trials (Furer, Cryz, Dosher, Nicole, Wanner, and Germanier 1982). Recently the determinant for the cholera toxin gene has been cloned by several groups from the chromosome of *V. cholerae* into *E. coli* K12. Strains of *E. coli* and *V. cholerae* that synthesize high levels of cholera B subunit in the absence of A subunit have been engineered and may be useful for cholera toxoid produc-tion (Mekalanos, Swartz, Pearson, Harford, Groyne, and de Wilde 1983; Kaper, Lockman, Baldini, and Levine 1984). The mutant strains of *V. cholerae* have been used to vaccinate orally human volunteers and they proved to be very effective vaccines, with efficacy calculated at over 90 per cent. Strains producing no enterotoxin or only the B subunit worked with similar efficiency, calling into question the requirement for an enterotoxin component of these strains. Some of the volunteers developed diarrhoeal symptoms shortly after ingestion of the vaccine. This may be a problem associated with strains that colonize the epithelial surfaces of the small bowel.

If colonization of the small bowel can in itself induce diarrhoeal symptoms it may be sensible to deliver toxoid antigen orally using alternative bacterial hosts. *Salmonella* species can infect the host in an invasive manner via the Peyer's patches found in the lining of the bowel. Once they have entered the

Peyer's patches these strains are ingested by reticuloendothelial cells but instead of being killed they survive and are transported throughout the body. Nevertheless, these strains actively stimulate the intestinal secretory immune system. Recently attenuated derivatives of *Salmonella typhi* and *S. typhimurium* have been developed that are useful as live oral vaccines (Hosieth and Stocker 1981). SL1344 is a mouse-virulent *S. typhimurium* strain that has an LD_{50} as low as 10^5 organisms following oral challenge. SL3261 is an avirulent derivative of SL1344 carrying a non-reverting deletion mutation in the *aro*A gene. The gene product of the *aro*A locus is involved in the metabolism of aromatic compounds and strains mutated at this site are unable to synthesize a number of essential aromatic compounds, including amino acids and enterochelin. These compounds are not freely available in mammalian tissues. Plasmids directing the expression of LT-B polypeptide can be introduced into SL3261, and such strains are still arivulent. Mice immunized with this strain are protected against subsequent challenge with SL 1344. Figure 17.2 shows the immune response in mice, both in terms of serum antibody and gut secretory antibody levels, to LT-B following infection and subsequent rechallenge of mice with SL3261 harbouring the LT-B plasmid. Clearly the mice mount a significant immune

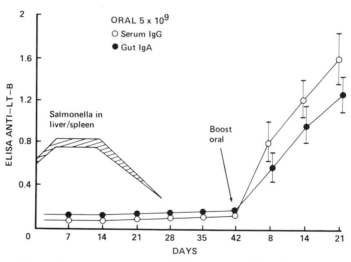

Fig. 17.2 Schematic representation of the pattern of the immune response in BALB/c mice infected with SL3261 pBR322-LT-B expressing LT-B immunogen. Immune response to LT-B is monitored using a GMI-ganglioside-based ELISA system. Mice were infected orally using a gavage tube and boosted at day 42. The hatched area represents the time viable salmonella could be isolated from the liver and spleen of the mice.

response to LT-B and the attenuated *Salmonella* strain is an effective means by which to deliver the enterotoxoid to the secretory immune system.

Conclusion

The application of recombinant DNA technology to the study of the major recognized enterotoxins of *E. coli* and *V. cholerae* has greatly speeded up the development of novel candidate immunogens, which deserve consideration as vaccines or vaccine components for the prevention of enteric diseases caused by these organisms. Already LT-B antigen has found use as a component of a commercially available vaccine. Safe attenuated live strains are showing great promise as future vaccines and candidate synthetic toxoid vaccines are ready to be assessed in humans. Nevertheless, controversy still exists as to whether toxoid components are required at all for the immunoprophylactic treatment of diseases caused by ETEC and *V. cholerae*, and carefully controlled clinical trials will be required to resolve this. It will be interesting to see how these questions are resolved over the next decade.

References

Burgess, N. M., Bywater, R. J., Cowley, C. M., Mullan, N. A., and Newsome, P. M. (1978). Biological evaluation of a methanol-soluble, heat-stable enterotoxin in infant mice, pigs, rabbits and calves. *Infect. Immunol.* **21**, 526–31.

Clements, J. D. and Finkelstein, R. A. (1979). Isolation and characterisation of homogenous heat-labile enterotoxins with high specific activity from *Escherichia coli* culture. *Infect. Immunol.* **24**, 760–90.

Dallas, W. S. and Falkow, S. (1979). The molecular nature of heat-labile enterotoxin (LT) of *Escherichia coli*. *Nature (Lond.)* **277**, 406–7.

—— and —— (1980). Amino acid sequence homology between cholera toxin and *Escherichia coli* heat-labile enterotoxin. *Nature (Lond.)* **288**, 599–601.

——, Gill, D. M., and Falkow, S. (1979). Cistrons encoding *Escherichia coli* heat-labile enterotoxin. *J. Bacteriol.* **139**, 850–8.

Dougan, G. and Morrissey, P. (1985). Molecular analysis of the virulence determinants of enterotoxigenic *Escherichia coli* isolated from domestic animals: applications for vaccine development. *Vet. Microbiol.* **10**, 241–57.

Finkelstein, R. A., Fujita, K, and Lospallutlo, J. J. (1971). Procholeragenoid: an aggregated intermediate in the formation of choleragenoid. *J. Immunol.* **107**, 1043–51.

Frantz, J. C. and Robertson, D. C. (1981). Immunological properties of *Escherichia coli* heat-stable enterotoxins: development of a radio-immunoassay specific for heat-stable enterotoxins with suckling mouse activity. *Infect. Immunol.* **33**, 193–8.

Furer, E., Cryz Jr., S. J., Dosher, F., Nicole, J., Wanner, M., and Germanier, R.

(1982). Protection against colibacillosis in neonatal piglets by immunization of sows with procholeragenoid. *Infect. Immunol.* **35**, 887–894.

Gaastra, W. and De Graaf, F. K. (1982). Host-specific fimbrial adhesins of non-invasive enterotoxigenic *Escherichia coli* strains. *Microbiol. Rev.* **45**, 129–161.

Gyles, F. L. 1974. Immunological study of the heat-labile enterotoxins of *Escherichia coli* and *Vibrio cholerae*. *J. Inf. Dis.* **129**, 277–88.

Hosieth, S. K. and Stocker, B. A. D. (1981). Aromatic dependent *Salmonella typimurium* are non-virulent and effective as live vaccines. *Nature (Lond.)* **291**, 238–9.

Houghten, R. A., Engert, R. F., Ostresh, J. M., Haffman, S. R., and Klipstein, F. A. (1985). A completely synthetic toxoid vaccine containing *Escherichia coli* heat-stable toxin and antigenic determinants of the heat-labile toxin subunit. *Infect. Immunol.* **48**, 735–40.

Kaper, J. B., Lockman, H., Baldini, M. M., and Levine, M. M. (1984). Recombinant non-enterotoxigenic *Vibrio cholerae* strains as attenuated cholera vaccine candidates. *Nature* **308**, 655–8.

Klipstein, F. A., Engert, R. F., and Houghten, R. A. (1983a). Properties of a synthetically produced *Escherichia coli* heat-stable enterotoxin. *Infect. Immunol.* **39**, 117–121.

——, —— and —— (1983b). Protection in rabbits immunized with a vaccine of *Escherichia coli* heat-stable toxin cross-linked to the B subunit of heat-labile toxin. *Infect. Immunol.* **40**, 888–93.

Lee, C. H., Moseley, S. L., Moon, H. W., Whipp, S. C., Gyles, C. L., and So, M. (1983). Characterisation of the gene encoding heat-stable toxin II and preliminary molecular epidemiological studies of enterotoxigenic *Escherichia coli* heat-stable toxin II producers. *Infect. Immunol.* **42**, 264–8.

Levine, M. M., Kaper, J. B., Black, R. E., and Clements, M. L. (1983). New knowledge on pathogenesis of bacterial enteric infections as applied to vaccine development. *Microbiol. Rev.* **47**, 510–50.

Lindholm, L., Holmgren, J., Wilkstrom, M., Karlsson, V., Andersoon, K., and Lycke, N. (1983). Monoclonal antibodies to cholera toxin with special reference to cross-reactions with *Escherichia coli* heat-labile enterotoxin. *Infect. Immunol.* **40**, 570–6.

Mekalanos, J. J., Swartz, D. J., Pearson, G. D. N., Harford, N., Groyne, F., and de Wilde, M. (1983). Cholera toxin gene nucleotide sequence, deletion analysis and vaccine development. *Nature (Lond.)* **306**, 551–6.

Morgan, R. L., Isaacson, R. E., Moon, H. W., Brinton, C. C. and To, C. C. (1978). Immunization of suckling pigs against enterotoxigenic *Escherichia coli* induced diarrhoeal disease by vaccinating dams with purified 987P or K99 pili, protection correlates with pilus homology of vaccine and challenge. *Infect. Immunol.* **22**, 771–7.

Moseley, S. L., Hardy, J. W., Imdadul Hug, M., Escheverria, P., and Falkow, S. (1983). Isolation and nucleotide sequence determination of a gene encoding a heat-stable enterotoxin of *Escherichia coli*. *Infect. Immunol.* **39**, 1167–74.

Nagy, L. K., Walker, P. D., Bhogal, B. S., and McKenzie, T. (1978). Evaluation of *Escherichia coli* vaccines against experimental colibacillosis. *Res. Vet. Sci.* **24**, 39–45.

Ørskov, I., and Ørskov, F. (1966). Episome-carried surface antigen K88 of *Escherichia coli* 1. Transmission of the determinant of the K88 antigen and influence on the transfer of chromosomal markers. *J. Bacteriol.* **91**, 69–75.

Ørskov, I., Ørskov, F., Smith, H. W. and Sojka, W. J. (1975). The establishment of K99, a thermolabile, transmissible K antigen, previously called 'KCO' possessed by calf and lamb enteropathogenic strains. *Acta path. microbiol. scand.* **83**, 31–6.

So, M. and McCarthy, B. J. (1980). Nucleotide sequence of transposon Tn 1681 encoding a heat-stable toxin (ST) and its identification in enterotoxigenic *Escherichia coli* strains. *Proc. nat. Acad. Sci. USA* **77**, 4011–15.

Williams-Smith, H. and Gyles, C. L. (1970). The relationship between two apparently different enterotoxins produced by enteropathogenic strains of *Escherichia coli* of porcine origin. *J. Med. Microbiol.* **3**, 387–401.

—— and Hall, S., (1967). Studies on *Escherichia coli* enterotoxin. *J. Pathol. Bacteriol.* **93**, 531–7.

—— and Linggood, M. A. (1971). Observations on the pathogenic properties of the K88 Hly and Ent plasmids of *Escherichia coli* with particular reference to porcine diarrhoea. *J. Med. Microbiol.* **4**, 467–85.

Winther, M. D. and Dougan, G. (1984). The impact of new technologies on vaccine development. In *Biotechnology and genetic engineering reviews* (ed. R. B. Russell), Vol. 2, pp. 1–39. Intercept Ltd, London.

The use of monoclonal antibodies to elucidate the antigenic structure and the mechanisms of neutralization of snake toxins

*André Ménez, Jean-Claude Boulain, Jean-Marc Grognet,
Eric Gatineau, Jacques Couderc, Alan Harvey, and
Pierre Fromageot*

Introduction

The immune system responds to exposure to foreign proteins by elaborating neutralizing antibodies (Boquet 1979). This property has been widely used to protect humans against the toxic proteins present in a number of natural poisons and venoms (Calmette 1907; Campbell 1979; Christensen 1979; Sawai 1979). The molecular basis of the mechanisms of the neutralization of toxins by their specific antibodies remains obscure and the use of antitoxin and antivenom is often little more than empirical. An understanding of the mechanisms involved in neutralization could be of importance in the development of a more rational therapy. As a first step, the nature of the antigenicity of the toxic proteins needs to be clarified. The advent of hybridoma technology (Köhler and Milstein 1975) to prepare monoclonal antibodies has provided new tools to investigate the antigenicity of proteins in general, and of toxic proteins in particular.

One approach for identifying an antigenic determinant consists in the examination of cross-reactivities of the antigen and a number of variants towards the specific monoclonal immunoglobulin (Boulain, Ménez, Couderc, Faure, Liacopoulos, and Fromageot 1982; Berzofsky, Buckenmeyer, Hicks, Gurd, Feldmann, and Minna 1982). Without doubt snake toxins, and in particular neuro- and cardiotoxins, are well-suited for such an investigation because:

(i) a large number of natural variants of the toxins with a single amino acid substitution are available (see reviews by Karlsson 1979 and Dufton and Hider 1983);

(ii) several derivatives of various toxins, chemically modified at a single amino acid residue, can be prepared. (Karlsson, Eaker, and Ponterius 1972; Hori and Tamiya 1976; Tsetlin, Arseniev, Utkin, Gurevich, Senyavina, Bystrov, Ivanov, and Ovchinnikov 1979; Faure, Boulain, Bouet, Montenay-Garestier, Fromageot, and Ménez 1983). In this chapter our recent findings concerning both the antigenicity and the molecular mechanisms of neutralization of the two major toxins present in the venom of *Naja nigricollis* are reviewed.

Venoms and toxins

The venom from *Naja nigricollis* was obtained from the Pasteur Institute (Paris). The crude venom contains at least three neurotoxins, among which toxin-α is the most abundant (Eaker and Porath 1967). It also contains one cardiotoxin, designated toxin-γ (Fryklund and Eaker 1975). These toxins have been purified using techniques described in detail by Karlsson, Eaker, and Porath (1966) and Fryklund and Eaker (1975).

Toxin-α is defined as a curaremimetic toxin. It binds specifically and with high affinity to the nicotonic acetylcholine receptor (Weber and Changeux 1974). Toxin-γ is defined as a cardiotoxin. It produces a direct depolarization of skeletal muscle fibres (Harvey, Hider, and Khader 1983). Toxin-α and toxin-γ are chemically homologous polypeptides, the sequences of which have been elucidated by Eaker and Porath (1967) and Fryklund and Eaker (1975), respectively. Figure 18.1 shows the amino acid sequences of both toxin-α and toxin-γ. The polypeptide chains have been folded according to a scheme based on the X-ray data of the homologous erabutoxin b from *Laticauda semifasciata* (Low, Preston, Sato, Rosen, Searl, Rudko, and Richardson 1976; Tsernoglou and Petsko 1976; Kimball, Sato, Richardson, Rosen and Low 1979), and *Naja mossambica mossambica* toxin V^{II}_4 (Rees, Moras, Thiery, Gillibert, Fischer, Schweitz, and Lazdunski 1983).

Chemical modifications were carried out on these toxins as described by Faure *et al.* (1983) and Grognet (1984). Toxin-α was labelled with tritium (Ménez, Morgat, Fromageot, Ronsseray, Boquet, and Changeux 1971). Toxin-γ was made radioactive by incorporating one ^{3}H-propionyl group per mole of toxin (Grognet 1984).

Monoclonal antibodies

Monoclonal antibodies were prepared according to the experimental procedure described by Köhler and Milstein (1975), but the high toxicity of the antigens necessitated some modification to the procedures usually used for immunization. Since our goal was to produce monoclonal antibodies against the *native* form of the toxins, we specifically avoided (unless otherwise

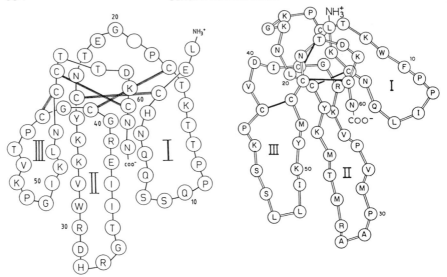

Fig. 18.1 Amino acid sequences of toxin-α (left) and toxin-γ (right) from the venom of *Naja nigricollis*. The polypeptide chain of each toxin has been folded according to a scheme based on the X-ray data of corresponding homologous toxins (Kimball *et al.* 1979; Rees *et al.* 1983).

indicated) the use of chemically detoxified toxins in the immunization experiments. As a compromise, we first injected subcutaneously, per mouse, approximately one LD_{50} of each native toxin in Freund's complete adjuvant. Increasing amounts of unmodified toxins were then injected into the survivors. Thus, in the case of toxin-γ, 2 μg, 10 μg and 20 μg of unmodified toxin were successively injected subcutaneously in the presence of complete Freund's adjuvant into Balb c mice at 2-week intervals. One month after the last injection, 20 μg of polyacetylated toxin-α (approximately 20 per cent as toxic as the native toxin) was injected intraperitoneally (i.p.). Four days later one mouse was killed and the spleen was removed. 10^8 spleen cells were mixed with 10^7 myeloma cells (X 63 NS) for fusion. Hybrid cells were then cloned. In the case of toxin-γ, 40 μg of unmodified toxin were injected three times at intervals of 10 days in Freund's complete adjuvant (total volume, 0.2 ml). One week after the last injection, 12 μg of unmodified toxin-γ in 0.9 per cent NaCl (0.3 ml) were injected i.p. Thereafter, the protocol adopted was similar to that described above for toxin-α.

The production of antibodies specific for toxin-α or -γ was confirmed by radioimmunassays, using either (^{3}H)-labelled toxin-α or (^{3}H)-propionyl toxin-γ. Positive wells were cloned into 96-well plates.

Two clones producing toxin-α specific antibodies (Boulain *et al.* 1982;

Trémeau *et al.*, in press) and two clones producing toxin-γ-specific immuno-globulins (Grognet 1984; Grognet *et al.* 1986) have been identified. Each clone (5×10^6 cells) was grown intraperitoneally in mice, and after one week 5–10 ml of ascites fluid per mouse were withdrawn. Each monoclonal antibody was purified from ascites fluid by affinity chromatography on a toxin-Sepharose column as described previously (Boulain *et al.* 1982). The two toxin-α-specific immunoglobulins were designated $M_{\bar{\alpha}1}$ and $M_{\bar{\alpha}2-3}$ while those specific for toxin-γ was designated as $M_{\bar{\gamma}1}$ and $M_{\bar{\gamma}2-3}$.

Table 18.1 shows some characteristics of the four monoclonal immuno-globulins. The two antibodies that are α-toxin-specific correspond to the same IgG2a isotypes. The dissociation constants (K_d) of the toxin–antibody complexes, derived from equilibrium binding experiments using radioactive toxins, are relatively small except in the case of the toxin-α–$M_{\bar{\alpha}2-3}$ complex, which is characterized by a K_d value substantially higher than others.

Identification of the amino acid residues belonging to the epitopes

For both toxins, the epitopes have been localized on the basis of cross-reaction experiments between the radioactive antigen and a series of deriva-tives of the same antigen, modified at a single amino acid residue (Faure *et al.* 1983; Grognet 1984), or a series of structurally homologous variants (Ménez, Bouet, Tamiya, and Fromageot 1976; Dufton and Hider 1983; Grognet 1984), toward the corresponding monoclonal antibodies.

Epitopes recognized by $M_{\bar{\gamma}1}$ and $M_{\bar{\gamma}2-3}$

Table 18.2 shows the amino acid sequences of the homologous variants of toxin-γ used in the cross-reaction studies, and Table 18.3 summarizes the IC_{50} values derived from competition experiments between radioactive toxin and the variants.

Naja mossabica mossabica toxins I and II have binding affinities similar to that of native toxin-γ toward $M_{\bar{\gamma}1}$, implying that their substituted pos-itions, 57 and 28, 30 and 31, respectively, are excluded from the epitope

Table 18.1 Some characteristics of monoclonal immunoglobulins specific for toxins-α and -γ. The dissociation constants were derived from Scatchard plots determined from direct binding experiments, using ^{3}H-labelled toxin-α and ^{3}H-propionyl toxin-γ (Boulain *et al.* 1982; Grognet 1984).

Monoclonal antibody	$M_{\bar{\alpha}1}$	$M_{\bar{\alpha}2-3}$	$M_{\bar{\gamma}1}$	$M_{\bar{\gamma}2-3}$
Isotype	IgG2a	IgG2a	IgG1	IgG2b
Dissociation constant (K_D, nM)	0.4	10	0.4	0.2

Table 18.2 Amino acid sequences of cardiotoxins that are structurally homologous to *N. nigricollis* toxin-γ as judged by circular dichroism analysis (Grognet 1984). Only the differences are shown.

	10	20	30	40	50	60
N. nigricollis toxin^γ	LKCNQLIPPFWKTCPKGKMNLCYKMTMRAAPMVPVKRGCIDVCXPKSSLLIKMCCNTDKCN					
N.m. mossambica toxin I	——N——					
N.m. mossambica toxin II	——————————————————————————————————— G–SK —————————————————————————					
N.m. mossambica toxin IV	——R———————E ————————————————————— L K ———————————————————N——					
N.h. annulifera CM 11	——K——————————————————— Y VSTLT ————————————N_ A V_V————N——					
N. nigricollis toxin^γ(NPS)	—————————•———					

The black mark indicates the position of the tryptophan side chain that incorporated a 2-nitrophenyl (NPS) moiety.

recognized by this immunoglobulin. Three of them, 28, 31, and 57, are also substituted in *N. m. mossambica* toxin IV, suggesting that one or both of the two remaining substitutions (located at positions 5 and 16) are responsible for the slight decrease in affinity of this toxin toward the antibody. Presumably, therefore, the epitope that is recognized by $M_{\bar{\gamma} 1}$ is on or in the proximity of loop I (see Fig. 18.1). Two lines of evidence support this view. First, when a large number of substitutions occurs away from this region, as in the case of *N. haje annulifera* CM 11 (Table 18.2), the binding affinity is not profoundly altered. The slight decrease in affinity observed with this toxin is possibly due to the substitution at position 5. Secondly, modification of Trp-11 induces a substantial decrease in affinity of the toxin for $M_{\bar{\gamma} 1}$. Clearly, this residue belongs to the epitope that is recognized by $M_{\bar{\gamma} 1}$.

Table 18.3 Relative affinities of the toxin-γ-specific monoclonal immunoglobulins for different cardiotoxins.

Toxins	IC$_{50}$ (nM)	
	$M_{\bar{\gamma} 1}$	$M_{\bar{\alpha} 2-3}$
Naja nigricollis toxin-γ	6 ± 2	5 ± 2
Naja nigricollis toxin-γ NPS	300 ± 10	8 ± 2
Naja mossambica mossambica toxin I	6 ± 2	5 ± 2
Naja mossambica mossambica toxin II	7 ± 3	60 ± 5
Naja mossambica mossambica toxin IV	40 ± 5	60 ± 5
Naja haje annulifera CM 11	40 ± 5	>1000

IC$_{50}$ values indicate the concentration of toxin derivatives required for 50 per cent inhibition of ^{3}H-propionyl toxin-γ to antibodies.

The affinity of the Trp-modified derivative for $M_{\bar{\gamma}2-3}$ is not significantly different from that of the native toxin. This clearly demonstrates that Trp-11 is excluded from the epitope specific for this antibody and also that $M_{\bar{\gamma}1}$ and $M_{\bar{\gamma}2-3}$ bind at topographically different epitopes. As shown in Table 18.2, the affinity of *N. m. mossambica* toxin II for $M_{\bar{\gamma}2-3}$ is weaker than that of toxin-γ. This toxin is substituted at three positions only (28, 30, and 31), all located at the tip of the central loop of the molecule. Presumably the epitope specific for $M_{\bar{\gamma}2-3}$ is located on or in close proximity to this region of the cardiotoxin. This is confirmed by the behaviour of *N. h. annulifera* CM 11 which is extensively substituted on loops II and III (see Table 18.2 and Fig. 18.1) and has virtually no affinity for $M_{\bar{\gamma}2-3}$.

In summary, we have prepared two monoclonal antibodies that clearly bind to topographically different epitopes on the surface of toxin-γ from *Naja nigrocollis*. One of these includes Trp-11 and is therefore located on loop I, whereas the other is located on or in close proximity to the tip of loop II and/or loop III (Fig. 18.2).

Epitopes recognized by $M_{\bar{\alpha}1}$ and $M_{\bar{\alpha}2-3}$

The preparation of six derivatives of toxin-α, selectively modified at a single amino group (NH$_2$-terminus, Lys-15, Lys-27, Lys-47, and Lys-51) or at Trp-29, was previously described by Faure *et al.* (1983). The relative affinities of

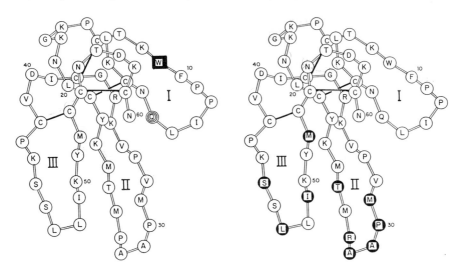

Fig. 18.2 Localization of two antigenic determinants on the surface of toxin-γ. The epitope on the left is recognized by $M_{\bar{\gamma}1}$. It definitely involves Trp-11, which has been emphasized by black caps, whereas Gln-5 is only assumed to be localized in its proximity. The other epitope shown on the right is recognized by $M_{\bar{\gamma}2-3}$. It involves one or more of the residues that are emphasized by black caps.

these derivatives for the two toxin-α-specific monoclonal immunoglobulins were determined from competitive binding curves (Boulain *et al*. 1982). Examination of the affinities (Table 18.4) indicates that:

1. In agreement with the data derived from direct binding experiments, $M_{\bar{\alpha}2-3}$ has a weaker binding affinity for toxin-α than has $M_{\bar{\alpha}1}$ (see Table 16.1).

2. The derivatives modified either at the NH_2-terminal group or at lysine 15 have lower affinities for $M_{\bar{\alpha}1}$ than the native toxin or other derivatives, implying that both the NH_2-terminal group and residue 15 belong to the epitope, which is recognized by this immunoglobulin.

3. The derivatives modified at residues 29 and 47 have a substantially weaker affinity for $M_{\bar{\alpha}2-3}$ than the native toxin or the derivatives modified at positions 1, 15 or 51. Thus, residues 29 and 47 belong to the epitope specific for $M_{\bar{\alpha}2-3}$. The derivative modified on Lys-27 displays a slight but quite reproducible decrease in affinity for $M_{\bar{\alpha}2-3}$; presumably this residue is included in the epitope that is recognized by $M_{\bar{\alpha}2-3}$.

Determination of the relative affinities of a series of natural variants of toxin (Boulain *et al*. 1982; Boulain and Ménez, in preparation), together with the examination of the spatial structure of the homologous erabutoxin b (Low *et al*. 1976; Tsernoglou and Petsko 1976) led us to propose, in addition, that Thr-16 and Pro-18 both belong to the determinant that is recognized by $M_{\bar{\alpha}1}$ (Boulain *et al*. 1982) and that Gln-7 belongs to the epitope to which $M_{\bar{\alpha}2-3}$ binds.

In summary, the two antigenic determinants that have been identified at the surface of *N. nigricollis* toxin-α are topographically different (Fig. 18.3). One is located at the edge of the first loop, whereas the other covers the three main loops.

Table 18.4 Relative affinities of the toxin-α-specific monoclonal immunoglobulin for different derivatives of toxin-α, chemically modified at a single amino acid residue.

Toxins	Relative affinities (K_D,nM)	
	For $M_{\bar{\alpha}1}$ (Boulain 1982)	For $M_{\bar{\alpha}2-3}$ (Trémeau *et al.*, in press)
Toxin-α	0.4 ± 0.1	9 ± 1
(1-acetyllysine) toxin-α	4.5 ± 2	9 ± 1
(15-acetyllysine) toxin-α	11.5 ± 2	5 ± 1
(27-acetyllysine) toxin-α	0.4 ± 0.2	61 ± 5
(29-nitrophenyl-tryptophan) toxin-α	0.3 ± 0.2	172 ± 8
(47-acetyllysine) toxin-α	0.5 ± 0.1	85 ± 6
(51-acetyllysine) toxin-α	0.5 ± 0.1	5 ± 1

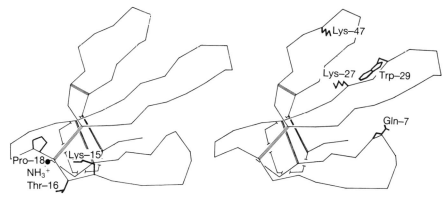

Fig. 18.3 Identification of some residues belonging to two antigenic determinants localized at the surface of toxin-α. The epitope recognized by $M_{\bar{\alpha}1}$ is on the left, while the epitope on the right is recognized by $M_{\bar{\alpha}2\text{-}3}$.

The antigenic determinants that have been identified in this paper are worthy of further characterization. It is essential that more tools, such as toxin derivatives modified at a single position, be prepared. To this end we are currently preparing derivatives of toxin-γ monoacetylated at a single amino group, using a procedure similar to that described by Faure *et al.* (1983). In addition, we have recently cloned the cDNA encoding a cura-remimetic toxin (Tamiya, Lamouroux, Julien, Grima, Mallet, Fromageot, and Ménez 1985) with a view to producing mutant proteins with single mutations by means of site-directed mutagenesis (Pielak, Mauk, and Smith 1985).

Neutralization of toxins-α and -γ by monoclonal antibodies

Toxin-γ-specific immunoglobulins

The neutralizing capacities of $M_{\bar{\gamma}1}$ and $M_{\bar{\gamma}2\text{-}3}$ were examined under *in vivo* and *in vitro* conditions. 30 μg of toxin-γ were injected (i.v.) in mice (18–20 g) in the presence and absence of 1 mg of toxin-specific monoclonal antibodies purified by affinity chromatography. In the absence of immuno-globulin, the mice died within 10 min of injection, whereas all mice survived when the toxin was preincubated with approximately a three times excess (on a molar basis) of either immunoglobulin (Table 18.5).

Toxin-γ depolarizes skeletal muscle fibres grown in cell culture from chick embryo muscles as previously described (Harvey *et al.* 1983). Cultures were exposed to a standard concentration of toxin (1 μM) either alone or prein-cubated for 4 h in the presence of 2 μM of $M_{\bar{\gamma}1}$ or $M_{\bar{\gamma}2\text{-}3}$. Toxin-γ induces a complete depolarization of the preparation within 20 min, whereas the

Table 18.5 Neutralizing effect of 1 mg ($\approx$7 nmol) of various monoclonal antibodies.

Mixture injected	No. of dead mice/No. of injected mice
3 μg toxin-α	10/10
3 μg toxin-α + 1 mg $M_{\bar{\alpha}1}$	0/10
30 μg toxin-γ	7/7
30 μg toxin-γ + 1 mg $M_{\bar{\gamma}1}$	0/7
30 μg toxin-γ + 1 mg $M_{\bar{\gamma}2-3}$	0/8

Toxins-α and -γ were injected intraperitoneally and intravenously, respectively, in the presence and absence of antibodies, into 18–20 g mice. Mixtures were injected in 0.9 per cent NaCl solutions (0.3 ml). Survivors were still alive 1 week after the injection.

mixture with either antibody has no depolarizing effect, even after several hours.

Toxin-α-specific immunoglobulins

Intraperitoneal injections made with 3 μg ($\approx$ 0.4 nmol) of toxin-α in the presence of approximately 1 mg ($\approx$14 nmol in toxin binding sites) of $M_{\bar{\alpha}1}$ reveal that the latter totally inhibits the lethal effect of the toxin (Table 18.5). By contrast, preincubation of one LD_{100} of toxin with a 50-fold molar excess of $M_{\bar{\alpha}2-3}$ does not abolish the lethal effect of the toxin, but clearly delays it. The weak neutralizing capacity of $M_{\bar{\alpha}2-3}$ may be related to its somewhat low affinity (compared with $M_{\bar{\alpha}1}$) for the toxin (see Table 18.1).

In contrast to the *in vivo* results, both toxin-α-specific monoclonal immunoglobulins appeared to be fully neutralizing under *in vitro* conditions. For example, addition of 1 nM (final concentration) of $M_{\bar{\alpha}1}$ to a mixture of (^{3}H)-labelled toxin (0.09 nM) and acetylcholine receptor (0.28 nM) completely inhibits the binding of the tritiated toxin to the receptor at equilibrium (Boulain *et al.* 1982).

We have demonstrated previously that $M_{\bar{\alpha}1}$ is capable of destabilizing the (^{3}H)-labelled toxin-α-receptor complex (Boulain and Ménez 1982), thus inducing a marked acceleration of the kinetics of dissociation of the complex (Boulain, Fromageot, and Ménez 1985). This effect has been investigated under *in vivo* conditions. Gatineau (1983) injected three times the LD_{50} of toxin-α into rats, which were then placed on artificial respiration for 12 h. Then 0.9 per cent Na Cl solution was injected into control rats while 6 mg of $M_{\bar{\alpha}1}$ was injected into others. Control and treated rats began to breath normally within 17 h and 70 min, respectively. Considering that neuromuscular transmission is normal when more than 60 per cent of the acetyl choline receptor sites are free of toxin (Barnard, Wieckowski, and Chiu 1971; Chang, Chuang, and Huang 1975) and also that the half time of dissocation for the toxin-receptor complex is approximately 15 h (Gatineau 1983), we propose that the rapid recovery of the respiratory capacity observed with treated animals results from a destabilization of the toxin-receptor complex by the immunoglobulin.

On the mechanisms of neutralization by monoclonal antibodies

An understanding of the molecular mechanisms associated with the neutralization of a toxin by a specific immunoglobulin requires an elucidation of the site, designated as the 'toxic' site, by which the toxin recognizes its physiological target. The 'toxic' site of cardiotoxins has not yet been clearly identified. All the models that have been so far proposed, however, suggest that it is localized on one or more of the three main loops I, II, and III (Lauterwein and Wuthrich 1978; Hider and Khader 1982; Dufourcq, Faucon, Bernard, Pezolet, Tessier, Bougis, Van Reitschoten, Delori, and Rochat 1982). These models agree well with our observation that masking either loop I with $M_{\bar{\gamma} 1}$ or loop II and/or III with $M_{\bar{\gamma} 2-3}$ inactivates the cardiotoxin molecule. However, some caution is required in the interpretation of the available data: neutralization of toxin after preincubation with antibody could also be the result of a conformational change induced in the toxin by the antibody (as demonstrated with $M_{\bar{\alpha} 1}$). Recently, Kfir, Botes, and Osthoff (1985) reported the preparation of another cardiotoxin-specific monoclonal antibody. This immunoglobulin, however, is not capable of neutralizing the cardiotoxin. The epitope recognized by this antibody is certainly different from those we have identified here.

In contrast to toxin-γ, the 'toxic' site of *N. nigricollis* toxin-α is well documented (Ménez, Boulain, Faure, Couderc, Liacopoulos, Tamiya, and Fromageot 1982; Faure *et al.* 1983; Rousselet, Faure, Boulain, and Ménez 1984). It comprises twelve invariant residues, which are essentially located on loops II and III and which point in the same direction (see Fig. 18.4). It is of special interest that three residues, Lys-27, Trp-29, and Lys-47, belong to both the 'toxic' site and the epitope recognized by $M_{\bar{\alpha} 2-3}$. Clearly these two surfaces overlap with each other. In principle therefore, the toxin cannot bind simultaneously to both the receptor and the immunoglobulin. This accounts for our observation that $M_{\bar{\alpha} 2-3}$ prevents the binding of the toxin to the receptor under *in vitro* conditions (see above). In contrast, $M_{\bar{\alpha} 1}$ binds at a site that is topographically different from 'toxic' site. Nevertheless, this immunoglobulin displays clear neutralizing capacities. Moreover, it can accelerate the dissociation of the toxin-receptor complex, implying the formation of a transient ternary complex between the antibody, the toxin, and the receptor (Boulain *et al.* 1985). Binding of the antibody possibly

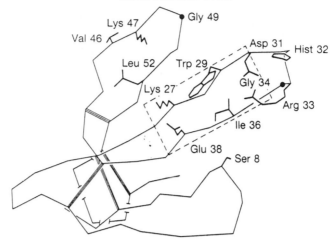

Fig. 18.4 The residues believed to be implicated in the toxic activity of *Naja nigricollis* toxin-α. These residues have been identified on the basis of various considerations, including their invariability among neurotoxins as well as a number of chemical modifications at single amino acid residues (Faure *et al.* 1983). The residues localized inside the dashed box mimic a structure that is similar to that of *d*-tubocurarine (Ménez *et al.* 1982). The structure of the polypeptide chain is from that of the homologous erabutoxin b (Kimball *et al.* 1979).

induces a conformational change of the toxin, in particular in the vicinity of the 'toxic' site, thus preventing the binding of the toxin to the receptor and/or destablizing the toxin-receptor complex.

Conclusion

Despite their relatively small size, toxins-α and -γ isolated from the venom of *Naja nigricollis* are immunogenic. Although they are highly toxic, specific monoclonal antibodies can be obtained without the neccessity to detoxify the toxins prior to immunization. Two monoclonal antibodies have been prepared against the native form of each toxin molecule. For both toxins, one immunoglobulin binds at a site located at the edge of loop I. For both toxins also, another monoclonal antibody binds at a site that overlaps loops II and III, extending to the tip of loop I in the case of $M_{\bar{\alpha}2-3}$. These antibodies are all neutralizing under *in vitro* conditions and three of them are neutralizing under *in vivo* conditions as well. It is of special interest that the mechanisms associated with the neutralization of a toxin may differ from one immunoglobulin to another. This is particularly clear in the case of α-toxin-specific immunoglobulins, where two different mechanisms have been considered. One of these correspond to a simple competition between the immunoglobulin and the receptor for overlapping sites. The other proposed mechanism implies a conformational change of the toxin subsequent to toxin-antibody complex formation. This would readily explain the inhibition of the binding of the toxin to the receptor and also the destabilizing effect of the immunoglobulin on the toxin-receptor complex.

Having localized some regions that elicit neutralizing antibodies, it would be of interest to reconstitute them chemically. A difficulty arises, however, that is related to the configuration of these epitopes. They are clearly composed of residues that are separated in the peptide sequence but are brought together by virtue of folding of the polypeptide chain. Particular structures, such as cyclic peptides, may have to be designed to mimic these structures. Without doubt, success in this field will lead to the improvement of existing antivenom therapies.

Acknowledgements — We are extremely grateful to Drs B. Moras, and J. C. Thiery (Strasbourg, France) for sending us the X-ray data on cardiotoxin prior to publication. We also thank Drs W. Guschlbauer and J. B. Harris for criticizing the manuscript. MRES, CNRS, INSERM, and CEA are gratefully acknowledged for financial support.

References

Barnard, E. A., Wieckowski, J., and Chiu, T. M. (1971). Cholinergic receptor molecules and cholinesterase molecules at mouse skeletal muscle junctions. *Nature (Lond.)* **234**, 207–9.

Berzofsky, J. A., Buckenmeyer, G. K., Hicks, G., Gurd, F. R. N., Feldmann, R. J., and Minna, J. (1982). Topographic antigenic determinants recognized by monoclonal antibodies to sperm whale myoglobin. *J. biol. Chem.* **257**, 3189–98.

Boquet, P. (1979). Immunological properties of snake venoms. In *Snake venoms* (ed. C. Y. Lee,). *Handbook of experimental pharmacology* Vol. 52, pp. 751–800. Springer, Berlin.

Boulain, J.-C. and Ménez, A. (1982). Neurotoxin-specific immunoglobulins accelerate dissociation of the neurotoxin-acetylcholine receptor complex. *Science* **217**, 732–3.

——, Fromageot, P., and Ménez, A. (1985). Further evidence showing that neurotoxin-acetylcholine receptor dissociation is accelerated by monoclonal neurotoxin-specific immunoglobulin. *Mol. Immunol.* **22**, 553–6.

——, Ménez, A., Couderc, J., Faure, G., Liacopoulos, P., and Fromageot, P. (1982). Neutralizing monoclonal antibody specific for *Naja nigricollis* toxin α : preparation, characterization and localization of the antigenic binding site. *Biochemistry* **21**, 2910–15.

Calmette, A. (1907). Les animaux venimeux et la sérotherapie antivenimeusé. In *Les venins*. Masson & Cie, Paris.

Campbell, C. H. (1979). Symptomatology, pathology and treatment of the bites of elapid snakes. In *Snake venoms* (ed. C. Y. Lee), Vol. 52, pp. 898–917. Springer, Berlin.

Chang, C. C., Chuang, S.-T., and Huang, M. C. (1975). Effect of chronic treatment with various neuromuscular blocking agents on the number and distribution of acetylcholine receptors in the rat diaphragm. *J. Physiol. (Lond.)* **250**, 161–73.

Christensen, P. A. (1979). Production and standardization of antivenins. In *Snake venoms* (ed. C. Y. Lee). *Handbook of experimental pharmacology* Vol. 52, pp. 825–42. Springer, Berlin.

Dufourcq, J., Faucon, J. F., Bernard, E., Pezolet, M., Tessier, M., Bougis, P., Van Rietschoten, J., Delori, P., and Rochat, H. (1982). Structure-function relationships for cardiotoxins interacting with phospholipids. *Toxicon* **20**, 165–74.

Dufton, M. J. and Hider, R. C. (1983). Conformational properties of the neurotoxins and cytotoxins isolated from Elapid snake venoms. *CRC crit. Rev. Biochem.* **14**, 113–71.

Eaker, D. and Porath, J. (1967). The amino acid sequence of a neurotoxin from *Naja nigricollis* venom. *Seventh international congress on biochemistry*, Tokyo, Col. VIII-3. Abstr. III, p. 499. Science Council of Japan, Tokyo.

Faure, G., Boulain, J.-C., Bouet, F., Montenay-Garestier, Th., Fromageot, P., and Ménez, A. (1983). Role of indole and amino groups in the structure and function of *Naja nigricollis* toxin α. *Biochemistry* **22**, 2068–76.

Fryklund, L. and Eaker, D. (1975). The complete covalent structure of a cardiotoxin from the venom of *Naja nigricollis* (African black-necked spitting cobra). *Biochemistry* **14**, 2865–71.

Gatineau, E. (1983). Etude *in vitro* et *in vivo* des effets neutralisants preventif et curatif des anticorps conventionnels et/ou monoclonaux spécifiques de la neurotoxine du venin de *Naja nigricollis*. Mémoire pour le diplome d'études approfondies de pharmacologie. Université René Descartes (Paris V) et Université de Paris-sud (Paris XI).

Grognet, J. M. (1984). Etude de la structure antigénique d'une neurotoxine de venin de cobra: la toxine gamma de *Naja nigricollis*. Thèse de 3ème cycle, Université R. Descartes, Paris.

——, Gatineau, E., Bougis, P., Harvey, A., Gouderc, J., Fromageot, P., and Ménez, A. (1986). Two neutralizing monoclonal antibodies specific for *Naja nigricollis* cardiotoxin: preparation, characterization and localization of the epitopes. *Mol. Immunol.* (In press.)

Harvey, A. L., Hider, R. C., and Khader, F. (1983). Effect of phosphilipase A on actions of cobra venom cardiotoxins on erythrocytes and skeletal muscles. *Biochim. biophys. acta.* **728**, 215–21.

Hider, R. C, and Khader, F. (1982). Biochemical and pharmacological properties of cardiotoxins isolated from cobra venoms. *Toxicon* **20**, 175–9.

Hori, H. and Tamiya, N. (1976). Preparation and activity of guanidinated or acetylated erabutoxins. *Biochem. J.* **153**, 217–22.

Karlsson, E., Eaker, D., and Porath, J. (1966). Purification of a neurotoxin from the venom of *Naja nigricollis*. *Biochim. biophys. acta* **127**, 505–20.

Karlsson, E. (1979). Chemistry of protein toxins in snake venoms. In *Snake venoms* (ed. C. Y. Lee), *Handbook of experimental pharmacology* Vol. 52, pp. 159–204. Springer, Berlin.

——, Eaker, D., and Ponterius, G. (1972). Modification of amino groups in *Naja*

naja neurotoxins and the preparation of radioactive derivatives. *Biochim. biophys. acta* **257**, 235–48.

Kfir, R., Botes, D. P., and Osthoff, G. (1985). Preparation and characterization of monoclonal antibody specific for *Naja nivea* cardiotoxin V II. 1. *Toxicon* **23**, 135–44.

Kimball, M. R., Sato, A., Richardson, J. S., Rosen, L. S., and Low, B. W. (1979). Molecular conformation of erabutoxin b; atomic coordinates at 2.5 Å resolution. *Biochim. biophys. Res. Commun.* **88**, 950–9.

Köhler, G. and Milstein, C. (1975). Continuous cultures of fused cells secreting antibody of predefined specificity. *Nature (Lond.)* **256**, 495–7.

Lauterwein, J. and Wüthrich, K. A. (1978). A possible structural basis for the different modes of action of neurotoxins and cardiotoxins from snake venoms. *FEBS Lett.* **93**, 181–4.

Low, B. W., Preston, H. S., Sato, A., Rosen, L. S., Searl, J. E., Rudko, A. D., and Richardson, J. S. (1976). Three-dimensional structure of erabutoxin b neurotoxic protein; inhibitor of acetylcholine receptor. *Proc. nat. Acad. Sci. (Wash.)* **73**, 2991–4.

Ménez, A., Bouet, F., Tamiya, N. and Fromageot, P. (1976). Conformational changes in two neurotoxic proteins from snake venoms. *Biochim. biophys. acta* **453**, 121–32.

——, Morgat, J. L., Fromageot, P., Ronsseray, A. M., Boquet, P., and Changeux, J.-P. (1971). Tritium labelling of the α-neurotoxin of *Naja nigricollis.* `FEBS Lett.* **17**, 333–5.

——, Boulain, J. C., Faure, G., Couderc, J., Liacopoulos, P., Tamiya, N., and Fromageot, P. (1982). Comparison of the 'toxic' and antigenic regions in toxin isolated from *Naja nigricollis* venom. *Toxicon* **20**, 95–103.

Pielak, G. J., Mauk, A. G., and Smith, M. (1985). Site-directed mutagenesis of cytochrome c shows that an invariant Phe is not essential for function. *Nature (Lond.)* **313**, 152–3.

Rees, B., Moras, D., Thiery, J.-C., Gillibert, M., Fischer, J.-C., Schweitz, A., and Lazdunski, M. (1983). Structure of a cardiotoxin isolated from snake venom. Eighth European Crystallographic Meeting, Liège, Belgium.

Rousselet, A., Faure, G., Boulain, J. C., and Ménez, A. (1984). The interaction of neurotoxins derivatives with either acetylcholine receptor or a monoclonal antibody. An electron spin resonance study. *Eur. J. Biochem.* **140**, 31–7.

Sawai, Y. (1979). Vaccination against snake bite poisoning. In *Snake venoms* (ed. C. Y. Lee). *Handbook of experimental pharmacology* Vol. 52, pp. 881–95. Springer, Berlin.

Tamiya, T., Lamouroux, A., Julien, J.-F., Grima, B., Mallet, J., Fromageot, P., and Ménez, A. (1985). Cloning and sequence analysis of the cDNA encoding a snake neurotoxin precursor. *Biochimie* **67**, 185–9.

Trémeau, O., Boulain, J. C., Conderc, J., Fromageot, P., and Ménez, A. A monoclonal antibody which recognizes the functional site of snake neurotoxins and which neutralizes all short-chain variants. *FEBS Letters.* (In press.)

Tsernoglou, D. and Petsko, G. A. (1976). The crystal structure of a postsynaptic neurotoxin from sea snake at 2.2 Å resolution. *FEBS Lett.* **68**, 1–4.

Tsetlin, V. I., Arseniev, A. S., Utkin, Y. N., Gurevich, A. Z., Senyavina, L. B., Bystrov, V. F., Ivanov, V. T., and Ovchinnikov, Y. A. (1979). Conformational studies of neurotoxin II from *Naja naja oxiana*. Selective *N*-acylation. Circular dichroism and nuclear magnetic resonance study of acylation products. *Eur. J. Biochem.* **94**, 337–46.

Weber, M. and Changeux, J.-P. (1974). Binding of *Naja nigricollis* (^{3}H)α-toxin to membrane fragments from *Electrophorus* and *Torpedo* electric organs. I Binding of the tritiated α-neurotoxin in the absence of effector. *Mol. Pharmacol.* **10**, 1–14.

Index